Contents

PART II: CONCEPTUAL APPROACHES
TO QUALITY OF LIFE

PART III: SOME CRITICAL ISSUES

Quality of Life in Health Promotion and Rehabilitation

Conceptual Approaches, Issues, and Applications

Edited by
Rebecca Renwick
Ivan Brown • Mark Nagler

SAGE Publications
International Educational and Professional Publisher
Thousand Oaks   London   New Delhi

For information address:

SAGE Publications, Inc.
2455 Teller Road
Thousand Oaks, California 91320
E-mail: order@sagepub.com

SAGE Publications Ltd.
6 Bonhill Street
London EC2A 4PU
United Kingdom

SAGE Publications India Pvt. Ltd.
M-32 Market
Greater Kailash I
New Delhi 110 048 India

Printed in the United States of America

Library of Congress Cataloging-in-Publication Data

Main entry under title:

Quality of life in health promotion and rehabilitation: Conceptual
   approaches, issues, and applications / editors, Rebecca Renwick,
   Ivan Brown, Mark Nagler.
      p. cm.
   Includes bibliographical references and index.
   ISBN 0-8039-5913-3 (acid-free paper).—ISBN 0-8039-5914-1 (pbk.:
acid-free paper)
      1. Health promotion. 2. Quality of life. 3. Medical
rehabilition. I. Renwick, Rebecca. II. Brown, Ivan, 1947- .
III. Nagler, Mark.
RA427.8.Q35' 1996
362.1'042—dc20   95-41770

96 97 98 99 10 9 8 7 6 5 4 3 2 1

This book is printed on acid-free paper.

Sage Production Editor: Diane S. Foster

**PART IV: APPLICATIONS OF QUALITY OF
LIFE IN HEALTH PROMOTION AND REHABILITATION**

A: CURRENT SOCIAL ISSUES

B: ABILITIES AND DISABILITIES

Foreword

Ron Draper

Health promotion has a close association with quality of life. It views health as being rooted in living and working conditions and sees itself as a contributor to the improvement of such conditions. Although this association has been recognized in general terms for a long time, it has not been systematically explored until now.

Health promotion is unique in the degree to which its short history is the result of deliberate political efforts to find a new paradigm for health policy. The experience in Canada is used here as an example of how health promotion is developing throughout the world, particularly in industrialized countries. Twenty years ago, Canada's Health Minister released *A New Perspective on the Health of Canadians* (Health and Welfare Canada, 1974). It used the health field concept to set a new framework for policy with health promotion as one of its major strategies. This was the first occasion on which the term *health promotion* was defined and given strategic significance.

A decade ago, Canada and the World Health Organization (WHO) co-sponsored the first International Conference on Health Promotion, which produced the *Ottawa Charter* (WHO, 1986). With WHO leadership, the charter has gained wide international recognition as an integrating and practical framework for health policy. On the occasion of the Ottawa Conference, Canada's Minister of Health released *Achieving Health for All: A Framework for Health Promotion* (Epp, 1986). The framework has played a major role in developing health promotion in Canada.

The *Ottawa Charter* is the political statement that goes the furthest in associating health promotion with quality of life. It recognizes the social as well as the physical and mental dimensions of health and sees health as a resource for life. It views health as grounded in "prerequisites for health," which are currently referred to as social, economic, and environmental determinants. It is committed to equity, which is to say equal opportunities to enjoy health. One of the five means of action identified in the charter is healthy public policy, which, simply stated, is the vehicle through which other sectors make their contribution to health. From the charter's perspective, a primary role of health promotion is to enable people to increase control over the influences on their health.

Viewed in retrospect, two broad streams of development can be seen in the practice of health promotion in Canada over the past two decades. One is primarily concerned with the individual and the other with the community and society. The first includes lifestyle campaigns that are long-standing parts of the Canadian landscape and health promotion services that are increasingly offered by local health departments or as an aspect of primary care. This stream of development grew out of biomedical models of disease prevention and risk reduction but has become increasingly concerned with positive aspects of individual functioning, including social ones.

The environmental stream is represented by the healthy communities movement (known in Europe as Healthy Cities). Its goals are to enlist citizen participation and the total spectrum of municipal services in the interest of health, assuming that improvements in urban living conditions will contribute to better health. This approach owes a great deal to ecological thinking and concern for environmental conservation and sustainable development. It views the home, the school, the workplace, and the community as settings for health.

Developments in other countries have in many ways been similar to those in Canada. The *Ottawa Charter* has been widely used as a planning framework and has reinforced trends that began some years earlier as a result of the WHO Health for All strategy with its emphasis on equity, participation, and intersectoral action. Lifestyle programs that began with a narrow focus on risk behaviors have become more positive, more strategic, and more concerned with the context within which life choices are made. Local action has been the predominant approach, reinforced by international networks concerned with health in different settings: Healthy Cities, Health Promoting Schools, and Healthy Workplaces. Serious attempts by regional and national governments to introduce healthy public policies have been limited and tentative. Health has not yet reached a realm of national and international debate comparable to the one concerning the environment, partly because of the continuing tendency to view health as synonymous with health care.

Individual and environmental lines of development are both essential to a comprehensive health promotion strategy and both will find comfort and food for thought in this book. For example, the quality of life framework described in the Renwick and Brown chapter offers a comprehensive entry point for examining influences on health in different settings supporting an ecological world view. The Raeburn and Rootman chapter, on the other hand, offers a means within this framework for sorting out those issues with which specific health promotion programs or services should be uniquely concerned.

Most direct health promotion action is local, and this is where the greatest progress has been made in Canada and other industrialized countries. The next big challenge for health promotion is to become more strategic. In practical terms, this will mean introducing working models of healthy public policy at the regional and national levels backed by the social consensus needed to sustain them. When this happens, policies in areas as diverse as agriculture, environment, employment, education, income support, and, dare we hope, trade and finance will be planned and applied with health considerations in mind. Their success or failure will be measured, in part, by the degree to which they contribute to the nation's health. Generally speaking, this is clearly not the case at present.

Although it is not widely recognized, the structural basis for moving toward healthy public policy is quietly being laid at the present time as a part of health system reform. Details vary from province to province in Canada, but, in general, these are two positive trends. Health councils appointed to advise on provincial policies are recommending that such policies be defined by goals and objectives that address a wide spectrum of health determinants. At the same time, the new health provincial infrastructure is being introduced to decentralize decision making, improve accountability, and coordinate the planning application of healthy public policy. Current preoccupation with controlling health care costs has precluded wide discussion of these hopeful signs.

Although much of this book is concerned with model building and measurement that is of interest to researchers, it will be useful to practitioners preparing for strategic challenges that lie ahead. Health promotion has often been hampered in the past by the absence of conceptual tools with which to plan its next move, but when they become available, progress follows. From the perspective of a practitioner, the quality of life models described in this book are additional valuable tools. Their strengths lie in their comprehensiveness, cohesiveness, and sensitivity to the realities and preferences of people—an entry point for thinking about healthy public policy.

People interested in policy will be struck by the great degree to which these models point toward structural issues that have to be addressed if health promotion is to contribute more to health gains. Of particular interest in this vein are the chapters by Raphael on application of one model to the concerns of adolescents and then to older people as well as the chapter by Shain on implications for labor relations.

The genius of the *Ottawa Charter* has been its capacity to set new directions for change without narrowing possibilities. This book illustrates another case in point. Given the philosophy of the charter, it has been widely assumed that its reference to reorientation of health services means improving the preventive and promotive capacity of primary care. This is certainly true, but now we know that there is more. The chapters concerned with rehabilitation services show the changes that will occur when they move away from a narrow focus on dimensions of individual functioning and think in terms of their effect on the quality of the lives of people with disabilities.

Introduction

J. David Baker

This book challenges us to look beyond our traditional perspectives and to reinvent the fields of health promotion and rehabilitation. Such challenges are not new. In 1894, Anatole France (quoted in Bartlett, 1980) issued a challenge to look beyond the superficial and examine the essence of how we treat each other: "The law, in its majestic equality, forbids the rich as well as the poor to sleep under bridges, to beg in the streets, and to steal bread" (p. 655). When unlawful activity is considered from this perspective, things that seemed self-evident and benign suddenly appear to be considerably more complex. Those who were concerned about their fellow humans could not help but be challenged to think about and act on the new insights this changed frame of reference gave them. Was the cause of their poverty any more just than the law that punished them for suffering it? What was to be done?

The editors of this book seek to pose a similar challenge. The phrase *quality of life* has been chosen to signal a change in perspective that is only just beginning to be evident in the fields of health promotion and rehabilitation.

The phrase is apt to cause disquiet. There have been those among us who have arrogantly judged, from a vantage point of power, the value of a human life. They have made decisions based on their assessment of a person's quality of life about providing supports to sustain that life. This attitude peaked in Nazi Germany, where such decisions were used as the basis for genocide. We like to think that we have moved well beyond this perspective, but important decisions about people's lives are still being made from positions of power. Such practice is difficult to combat, especially in a period when responsibility of government in the areas of human and environmental services is being cut back.

This book is not about judging the value of lives but, rather, about how we can enhance the quality of each person's life. A major theme running through the book is the fundamental importance of listening to, and acting on, people's own judgments about quality. It is not coincidence that many of the authors have experience working with persons with developmental disabilities. This group has been among the most vulnerable to having their own judgments and wishes disregarded.

The editors are acutely aware of how the emergence of three trends all coincide: consumer movements among disadvantaged people, the broadening of legal guarantees of equality to remove barriers that contributed to their disadvantage, and the broadening of the perspective of human service professionals to take into account the aspirations of their clients. Only when change occurs in all these areas can it be expected that societal attitudes and institutions will undergo fundamental change.

These and other trends have brought about changes in our perspective on health and health services in recent years. Within the traditional medical model, the doctor was charged to "do no harm." The patient was presumed to control the relationship through the giving or withholding of consent to treatment. This model disregarded the enormous imbalances in power and information that exist between the doctor and the patient. New models have emerged that attempt to redress this imbalance or at least take it into account. Health is increasingly being considered as a much broader concept than simply the treatment of illness, and the emphasis on health promotion has fostered the view that health, in its broad sense, can be influenced through positive action based on decisions at the personal level.

Likewise, rehabilitation has been evolving and redefining itself. The recognition that barriers created by society prevent persons with disabilities from realizing their goals has begun to propel this change. Increasingly, those in the rehabilitation field will find themselves working as partners with persons with disabilities in seeking strategies, including advocating for laws that will dismantle these environmental barriers and prevent the creation of new ones.

This book contains important ideas about how these and other changes will come about. In particular, it puts forward *quality of life* as an interesting and new perspective for considering, planning, and implementing such changes within the fields of health promotion and rehabilitation. It challenges us as professionals, and as members of society, to think about our responsibility for others, particularly those who are disadvantaged. But most of all, this book demands that we hear what is being said by those in the best position to judge quality—namely, those for whom professionals have presumed to speak up until now.

Acknowledgments

We would like to acknowledge our students and research assistants—Christine Grekos, Azmina Habib, and Anne Muegge—who helped to prepare the manuscript as well as Sharon Nagler, who provided editorial comments. We also thank Christine Smedley, our editor at Sage Publications, who offered advice and encouragement at every stage of preparation. This book has benefited from the work of our fellow contributors. They are scholars and professionals, some of whom bring the added dimension of personal experience of their own disabilities or a family member's to the material presented.

We are grateful for the resources and facilities provided by the Department of Occupational Therapy and the Centre for Health Promotion at the University of Toronto; Renison College, University of Waterloo; and Ryerson Polytechnic University. Preparation of this manuscript was supported in part by a grant from the Social Sciences and Humanities Research Council, awarded through the University of Waterloo.

PART
I

QUALITY OF LIFE
IN HEALTH PROMOTION
AND REHABILITATION

1

The Centrality of Quality of Life in Health Promotion and Rehabilitation

Ivan Brown
Rebecca Renwick
Mark Nagler

Quality of life is currently receiving significant attention in the health and other human service fields internationally. This attention is part of a strong general interest in (a) the quality of a wide variety of services, (b) the quality of outcomes that result from those services, and (c) optimizing quality within the lives of individuals at a personal level. Taken together, these amount to what Schalock (1994b) has termed the "quality revolution" (p. 2).

The interest in quality of life appears to have stemmed from trends toward greater attention to the personal needs and wishes of individuals within the health and social services and getting better results with fewer resources, rather than from clear, thorough conceptualizations of quality of life (see Parmenter, 1994). Some coherent, detailed conceptualizations have emerged in recent years, but considerable work still needs to be accomplished to expand and solidify our understanding of this concept. Such work is particularly needed in health and other human service fields in which the goal is to improve people's lives and the ways they live.

The overall purpose of this book is to further the work of understanding quality of life in the fields of health promotion and rehabilitation, two multidisciplinary subfields of health and other human services. These subfields pay particular attention to improving not only health, functioning, and other specific aspects of life but also the more general quality of the lives that people lead. The central theme of this book is that quality of life is a construct that is at the heart of both health promotion and rehabilitation.

The two fields already share many goals and methodologies, but quality of life is the common ground and the concept that closely links them. Maintaining or enhancing quality of life of individuals is the overriding principle inherent in the rehabilitation process (Johnson & Jaffe, 1989; Seton, 1993). It is also the cornerstone of health promotion, which seeks to empower people to take charge of and improve their own health (Epp, 1986; Raphael, Brown, Renwick, & Rootman, 1994b; World Health Organization [WHO], 1986).

For this reason, this book presents quality of life as an important focus for research and as a proactive force in health promotion and rehabilitation theory, policy development, and practice. Both fields continue to develop and evolve, clarifying and reshaping their ranges of interest and foci of study. It is our contention that the extension of the knowledge base concerning quality of life in the context of health promotion and rehabilitation carries with it considerable promise for advancing both fields.

The Social Context for Quality of Life

Quality of life has been described as a predominant theme for this decade (Goode, 1994b; Lawton, 1991; Schalock, 1990b). The emergence of this theme has not occurred in isolation but, rather, is related to, and has occurred within, the context of a number of interrelated social and cultural trends.

THE MOST IMPORTANT TRENDS

Development of Social Welfare. Over the past several decades, there has been tremendous movement toward establishing comprehensive social welfare in most Western countries. This movement has focused attention on protection, access, and increasingly expanded roles for numerous institutions and areas of life, including housing, education, rehabilitation and care, health services, and other social services. Among the growing recognition that social welfare cannot expand indefinitely, attention has turned to improving quality within the services that do exist.

Equality and Human Rights. The equal treatment of people and other rights of all human beings have been recognized and specified by most developed countries. Equality values and human rights increase the possibilities for individuals and groups of individuals to lead lives of higher quality because they draw particular attention to inclusion of disadvantaged groups of people, such as people with disabilities (but see Rioux, Chapter 10, this volume, for a discussion of the concept of equality).

Legislation and Policy. In all Western countries, entitlements and rights were expanded through significant legislative thrusts. These directly affect a wide variety of disadvantaged groups of people and, more indirectly, through numerous policies that were subsequently developed. Legislation such as the Americans with Disabilities Act of 1990 and policies such as deinstitutionalization have added impetus to the need to conceptualize and study quality of life in a more thorough way, to evaluate existing policies, and to apply new knowledge to providing quality programs and services.

Normalization. This term emerged from the field of developmental disabilities in response to closing institutions and moving residents to "normal" community settings, where they could live life in "normal" ways. Although the term has been interpreted in various ways and has not been without controversy, its thrust has reached and affected other populations. The trend toward normalization has occurred within other disability groups, people who have experienced sexual abuse, people with mental illness, and many others. For such populations, centering on normalization usually means expanding the supports that increase the possibility of enjoying the things that the general population enjoys, thereby, presumably, increasing the quality of life.

Holism. Holism, which views human life and environments as functioning in complex, interrelated patterns, is a paradigm that has become more closely regarded in recent decades. Holism places emphasis on quality of the whole person in interaction with his or her environments rather than simply on specific aspects of his or her life. The growth of holism has carried with it an interest in what quality of life as a whole constellation of dimensions means to people and groups of people.

Economic Constraints. Over the past several decades, people in developed countries have enjoyed many benefits that arose from positive economic expansion. This expansion has resulted in increases in the general standard of living and has allowed for many improvements in the way people lead their lives. One interpretation of these improvements is that they constitute increases to overall quality of life. More recently, however, economic constraints in most countries have turned attention away from the probability of effecting major positive changes to the standard of living and, instead, toward seeking out quality within the standard of living we have and reevaluating the standard of living we thought we wanted. Economic constraint has pushed us to reexamine the meaning we attach to quality within our lives.

Quality of Life and Related Concepts

QUALITY OF LIFE

Quality of life is a social construct and, as such, has no inherent substance but, rather, has only the meaning that it is accorded (see I. Brown, Chapter 15, this volume; Labonté, Chapter 11, this volume). On the one hand, the word *quality* is a simple enough concept, generally understood to mean excellence or superiority, that can be applied to one's whole life. *Quality of life,* then, means how excellent or superior one's life is, as a whole. The problem is that although the general meaning of quality may be commonly understood, the specific meaning, when applied to people's lives, consistently varies among individuals and groups of people. Brown (1994) explained as follows:

> It is highly likely that no two people, from their own perspectives, think of excellence [and] superiority . . . in precisely the same way. . . . The essential meaning of quality may be understood by all, but when it is related to real people's lives, it is interpreted in any number of ways. (p. ii)

Thus it seems apparent that we already know what quality of life means in general, through our common usage of the word *quality,* but the meaning of quality varies among individuals and groups of people. The question for quality of life, then, becomes what people *think* constitutes quality within their lives. Someone asking this question assumes that "there are many means to the same [commonly understood] end" (Brown, 1994, p. ii), seeks to discover what those means are, and attempts to understand their meanings when applied to the lives of people.

That there are many means to the same end has not typically been made explicit or even understood in the academic literature, and interpreting quality in any number of ways has sometimes been thought to represent a problem in conceptualization. At other times, it has simply been accepted as the nature of the concept, and different interpretations are seen to reflect the specific purposes to which the concept is applied (Schalock, 1991).

OTHER RELATED CONCEPTS

Understanding the meaning of the concept *quality of life* is a conceptual challenge that can be addressed separately from examining the interrelationships between the general concept and other closely related ones, such as life satisfaction, happiness, morale, and well-being. It may be that the former challenge needs to precede the latter. Alternatively, it may be that the two challenges need to be explored simultaneously. It may also be that quality of life and other related concepts represent different levels of abstraction. If so, these different levels of abstraction may present an additional challenge to the ways that they interrelate.

One factor makes such exploration essential, for it has complicated our understanding of quality of life in recent years: Our haste to jump on the quality of life bandwagon has often led to liberal borrowing from other concepts that are related to it. Life satisfaction, happiness, morale, and well-being have been among the concepts from which quality of life has borrowed, because, like it, they are "global concepts, referring to life as a whole rather than to specific aspects of it" (Bowling, 1991, p. 151). Yet even these concepts have not been used in a consistent way (Stones & Kozma, 1980; Stull, 1987). In fact, it seems safe to say that all of these concepts have been used inconsistently in the literature and that many of them have been used interchangeably.

Quality of life appears to be a broader concept than the others from which it borrows (McDowell & Newell, 1987). This provides some reasonable grounds for such adoption because quality of life may subsume concepts such as happiness, morale, and life satisfaction. Still, there is overlap among these concepts, and there is equally a need to explore the nature of these overlaps and the relationships among them. Some of this exploration is begun within this book (e.g., Labonté; Rioux & Bach) but more will need to follow in future endeavors.

QUALITY OF LIFE AND HEALTH

Health is another concept that is closely related to quality of life and from which quality of life has borrowed (Renwick & Friefeld, Chapter 3, this volume). Quality of life is usually thought of as a broader concept than health, and health is sometimes thought to be subsumed by quality of life (McDowell & Newell, 1987; Raeburn & Rootman, this volume). But it seems likely that the relationship between the two concepts is considerably more complex than has been depicted to date for at least two reasons.

First, health is often cited as "one of the most important determinants of overall quality of life" (McDowell & Newell, 1987, p. 205), but conversely, quality of life is also thought of as a determinant of overall health (Raphael et al., 1994b). Good health is a universally held indicator of quality in life, but having a good overall life is likely to result in people being more healthy as well. The relationship between the two concepts needs to be explored further.

Second, although both health and quality of life are social constructs, quality of life may be more abstract in its conceptualization. Health is more readily understood to relate to concrete things, such as activity level, functional ability, absence of disease, and absence of pain. In its broader sense, where it relates to physical, psychological, and social well-being (WHO, 1986), health is more abstract but still relates to specific aspects of well-being. Quality of life, on the other hand, is not related to concrete things at the conceptual level at all. Only when it is applied to individuals and when those individuals disclose what they mean by and value as quality, can quality of life be tied to concrete indicators. This difference in the two concepts makes direct comparisons difficult and makes relationships between them harder to tease out.

A term that has gained considerable usage in recent years is *health-related quality of life*. This term is typically used in a narrow sense within the field of medicine among those who are primarily interested in the quality of changes that occur as a result of medical interventions (e.g., Schipper, Clinch, & Powell, 1990). Recently, some researchers in the medical field (e.g., Spilker, 1990) have begun to look beyond this reductionistic perspective to consider the relationship between health and more general well-being within people's lives.

Health promotion, which is based on a broader view of health that includes physical, psychological, and social well-being, also appears to view health-related quality of life in a broader way. For example, health is viewed as a resource for daily living, and overall quality of life has been described as the "true bottom line for health promotion" (Green & Kreuter, 1991, p. 48). To date, though, work on quality of life in health promotion has begun to be explored by only a few authors (e.g., Green & Kreuter, 1991; Raeburn & Rootman, 1995; Raphael et al., 1994b), who have set the stage for further developments. In this volume, the relationship between health and quality of life from the health promotion perspective is furthered by Raeburn and Rootman and others.

Rehabilitation has placed an emphasis on quality of life (Seton, 1993) and has also used the term *health-related quality of life*. The general field has placed an overwhelming emphasis on outcome measures rather than on theory (Parmenter, 1994) and has tended to use functional status and health status as substitutes for quality of life (Bergner, 1989; Renwick & Friefeld, this volume). By contrast, the subfield of rehabilitation that focuses on developmental disabilities has, interestingly, made a solid contribution to the overall quality of life literature (e.g., Goode, 1994b; Schalock, 1990b). Brown (1994) claimed the following:

> The field of developmental disabilities appears to be playing a substantial role in the development of a more general understanding of what quality means, how it might be assessed and measured, and how it might be fostered in service delivery and other systems. (p. i)

The contribution of knowledge about quality of life from the developmental disabilities field to our understanding and use of health-related quality of life has not been explored up to now. A number of the authors in this book, however, have begun to make that contribution.

Quality of Life in Health Promotion and Rehabilitation

There are similarities as well as differences between the fields of health promotion and rehabilitation. Both fields are multidisciplinary, as reflected in the backgrounds of the contributors to this volume. Both fields are evolving rapidly (e.g., see Pederson, O'Neill, & Rootman, 1994; Renwick & Friefeld, this volume). They are also concerned with many of the same life domains. Both are committed to prevention of illness and disability (McComas & Carswell, 1994), although health promotion places a greater emphasis on prevention than rehabilitation does. Further, both fields are increasingly concerned with environmental factors that contribute to health (Green & Kreuter, 1991; Roessler, 1990).

Rehabilitation has concentrated on restoring, maintaining, and increasing function (although it is now more oriented to community integration) of persons with disabilities. Within rehabilitation, improving function is often viewed as enhancing the quality of life for people who use its services. This field is concerned primarily with individuals and has not often focused on interventions for populations (McComas & Carswell, 1994). Health promotion seeks to enhance people's control over their own health (WHO, 1986) and thus over their lives. This field is concerned with the health of individuals (e.g., lifestyle issues) but it is more focused on the health of populations (e.g., communities, neighborhoods, the general population, and particular populations such as smokers, cyclists, and pregnant women).

The most striking area of commonality between the two fields is their shared, overarching goal: to improve quality within the lives of people and groups of people, with and without disabilities (Epp, 1986; Raeburn & Rootman, 1995; Raphael et al., 1994b). Bonds between the two fields have already been forged by previous efforts to integrate principles of health promotion and rehabilitation (e.g., Johnson & Jaffe, 1989; Jongbloed & Crichton, 1990; McComas & Carswell, 1994). It is through future developments in the theory, research, practice, and policy on quality of life, however, that there is the greatest potential for drawing the two fields closer together.

Guiding Principles of This Volume

Several basic assumptions or themes concerning quality of life were used as guiding principles for the content of the book. Our intention in proposing them is to suggest that they be adopted as guiding principles in future considerations of quality of life in health promotion and rehabilitation. These guiding principles are as follows:

- Quality of life is a multidimensional construct.
- Every individual is biopsychosocial in nature (i.e., has physical, psychological, and social aspects) and is in continual interaction with his or her environment.
- Because quality of life arises out of this complex person-environment interaction, a holistic approach is necessary for understanding it.
- The components of quality of life are the same for people with and without disabilities.
- Disability or any other handicapping condition, by itself, does not necessarily lead to increased or decreased quality of life for a person.
- The basic components of quality of life are those things that are common to all people and that constitute the human condition.
- Although the basic components of quality of life are the same for all people, the meaning attached to quality will differ to varying degrees from one person to another. This is because individuals attach differing relative importance to the

basic components of quality of life and have differing opportunities and constraints within their lives.

Overall Foci For Quality of Life

Four foci emerge as central to ongoing inquiry about quality of life as a key
common concept in the fields of health promotion and rehabilitation:

- The degree to which health promotion research and practice can and do contribute
  to improved quality of life of people
- The degree to which rehabilitation research and practice can and do contribute
  to improved quality of life of people
- The degree to which our understanding of quality of life influences health
  promotion activities
- The degree to which our understanding of quality of life influences rehabilitation
  activities

The first two foci are primarily (but not exclusively) concerned with
research and practice; the second two are primarily (but not exclusively)
concerned with theory and policy. There is considerable overlap among the
four and they interweave in the common ground between the two fields. The
intent in setting them out in this manner is to assist in clearly understanding
the challenges ahead.

Structure of this Book

In its first three parts, this book focuses on theory and research that
supports and acts as a guide to policy development and service practice. In
the fourth part, a number of applications are addressed. It is not the intention
that these applications be comprehensive but, rather, that they serve as
examples of some of the areas in which theory and research in quality of life
can be applied to policy development and service practice. The final section
of the book, Part V, ties together some of the major themes that arise from
the preceding sections and gives some overall directions for quality of life
theory, research, and applications in the future. A short summary of each part
is provided here.

Part I: Quality of Life in Health Promotion and Rehabilitation. These first
three chapters set out an argument for using quality of life as a central focus

in the fields of health promotion and rehabilitation. They introduce some key themes and concepts that are explored further in the other sections of the book. They also provide a general framework within which to understand the contributions of the book's other authors.

Part II: Conceptual Approaches to Quality of Life. Collectively, the chapters in this part review past and current conceptual perspectives on quality of life and consider their relevance and usefulness to health promotion and rehabilitation. These chapters also present new conceptual frameworks that can guide research, policy, and practice in both fields. The conceptual models presented can also serve as the underpinnings or catalysts for new frameworks relevant to both fields.

Part III: Some Critical Issues. This section examines quality of life issues of current importance that pertain to ethics, policy, quality assurance, and measurement.

Part IV: Applications of Quality of Life in Health Promotion and Rehabilitation. This section is organized into three subsections: (a) current social issues, (b) abilities and disabilities, and (c) major life activities. Together, these three subsections represent applications of quality of life concepts, principles, and perspectives to various populations (e.g., adolescents, older persons, workers, homeless persons, persons with disabilities and chronic illnesses, and persons who have experienced sexual abuse). Among these applications, research, assessment methodology, and critical analyses are highlighted, and implications for assessment, intervention, and policy development are outlined.

Part V: Future Directions. The final section of the book summarizes the key themes presented and discusses their implications for future conceptualization, research, service practice, and policy development in health promotion and rehabilitation.

Conclusion

The fields of health promotion and rehabilitation are both evolving rapidly. Both are multidisciplinary in nature and have similar overall goals. A better understanding of quality of life theory, research, and applications will advance both fields, draw them closer together, and help them evolve further.

The authors of this book represent a spectrum of disciplines that is typical of both fields. Such a range of perspectives can stimulate new ideas in theory, research, and practice because it brings together people from a variety of backgrounds. But it can also be something of a disadvantage because there is not always agreement among the various perspectives offered. For this reason, it is all the more important to have a clear understanding of the concepts that are central to the fields. It is our belief that this book represents a strong start to understanding clearly that quality of life is a central concept tying together the fields of health promotion and rehabilitation.

2

Quality of Life and Health Promotion

John M. Raeburn
Irving Rootman

Quality of life and *health promotion* are two concepts that have achieved considerable prominence over the past decade or so. Although they have been related to one another in significant health promotion documents (e.g., Epp, 1986; Lalonde, 1974; World Health Organization [WHO], 1986), the nature of their relationship has not been examined to any great extent (exceptions being Green & Kreuter, 1991; Raphael, Brown, Renwick, & Rootman, 1994b). This chapter attempts to examine this relationship and proposes a model to summarize the approach taken here.

This chapter discusses the concepts of health and health promotion. It examines the concept of quality of life and discusses its relationship to health and health promotion. It then presents a conceptual model showing the potential relationships between the three concepts. The chapter concludes with a discussion of applications of the conceptual framework in health promotion and a brief summary.

Health

The concept of health is discussed in depth elsewhere (Rootman & Rae-burn, 1994) from a number of different perspectives (e.g., historical, lay, medical, nursing, academic, international). There are significant differences in definitions of health depending on the perspective taken and the social and political context. For example, the Old English version was *haelth,* meaning safe, sound, or whole, whereas medical and popular Western definitions tend to relate to the absence of disease. Nursing and academic definitions, on the other hand, tend to be multidimensional, sometimes referred to as *biopsychosocial.*

The most commonly cited definition, however, is the one put forward by WHO in the charter that created it as an organization—namely, "a state of complete physical, mental and social well-being and not merely the absence of disease" (WHO, 1948, p. 1). Although this definition has been repeatedly criticized, it is attractive to people working in health for a number of reasons. In particular, it is positive and it suggests that health has other dimensions besides the physical. It is thus an expansive definition and one that challenges us to find new ways to promote health. For these reasons and because it is still the most widely accepted definition, we will use it in this chapter in relation to the concept of quality of life.

Before doing so, however, it should be noted that the definition was elaborated in a more recent document arising from the First International Conference on Health Promotion in 1986—the *Ottawa Charter for Health Promotion.* There, it was noted that for people "to reach a state of complete physical, mental and social well-being, an individual or group must be able to identify and realize aspirations, to satisfy needs, and to change or cope with the environment" (WHO, 1986, p. 1). In other words, health is not an end in itself but, rather, a resource for living, and the concept can be applied to individuals, groups of people, communities, or whole populations.

Health Promotion

Although the concept of health promotion also has many different defini-tions, the most widely cited and accepted one was also contained in the *Ottawa Charter for Health Promotion.* Building on earlier discussions within WHO, it was defined in the charter as "the process of enabling people to increase control over, and to improve, their health" (WHO, 1986, p. 1). Central to this concept of health promotion is the underlying notion of *empowerment.*

There is a growing body of literature on empowerment, but one of the most thorough discussions is presented by Labonté (1993). On the basis of a discussion by Morriss (1987), he suggests that empowerment can be said to exist simultaneously at three interpenetrating social levels:

1. At the intrapersonal level, it is the experience of a potent sense of self. . . . It is *power within,* the experience of choice.
2. At the interpersonal level, it is *power with,* the experience of interdependency.
3. At the intergroup level, it is the cultivation of resources and strategies for personal and sociopolitical gains, enhancing advocacy and participatory democracy, creating greater social equity; it is *power between,* [all italics added] the experience of generosity. (Labonté, 1993, p. 52)

The role of health promotion is to enable people to become empowered at each of these levels and a number of strategies have been developed to this end. According to Labonté, the key ones are personal care, small group development, community organization, coalition building and advocacy, and political action (Labonté, 1993). Labonté discusses empowerment in detail in a subsequent chapter in this volume.

The Ottawa charter (WHO, 1986) also suggests the following areas of action for health promotion: building healthy public policy, creating supportive environments, strengthening community action, developing personal skills, and reorienting health services. Although these are not identical to the strategies proposed by Labonté, they are certainly compatible. In any case, both views make it clear that health promotion involves action, presumably on those factors that exert an influence on people's health.

Quality of Life

As is made clear in this book, the concept of quality of life has been conceptualized in many different ways, although most would agree that it is an expression of "how good life is" for individuals or groups of people. For the purposes of this chapter, we accept the conceptual framework as well as the definition of quality of life advanced in detail in the Renwick and Brown chapter of this book. They define quality of life as "the degree to which a person enjoys the important possibilities of his or her life." We furthermore accept the idea that there are nine key areas of life in which people can achieve various degrees of quality of life. We also accept the notion that there are moderating conditions, including "control," which affect the quality of life of people.

There are a number of reasons why we accept this conceptualization of quality of life, aside from the fact that the second author of this chapter was involved in its development. Among other qualities, it is comprehensive, it is designed for individuals but can be aggregated for groups, it includes elements of social indicators, but perhaps most important, it is contextual.

Given the concepts of health, health promotion, and quality of life as defined here, can they be integrated into an overall conceptual framework? And if so, how? Our view is that they can, and we present one way of doing so following a brief review of the limited literature on the relationship of quality of life to health and to health promotion.

Quality of Life and Health

Over the past two decades, there has been more and more literature linking the concept of quality of life with that of health. In the health area, quality of life has traditionally been used as an outcome variable to evaluate the effectiveness of medical treatments (Hollandsworth, 1988) and rehabilitation (Livneh, 1988).

A number of the researchers in this field, however, explicitly reject the WHO definition of health. For example, Schipper, Clinch, and Powell (1990) argue as follows:

> This is a commendable definition, but it includes elements that are beyond the purview of traditional, apolitical medicine. Opportunity, education, and social security are important overall issues in the development of community health but they are beyond the immediate goal of our assessment, which is treating the sick. (p. 16)

Others, such as Kaplan and Bush (1982) and Torrance (1982), take the same view. On the other hand, some researchers working in this field have more sympathy for the WHO definition of health in relation to quality of life. For example, Bowling (1991) points out that only when one takes the WHO definition seriously does one begin to focus on indicators of positive well-being as worthy of attention. In practice, however, she avoids defining quality of life independent of the effects of illness on functioning. And in fact, this is the approach of most researchers using the concept of quality of life in the medical or health fields.

In contrast, the approach suggested here and in the chapter by Renwick and Brown defines quality of life explicitly and integrates it with the WHO definition of health.

Quality of Life and
Health Promotion

To date, there has been an even more limited literature on quality of life and health promotion than on quality of life and health. This is somewhat surprising given the fact that the *Ottawa Charter for Health Promotion* uses the concept of quality of life, noting that "good health is . . . an important dimension of quality of life" (WHO, 1986, p. 1).

A notable exception to this paucity of literature is found in the work of Green and Kreuter. In their health promotion model, assessing quality of life concerns is part of the social diagnosis phase of program development (Green & Kreuter, 1991). These concerns consist of the actual views held by community members about relevant issues, which provide the context for understanding how health issues could be raised at the community level. However, Green and Kreuter do not define quality of life explicitly before proceeding to discuss measurement.

In contrast, Raphael and his colleagues (Raphael et al., 1994b) do define quality of life using the definition adopted in this chapter. They suggest that it can be viewed as a determinant of health, as an outcome of health promotion interventions, or as an indicator of need. This is our view as well.

Quality of Life, Health,
and Health Promotion

This brings us to our proposed conceptual model for showing the relationships among the concepts of quality of life, health, and health promotion in an integrated fashion. This is not to suggest that our model is the only or necessarily the best model for doing so. We feel that it is a step in the right direction, however, and is helpful for understanding issues of concern in health promotion and rehabilitation.

To this end then, Figure 2.1 shows the relationship between the concept of quality of life as explicated in the Renwick and Brown chapter and the concept of health as defined by WHO. As can be seen, health is viewed here as encompassing three of the nine components of quality of life—namely, *physical being, psychological being,* and *social belonging,*

It could be argued that other quality of life components, such as *spiritual being* and *community belonging,* should also be included under the term *health.* And indeed, some of the other contributors to this volume discuss these kinds of factors in relation to health. Most of the criticisms of the current WHO definition, however, are that it is too broad and all-encompassing.

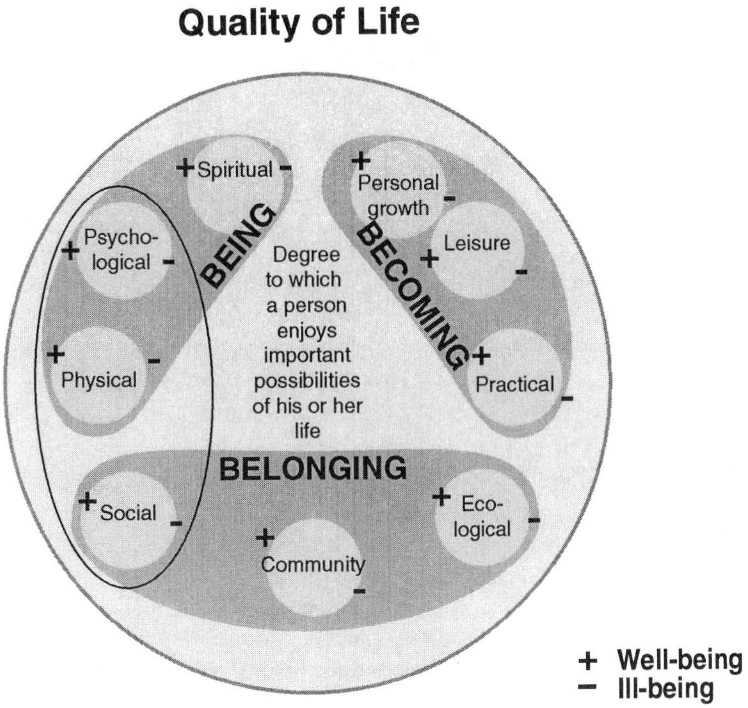

Quality of Life

Figure 2.1. Health as a Component of Quality of Life

Furthermore, the authors believe that one of the most valuable products of an attempt to look at the relationships between health and quality of life is to draw boundaries around what is understood to be health as opposed to "life." This has a purely pragmatic aspect to it. As economies contract and health budgets are compressed, an area such as health promotion is likely to lose its credibility if it is seen as trying to include "the whole of life." The authors believe it is wiser to keep a relatively broad definition of health and especially to have a positively oriented one but also to limit it to an area that is unambiguously health and allow other sectors (such as welfare and justice) to deal with other issues. However, this does not preclude communication and collaboration between those concerned with health promotion and these other sectors.

Another notable feature of Figure 2.1 is the specification of positive and negative ends of a continuum of well-being on all of the components of quality of life. The positive end might be called *well-being* and the negative, *ill-being.* This captures the idea proposed in the Renwick and Brown chapter that there can be differences between components of quality of life in terms of where individuals find themselves at any one time. Thus it is preferable to produce a quality of life "profile" rather than an overall score on quality of life (i.e., a multidimensional rather than unidimensional approach).

Before we can address the question of where health promotion fits into this conceptual framework, we must first deal with the issue of what factors contribute to quality of life and to health. Figure 2.2 graphically represents our analysis of this.

As Figure 2.2 indicates, quality of life is viewed as being the result of identifiable quality of life determinants in interaction with moderating conditions. These quality of life determinants, as distinct from those labeled "moderating conditions" in the central ellipse, are permanent or at least long-term factors that are the "givens" of an individual's or group's life. These long-term factors are divided into two categories: environmental and psychological.

Environmental determinants are subdivided into *macro* and *immediate* components. Macro environmental determinants are those associated with terms such as *biospheric, economic, societal, cultural, political,* and *national.* These are wider system factors affecting, but somewhat remote from, the immediate and everyday control and experiences of people in the community. Immediate environmental factors are those such as family, neighborhood, workplace, school, house, community association, and so on—environmental aspects close to the everyday lives and experiences of ordinary people, where there is more likelihood of at least some control at a local level.

Personal determinants are those associated with attributes of individuals and are subdivided into two subcategories: biological and psychological. Biological determinants are aspects of the body, brain, and behavior that are present due to genetic inheritance, somatic illness, accidents, and so on and are relatively unchangeable. Psychological determinants have to do with habits, cognition, emotions, perceptions, and experiences, which represent the individual's characteristic ways of dealing with the world and which may or may not be relatively changeable.

Obviously, this analysis is rather simplistic. Macro and immediate environmental aspects overlap and interact, as do environmental with personal and biological with psychological factors. The aim here is not to provide a pedantic or ultimate analysis but, rather, to state simply that there are a range of determinants with different dimensions that are capable of being conceptualized in terms of manageable chunks that are then amenable to change or attention, when and where this is appropriate. It should also be noted that the determinants circle in Figure 2.2 is seen as representing the situation for a person or group at any given time.

Quality of Life Field

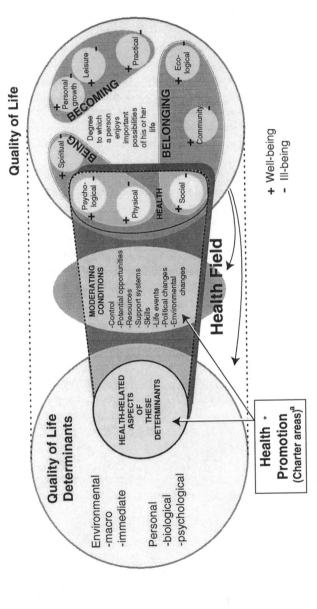

Figure 2.2. Comprehensive Health, Well-Being, and Quality of Life Framework, With Role of Health Promotion Shown

These determinants are in turn influenced by moderating conditions as illustrated in the ellipse between the Determinants circle and the Quality of Life circle. That is, given that people find themselves in a set of determining conditions (the left-hand circle), both environmental and personal, then, to the extent that these conditions are likely to have negative quality of life effects (as measured in the right-hand circle), they can be moderated by a number of variables. For example, someone might live in an oppressive macro environmental situation (e.g., war, poor housing, unemployment, crime), but if he or she feels there is some opportunity to exercise control over the situation (e.g., by leaving, joining a resistance group, or some other constructive action), then the quality of life effect of the oppressive situation could well be moderated in a positive direction. Certainly, there is evidence from the literature on stress that factors such as social support can positively affect well-being in otherwise noxious or pressured situations (Steptoe & Appels, 1989). These moderating conditions can either be environmental (e.g., opportunities or resources provided to do something about a situation) or be personal (e.g., skills developed to deal with a situation). They can also be a combination of the two (e.g., a support group organized that then enhances well-being).

One problem with showing moderating conditions as a separate entity is that, in practice, it may be difficult to differentiate quality of life determinants from moderating conditions. For example, a community (immediate environment, quality of life determinant) may be oppressive but also offer opportunities and resources to change the situation. On the whole, the distinction between the two is, as mentioned, that determinants refer mainly to long-term existential conditions of a general nature, whereas moderating conditions are those external to the situation that alter the normally expected negative effects of various determinants in a positive direction. The distinction between determinants and moderating conditions makes the point that the effect of existing conditions is not "pure" but can sometimes be changed dramatically by the presence or absence of moderating factors.

As can also be seen from Figure 2.2, there is a feedback loop going from the Quality of Life outcome ellipse to the Moderating circle and another one to the Determinants circle because changes in outcomes could in turn result in changes in the moderating conditions or determinants. All of this can be referred to as the *quality of life field*.

The other element of this figure that deserves comment is the *health field*. In the left-hand Determinants circle, health is seen as being affected by many or all of the same factors as those that affect quality of life. In short, almost anything can affect health, as can almost anything affect quality of life. Because health and quality of life domains each has its own set of preoccupations and emphases, however, we feel it is important to distinguish the health-related aspects of the overall quality of life components from the larger array simply because in discussions of health (as distinct from quality of life), different considerations obtain. For example, if one is looking at overall quality of life from a developmental disability perspective, then determinant items such as transportation, recreational facilities, supportive halfway houses, and so on might be important considerations. If one is looking at health in terms of a given community, however, then although matters such as transportation, recreational facilities, and specialist housing will all impinge on health, they are unlikely to be as central as other concerns, such as adequate food, presence or absence of violence, lifestyle habits, and so on. So quality of life and health share the same general array of determinant factors, but they take on a special aspect when considered in a health context.

Similarly, the moderating conditions need special consideration when one is considering a health field distinct from a quality of life field. Again, many of the same kinds of moderators are likely to apply in both areas, but the emphases are likely to be different when the concern is health. For example, there is a whole literature on the issue of personal control as related to specific physical health conditions (Steptoe & Appels, 1989), whereas the same arguments do not yet appear to have been made for more general quality of life outcomes.

In summary then, the health field is a subfield of the quality of life field but has more limited outcomes and a different set of emphases in the areas of determinants and moderating conditions. The overall paradigm is the same for both, however.

This brings us to the role of health promotion in this overall conceptualization. As noted in Figure 2.2, the term *health promotion* is based on the Ottawa charter (WHO, 1986), and the "inputs" are the five action areas outlined in it. That is, health promotion is a broad-spectrum, wide-ranging endeavor with dimensions (outlined earlier) ranging from the individual skills level through community action and health service change to wider environmental, policy, and ecological concerns. Here, health promotion actions are seen as being applied to two components of the health field— namely, the Determinants circle and the Moderating Conditions ellipse. That is, on the one hand, health promotion is concerned with the creation of both a general healthy environmental climate in which people operate and of a culture for helping to determine healthy behavior (determinants). On the other hand, it also involves deliberate, planned interventions designed to create new environments and changes in personal factors (moderating conditions).

The outcomes of health promotion will hopefully be reflected as positive changes in the three health subareas of the right-hand Quality of Life output circle. The placement of the health area in a wider quality of life context emphasizes that the context for this health is a quality of life context. Furthermore, our overall concern is with "social health in a positive quality of life context." Also, it is quite likely that effective health promotion interventions will have a positive effect on some or all of the other quality of life indicators. The real strengths of this conceptualization are that (a) health is a clearly specified domain within a larger quality of life domain and (b) the emphasis is on positive outcomes oriented toward well-being, not just prevention of disease or other negative indicators.

Application of Quality of Life in Health Promotion

There are a number of ways in which this conceptual framework might be applied in health promotion. For one, it helps to place in context and at the same time delimit the role of health promotion. That is, it makes it clear that health promotion, although it may affect larger domains of quality of life, is not solely responsible for doing so. In fact, its main focus of action should be on the determinants and moderators that are most likely to affect health. It is hoped that this will prevent health promotion practitioners from becoming overwhelmed by the enormity of their responsibilities.

The framework can also be helpful in providing a checklist of the key elements to be considered in developing any health promotion intervention. That is, it makes clear that macro and immediate environmental as well as biological and psychological personal factors need to be considered along with key moderating conditions such as control, potential opportunities, resources, support systems, skills, political changes, and environmental changes. Any specific initiative may emphasize a few of these elements but will be enriched by paying some attention to the others.

We believe the framework is also helpful in drawing attention to the fact that all of the factors involved are interrelated and that they exert influence in both directions. It reminds us that we must not engage in simplistic unidirectional thinking with respect to cause but, rather, consider it in its full complexity. This in turn can help us in developing initiatives that are realistic in terms of expectations of success.

Finally, given the focus of this book on rehabilitation, this framework should make it clear to those who are concerned about issues of rehabilitation that they have much in common with those who are concerned about promoting health. Many of the issues and ways of thinking about them are similar and we can continue to benefit from one another as we address them. Furthermore, health promotion can be intrinsic to rehabilitation research and practice. Health promotion and quality of life are key issues for people with and without disabilities.

Summary

We have presented what we consider to be an innovative framework for considering the relationships between quality of life, health, and health promotion and have made some suggestions regarding how this framework might enhance practice in health promotion and rehabilitation. Health was viewed as a subfield of the quality of life field, well-being as the positive aspect of experienced quality of life, and health promotion as that set of actions that alters the determinants and moderators of health as defined here.

Although we think that this is a valuable and workable framework, we would not like to leave the impression that this is the last word on the topic. It appears to us that, although we are advancing toward a better understanding of the relationship between the concepts discussed, there is more that needs to be done.

For one thing, we need to undertake an analysis of the concepts at different levels of aggregation. We have tended to concentrate on the individual level in this analysis. However, the definitions and concepts may apply equally well at the group, community, and societal levels. This requires further analysis and research.

Similarly, we need continuing discussion and debate about the relationship between the concepts of quality of life, health, and health promotion. Although we feel that the ground we have covered here permits us to plan for and take sensible action, it is important that we not assume that the conceptual problems have been fully addressed and that there are not other equally legitimate approaches that may have different emphases.

Finally, we are left with the challenge of defining and enhancing the relationship between health promotion and rehabilitation. We believe this chapter helps in that regard but it is only a small beginning. Other chapters in this book contribute further to an understanding of this relationship.

3

Quality of Life
and Rehabilitation

Rebecca Renwick
Sharon Friefeld

Enhancing quality of life is usually the inherent, overarching goal of rehabilitation interventions and programs (e.g., Fabian, 1991; Roessler, 1990; Sartorius, 1992). Thus, quality of life should be an important focus for theory, research, and practice in rehabilitation. The quality of life of individuals receiving rehabilitation services, however, is often not assessed directly. Rather, it is assumed to be enhanced if progress or improvement occurs in individuals' level or patterns of functioning (e.g., functional performance, limitations, strengths, independence, or adjustment) or overall health. When it is assessed clinically or in the context of rehabilitation research, quality of life is most commonly measured in terms of functional status in one or more areas (e.g., Turner, 1990) or health status (e.g., Bergner, 1989). Frequently, the literature in this area offers no clear conceptualization of quality of life

AUTHORS' NOTE: The authors thank Azmina Habib for her assistance in preparing this chapter and Ivan Brown for his helpful comments.

(Fabian, 1991) and treats the construct as if it were interchangeable with other constructs—in particular, functional status and health status (Bergner, 1989). Furthermore, the relatively few conceptualizations of quality of life that do appear in the rehabilitation literature are typically not detailed or well developed. In fact, most approaches are operational in nature; that is, they are concerned with measures used to assess quality of life rather than with its conceptual foundations (Renwick, 1993).

To provide a context for the material presented in this chapter, the evolution of rehabilitation and its changing focus are considered. Recent trends that have implications for approaches to quality of life in the context of rehabilitation are also discussed. Then, the major approaches to quality of life currently used in rehabilitation are briefly reviewed. Finally, the chapter suggests future directions concerning the quality of life construct and its applications within the context of rehabilitation.

The area of developmental disabilities is often viewed as constituting a subfield within rehabilitation. Recent conceptualizations of and research on quality of life in this subfield (e.g., Goode, 1994b) have made a strong contribution to our overall understanding of quality of life. Several other chapters in this volume discuss some of these contributions in the area of developmental disabilities (e.g., the chapters by R. Brown, Ouellette-Kuntz & McCreary, and Schalock). Therefore, the current chapter concentrates on rehabilitation with other populations.

Rehabilitation:
An Evolving Field

The term *rehabilitation,* as employed in this chapter, refers to a multidisciplinary field that is concerned with physical, emotional, cognitive, and social aspects of functioning in the major areas of life (e.g., mobility, communication, activities of daily living, vocational activities, social relationships, and leisure and recreation) across the lifespan. Since the early years of this century, rehabilitation has continued to evolve (Turner, 1990). Traditionally, it focused on compensatory programs (Frey, 1984) but in recent years it has begun to concentrate more and more on facilitating adjustment to disability as well as social and community integration of persons with disabilities (Kerr & Meyerson, 1987; Turner, 1990; Wood-Dauphinée & Williams, 1987). Some of the newest approaches emphasize the participation of individuals with disabilities in the aspects of community life in which they choose to be involved (Emener, 1993). The most contemporary perspectives on rehabilitation also include attention to health promotion as well as primary and secondary prevention of disability (Johnson & Jaffe, 1989; Stuifbergen & Becker, 1994; Teague, Cipriano, & McGhee, 1990).

This change in perspective in the field of rehabilitation has meant that there is increasing attention to the interaction between persons and their environments (Turner, 1990). Current developments in the field are not typically reflected explicitly enough in rehabilitation approaches to quality of life. As Roessler's (1990) analysis suggests, however, quality of life is a construct that makes provision for more clearly understanding both personal and environmental factors in the context of rehabilitation. It can also provide a framework for understanding the interactions between persons and their environments.

Influential Current Trends

Rehabilitation, like other fields, evolves over time in response to advances in knowledge and social change. The past two decades have given rise to some important trends that have influenced the evolution of rehabilitation or are likely to do so in the immediate future. In particular, they have implications for which approaches to quality of life are employed within the field. These developments are beginning to inform and could significantly advance conceptual perspectives on, measurement of, and interventions that focus on quality of life. To date, however, the relationships between these influential trends and quality of life have not been made sufficiently explicit. Similarly, the ways in which quality of life conceptualizations can contribute to rehabilitation theory, research, and practice have not yet been adequately explored.

ACTIVISM FOR INCLUSION
OF PERSONS WITH DISABILITIES

One of these developments is the flourishing and dynamic activism within the independent living movement and the consumer movement. At the heart of these sociopolitical movements are several well-articulated themes: inclusion and participation in all aspects of society, equal status and opportunity with nondisabled persons, empowerment, and personal control for individuals with disabilities (Carpenter, 1991; McPherson, 1990; Zola, 1994). These movements also advocate for participation of persons with disabilities in defining key issues in research and policy formulation that pertain to their lives (Bach, 1994; Woodill, 1992).

The common thread linking these issues and themes expressed by persons with disabilities is the realization that environmental factors (e.g., social, political, cultural, and physical) continue to pose significant obstacles to their opportunities for participating in and contributing to society. Clearly, this could affect the quality of life experienced by individuals with disabilities.

DISABILITY AND ENVIRONMENTAL FACTORS

These ideas concerning the full and equal participation of persons with disabilities in society have profoundly influenced current thinking about and definitions of disability. Specifically, disability is viewed more and more in environmental terms rather than simply as an attribute of individuals, as has traditionally been the case (see Fougeyrollas, 1992; Jongbloed & Crichton, 1990; World Health Organization [WHO], 1980b). In essence, this contemporary perspective on disability "asserts that environmental barriers are as (or more) important than personal characteristics in determining disability outcomes" (Jongbloed & Crichton, 1990, p. 34). This implies that rehabilitation professionals and researchers need to accord more attention than they currently do to such environmental issues as social support, access to vocational and leisure programs and resources, and attitudes toward disability (DeJong, 1979; Jongbloed & Crichton, 1990). One way to better address such issues is to make use of conceptualizations of quality of life that provide frameworks within which to examine the person-environment interaction and the potential of environments to foster quality of life. Another advantage of using such conceptualizations of quality of life is that they serve as a means of making explicit, measuring, and evaluating the ultimate goal of rehabilitation—to improve the quality of specific aspects of life, especially as they pertain to the whole life of the individual.

HEALTH PROMOTION,
DISABILITY, AND QUALITY OF LIFE

The growing emphasis on principles of health promotion constitutes another recent trend that could significantly enrich approaches to quality of life within the field of rehabilitation. Health promotion is a multidisciplinary field that is concerned with the exercise of personal control—in particular, "enabling people to increase control over and to improve their health" (WHO, 1986, p. 2). This focus of concern applies to persons with and without disabilities (Epp, 1986; Health and Welfare Canada [HAWC], 1988; Johnson & Jaffe, 1989; McComas & Carswell, 1994). This concept of empowerment is one shared by both the independent living movement and the field of health promotion (Brooks, 1984) and has recently begun to be discussed in the context of rehabilitation (Emener, 1993; McComas & Carswell, 1994).

Health promotion embraces a broad perspective on health (Epp, 1986; HAWC, 1988; Johnson & Jaffe, 1989; WHO, 1986) that recognizes that environmental factors (e.g., financial, legal, cultural, social, physical) exert significant influence on people's health and quality of life. Furthermore, health is seen as "part of everyday living, an essential dimension of quality in our lives. 'Quality of life' in this context implies the opportunity to make choices and to gain satisfaction from living" (Epp, 1986, p. 5). Health is conceptualized as a resource people can use to cope with or modify their environments—that is, their most immediate living and working environments as well as their neighborhoods and communities. Furthermore, health is envisioned as encompassing the "energy, strengths and abilities of the individual interacting effectively with those of the group and with opportunities and influences in the environment" (HAWC, 1988, p. 7) in ways that foster quality of life. These principles imply that health, as defined in a broad sense, is a major aspect of quality of life and that it can be promoted at both the individual and population levels.

The powerful themes implicit in the current trends outlined here have considerable significance for the way in which quality of life is conceptualized and measured in the context of rehabilitation as well as for the focus of rehabilitation interventions and programs. The implications of these themes are discussed in the final section of the chapter.

Current Rehabilitation
Approaches to Quality of Life

Before examining how the developments discussed in the previous section could contribute to the evolution of approaches to quality of life in the field of rehabilitation, it is helpful to review some of the major approaches currently employed. The rehabilitation literature on quality of life is quite diverse, and many operational approaches to the construct have been developed for specific purposes or for use in specific settings or situations (Bergner, 1989). Thus, it is often difficult to group these operational approaches except within broad categories.

As previously noted, there have been very few attempts to define and conceptualize quality of life within the field of rehabilitation. When conceptual definitions of quality of life are presented, they usually portray the construct in terms of the function or functional patterns (e.g., Schipper & Levitt, 1985; Turner, 1990) or health status (Bergner, 1989) of individuals. The conceptualizations that do appear in the literature are typically general and restricted to listing the domains that are relevant to quality of life (e.g.,

Bergner, 1989; Schipper & Levitt, 1985). Usually, these domains pertain to function or performance in the following areas: physical, cognitive, emotional, and social (i.e., role and interpersonal). These conceptualizations, however, do not specify the relationships among their various components.

Almost all rehabilitation approaches to the construct are measurement-oriented or operational ones that are not explicitly based on any developed theoretical framework of quality of life (Parmenter, 1994). A number of these operational approaches have been reported in the literature. However, because many of them are described and reviewed elsewhere (Bergner, 1989; Bowling, 1991; McDowell & Newell, 1987; Turner, 1990), only a brief overview of the major ones (and some exemplars of each) used in rehabilitation are presented here. Although, as Bergner (1989) observes, the terms *functional status* and *health status* are frequently used as synonyms for *quality of life,* it is possible to distinguish between functional status and health status operational (measurement) approaches. There are other approaches to quality of life measurement within rehabilitation (for brief reviews see the Day & Jankey chapter and Fabian, 1991) but the functional status and health status measures are the ones most commonly used (e.g., see Bergner, 1989; Turner, 1990).

FUNCTIONAL STATUS APPROACHES

Most of these operational approaches to functional status have not been developed for the specific purpose of assessing quality of life and are not based on any explicit conceptual formulation of the construct. They have come to be used as measures to assess or make inferences about quality of life, however.

The content of operational approaches to functional status concentrates primarily on individual function within selected areas of life. Some of these measures do include scales or items that tap various aspects of mental or emotional health or selected physical symptoms (e.g., fatigue) but this is a more minor focus. The measures outlined here exemplify the functional status approach.

The Barthel Index (BI) (Mahoney & Barthel, 1965) consists of 10 items concerning activities of daily living and is rated by a rehabilitation professional on the basis of observation or medical records. Ratings are made on the level of independence in each of the 10 functional activities assessed. The major emphasis is on physical performance of each activity.

Jette's (1980) Functional Status Index was constructed for use with persons who have chronic diseases. It assesses 45 daily activities in five areas: gross mobility, personal care, hand activities, home chores, and interpersonal activities. Each item is rated along three dimensions: levels of dependence, pain, and difficulty in performing the activity. The ratings are determined on the basis of the respondent's answers (in the context of an interview) to the instrument items.

The Functional Activities Questionnaire (Pfeffer, Kurosaki, Chance, Filos, & Bates, 1984) was originally designed for use with older adults living in the community. The 10 items are concerned with higher-level mental and social functioning inherent in daily independent living activities (e.g., organizing appointments and financial matters, shopping and transportation, meal preparation). All items are rated, according to the individual's level of dependence or independence, by a close other person (e.g., a friend, relative, or child of the target person).

HEALTH STATUS APPROACHES

Health status approaches to quality of life tend to have a wider scope than the functional status approaches. They usually include items that pertain to functional abilities, however. The content of health status approaches has frequently been based on conceptual formulations concerning health, not on conceptualizations of the quality of life construct (Bergner, 1989). These approaches do not attempt to explicate the relationship between the health status and quality of life constructs.

Some health status approaches can be characterized as being applicable to a variety of populations. Several examples are briefly considered here. The Sickness Impact Profile (SIP) (Bergner, Bobbitt, Carter, & Gilson, 1981) is one of the best known operational approaches used to assess quality of life. It was designed to evaluate perceived health status and "detect changes or differences in health status that occur over time and between groups" (Bergner et al., 1981, p. 787), including changes following interventions. Its major dimensions encompass psychological and physical health, sleep and rest, eating, work, and home management, as well as recreation and pastimes. The SIP is rated on the basis of the respondent's answers to 136 items concerning health-related behaviors and activities (in either a self-report or interviewer-administered format).

The Nottingham Health Profile (NHP) (Hunt, McKenna, McEwen, Williams, & Papp, 1981) focuses on individuals' subjective assessments of their physical, emotional, and social health through responses to questions about "feelings and emotional states" (McDowell & Newell, 1987, p. 286). The NHP consists of 38 self-administered items concerning six major aspects of health: mobility, pain, sleep, social isolation, emotional reactions, and energy level.

A few health status operational approaches concentrate on specific populations. Arthritis has been the focus for the development of a variety of measures. The Arthritis Impact Measurement Scale (AIMS) (Meenan, German, Mason, & Dunaif, 1982) is one of the most frequently cited and best-known operational approaches to health status that has been used to assess quality of life of a specific population. It consists of nine scales (45 items) that evaluate the physical, social, and emotional well-being domains of health for persons with arthritis. Nineteen additional items deal with health and the individual's perceptions about it as well as demographic information. Most of the self-administered items of the AIMS ask respondents about their health-related behaviors and activities, but the items concerning emotional well-being include questions about depression and anxiety.

LIMITATIONS OF FUNCTIONAL STATUS
AND HEALTH STATUS APPROACHES

These approaches are, understandably, not tied to well-developed conceptual frameworks of quality of life because they were originally developed as measures of function and health. Still, they continue to be used, partly because there is a dearth of such frameworks in the rehabilitation literature on which to base quality of life measures. Although there appears to be some conceptual overlap of functional status and health status with quality of life, it cannot be assumed that measures of functional status or health status adequately tap quality of life experienced by individuals. For instance, it is often assumed that quality of life and measures of functional status are positively correlated; however, the research that addresses this issue is sparse and the findings equivocal at best (Fabian, 1991).

Another limitation is that the content of the major approaches considered here does not reflect to any great extent the major themes implicit in the current trends influencing rehabilitation that were previously discussed. This may be due, in part, to the fact that some of these approaches have been in use for some time and many have not been recently updated and revised. To a large extent, continuing use of these measures is likely to be based on their demonstrated psychometric properties (e.g., see Bowling, 1991).

The most noticeable common characteristic of these approaches is the preponderance of attention accorded to the individuals' characteristics, reactions, and behaviors (i.e., functional strengths, weaknesses, skills, independence, or adjustment) in various areas of life. Environments in which individuals live, work, and recreate and the contributions these environments make to quality of life receive little direct consideration. Even when the interaction between the individual and the environment is the purported variable of interest, the focus remains primarily on the characteristics, reactions, and behaviors of the person.

These operational approaches do not appear to acknowledge the concepts of empowerment and the importance of the individual's own perspective. In fact, some of the approaches do not even elicit responses from the consumer and rely instead on ratings by the professional or others. Most of them were not developed with input from consumers, but even those that were (e.g., Hunt et al., 1981) relied on specific data collected and analyzed by the researchers rather than an ongoing process of consultation and review by persons with disabilities. Furthermore, they do not make provision for identifying which aspects of daily living and function are more important than others and which are relatively unimportant to particular individuals with disabilities. They do not illuminate how satisfactory these various aspects of function and daily living are for the individual. They also do not examine the extent to which choices and opportunities for enhancing quality of life are available in individuals' environments.

Future Directions

There is a pressing need for new conceptual frameworks of quality of life that are relevant to the evolving focus and concerns of rehabilitation as well as the current influential trends discussed earlier in this chapter. New conceptual frameworks should provide opportunities for understanding how the evolving field of rehabilitation fits with the overall goal of improving the quality of people's lives. In addition, they should provide broad frameworks within which current and future developments in the field can be coherently integrated. By way of specific examples, new conceptual frameworks should provide the basis for development of quantitative instruments and qualitative methods (e.g., interview formats) for use in rehabilitation research and clinical assessment (e.g., see Raphael, Brown, Renwick, & Rootman, in press; Rudman, Renwick, Raphael, & Brown, 1995). They would also serve as guides for program planning and intervention (e.g., see Renwick, Brown, & Raphael, 1994). Such conceptual models would enable researchers and practitioners to concentrate more clearly and directly on quality of life as a focus for assessment, intervention, and outcomes in rehabilitation. At present, despite their higher-order goal of enhancing quality of life (Roessler, 1990), most interventions in rehabilitation are focused on increasing function instead of being directly targeted to enhancing quality of life. Having detailed conceptual frameworks around which to plan and evaluate quality of life interventions, however, would encourage and facilitate their use in rehabilitation (see Sartorius, 1992).

Ideally, these new conceptual approaches should be detailed and specify the relationships among their component parts. The potentially most useful frameworks would also take into account the evolutionary changes in the field as well as the current influential trends and the emergent themes associated with these. For instance, because the major consumers of rehabilitation services are persons with disabilities, it is important for these conceptual frameworks to incorporate, or at least take account of, principles and concepts for which consumers are advocating. This would include concepts and principles related to exercise of personal control and decision making as well as independent living (Carpenter, 1991; DeJong, 1979; Zola, 1994). It would also be appropriate to build in some consideration of which areas of daily life are relatively important and unimportant for individuals, as this will vary from person to person. New quality of life models could guide research, assessment, intervention, and outcome evaluation. Therefore, developing them in partnership with persons with disabilities could help to make most aspects of rehabilitation more clearly relevant to the lives of persons with disabilities.

Current developments in health promotion could also inform the development of new conceptual models of quality of life within the field of rehabilitation. Its broader perspective on health, which includes explicit attention to such environmental factors as its social determinants (HAWC, 1988), would be useful in this regard. New frameworks for use in rehabilitation would benefit from incorporating this perspective because it would enable an understanding of the larger context within which individuals interact as they live their everyday lives. Frameworks incorporating this perspective could also be used to guide rehabilitation research and assessment aimed at determining specific environmental factors that contribute to quality of life. Such an understanding is necessary if rehabilitation is to be truly effective in facilitating improved quality of life. This kind of attention to the contributions of environments to quality of life would also encourage rehabilitation professionals and researchers to bridge gaps between their own field and others (e.g., education and social services) (see Sartorius, 1992). Cooperation between researchers and professionals in rehabilitation and these other fields could serve to focus joint efforts on a wide spectrum of environmental issues that affect life as a whole for persons with disabilities. Such an holistic approach has the potential to more effectively promote quality of life for persons with disabilities than the more fragmented approaches currently used.

The concepts of opportunities to exert personal control by making choices and of deriving satisfaction from living are inherent in quality of life, according to at least one health promotion framework (Epp, 1986). The degree to which individuals find various aspects of daily living satisfying and the extent to which opportunities for making choices and changes in their environments could be useful additions to rehabilitation frameworks of quality of life.

Health promotion also emphasizes the importance of both individual and population approaches to enhancing health and, ultimately, making a positive contribution to quality of life. Conceptualizations of quality of life for use in rehabilitation would benefit from the recognition of this principle. Models that could guide interventions at the community and population levels are rarely employed in rehabilitation (but for an example, see McComas & Carswell, 1994). New models of the kind being suggested here might be used effectively in large-scale programs targeted to enhancing quality of life for persons with disabilities (e.g., in schools, the workplace, and public areas such as shopping centers and recreational facilities).

The development of conceptual approaches to quality of life in the context of rehabilitation is in its infancy. A number of conceptual frameworks of quality of life that have been developed recently, however, have particular relevance for rehabilitation. These frameworks encompass many of the ideas discussed in this chapter and have the potential to contribute significantly to further development in this area. Several of them are discussed in other chapters of this volume, particularly in Section II that follows. They can serve as valuable springboards for, and contribute useful insights and concepts to new approaches to quality of life that include attention to the relationship between functioning and the broader issue of enhancing the quality of life for persons with disabilities. When these new conceptualizations of quality of life are developed and applied, they should contribute significantly to rehabilitation theory, research, and practice and thus to the evolution of the field as a whole.

PART

II

CONCEPTUAL APPROACHES
TO QUALITY OF LIFE

4

Lessons From the Literature

Toward a Holistic Model
of Quality of Life

Hy Day
Sharon G. Jankey

There is an ancient Indian fable that tells of seven blind men who went to investigate an elephant. But being blind, they were able to explore it only by touch. So they each touched a different part of the elephant and, basing it on their own experiences, perceived the concept of elephant differently. To the man who felt the tail, an elephant was like a rope; to the man who felt the leg, it was a tree trunk; to one a wall, and so on. Each blind person perceived the concept in a restricted manner. But none of them really experienced the totality of the elephant.

In this chapter we will argue that some earlier, influential theoretical approaches to quality of life were formulated by people who perceived the concept from a restricted spectrum and defined it such that it lacked totality. Using qualitative methodology, we asked people from different walks of life what quality of life means to them and, from their responses, generated a holistic model that is more inclusive than other definitions. But first we examine the history of the concept as it has developed in North America and illustrate the narrowness of previous models.

The Social Indicators Approach:
The Roots of Quality of Life

The term *quality of life* was popularized in the 1960s by politicians interested in providing a platform to trumpet the success of their administrations. U.S. President Lyndon Johnson has been quoted as using the quality of life term in a speech in 1964 at the University of Michigan that deals precisely with a concern for the "good life" or a "quality life":

> The task of the Great Society is to ensure our people the environment, the capacities, and the social structures that will give them a meaningful chance to pursue their individual happiness. Thus the Great Society is concerned not with how much, but with how good—not with the quantity of the goods, but with the quality of their lives. (quoted in Campbell, 1981, p. 441)

Later, in 1969, U.S. President Richard Nixon took much the same approach when he established the National Goals Research Staff, which was to have been involved in "developing and monitoring social indicators that can reflect the present and future quality of American life and the direction and rate of its change" (quoted in Campbell, 1981, p. 441). It appeared that the adoption of the goal that everyone has the right to a quality life brought the quality of life term into common usage (Schuessler & Fisher, 1985). Politicians' use of the term appeared to be a demonstration that they were interested in the actual well-being of their electorates. Thus, enhancing quality of life became a goal for politicians concerned with being reelected.

Politicians were familiarized with the concept of quality of life through groundbreaking research by a handful of major research institutions in the United States, including the Russell Sage Foundation, the Institute of Social Research at the University of Michigan, and the National Opinion Research Center at the University of Chicago. At these institutions, researchers used a social indicators approach to define what quality of life meant to them. This approach replaced the economic one that had, in the past, been the way the success of a nation's health had been conceptualized. The climate for the emergence of the social indicators approach was ripe in the 1960s because, along with an unprecedented rise in national income, came the opportunities and material benefits it brought. But with it also came rising rates of violence, crime, and public disorder (Campbell & Rodgers, 1972). The new problems that were emerging despite increased societal wealth suggested that there was more to society than economic growth, and the social indicators gauged the rising importance of the social welfare of the nation.

But the social information being collected at that time lacked one important aspect. Only objectively oriented information was being collected, with a focus on external factors. These were presumed by the researchers to constitute quality of life and consisted of external conditions such as education, income, housing, and neighborhood domains. Research centered primarily on finding effective ways to measure quality of life and then applying these measures to broad general populations in various U.S. cities and states as well as various West European countries and the United States (Andrews, 1986). This approach to quality of life measurement is still popular today. However, even though early work found statistically significant relationships between sociodemographic variables and people's quality of life, these relationships were weak. Thus, it became clear that there was more to quality of life than simply the objective circumstances in which people lived. All the measures consisted of a researcher-selected set of conditions, or domains, that were then pooled to form an index of quality of life. But the selection of the domains, being researcher-driven, reflected the priorities and interests of each individual researcher, and so the indicators were far from identical and, in fact, barely resembled each other.

The Psychological Indicators Approach

The seminal work of Campbell and Rodgers (1972) redirected the course of quality of life research. They advocated that social or objective indicators are limited in their function in that they serve only as indirect indicators of the quality of a person's life. Moreover, they showed that social indicators rarely account for more than 15% of the variance in an individual's quality of life. Psychological or subjective indicators, on the other hand, were purported to be direct measures and were seen by them as accounting for additional variance not predicted by objective measures.

Psychological indicators refer to an individual's subjective reactions to life experiences. Such subjective measures depend primarily on the direct experience of the person whose life is being assessed and indicate how people perceive their own lives. Happiness, satisfaction, and related attitudes become worthy of measurement in the psychological or subjective approach. The importance of these psychological indicators was demonstrated dramatically by Campbell and Rodgers (1972), who found that these indications accounted for over 50% of the variance in quality of life. They concluded that quality of life is a psychological experience that may not correspond closely to external conditions.

The psychological indicators approach is not without its detractors, however. Zautra and Goodhart (1979) pointed to three good reasons why some researchers are skeptical of psychological indicators. One is the possibility of social-desirability-response bias. Many studies (cf. Campbell, Converse, & Rodgers, 1976; Klassen, Hornstra, & Anderson, 1975) have found social desirability to exert a small but nonetheless pervasive effect on reports of satisfaction, mood, and symptomatology. A second reason involves idiosyncrasies in reports of feeling states between persons. For example, two individuals may mean different things in their response of "very satisfied," and individuals' responses on one day may be different from their responses on another day. Inherent in all self-report measures is the variability of response patterns within the same individuals, depending on their mood, external conditions, and the like (Diener & Emmons, 1984). A third reason is the possible inadequacy of social indicators as measures of quality of life, particularly as reflected in the realities of environmental conditions. Thus, certain aspects of quality of life can be assessed only by external, objective measures.

The Comparison Approach

Alex Michalos (1986) advocated a "gap" approach to quality of life, wherein the salient feature is the gap between one's present life and a standard to which one is comparing oneself. His multiple discrepancies theory combined aspects of six gap-theoretical hypotheses that had been reported in the literature; a summary of Michalos's review follows. One goal-achievement-gap theory refers to the perceived gap between what one actually has and what one wants to have. A second type of gap theory involves the perceived gap between what people actually have and what they consider to be the real ideal. A third type involves the perceived gap between present circumstances and what one expects, or expected, to become. Yet a fourth type concerns the perceived gap between one's present quality of life and the best one has ever had in the past. A fifth suggests that there is an important perceived gap between what one has and that possessed by a reference person or group. These latter theories have been termed *relative deprivation theories, social comparison theories,* and *reference class theories.* A sixth type focuses on the gap between a personal attribute and an attribute of one's environment—that is, person-environment fit or congruence theory. Michalos's approach, acknowledging all six of the gap theories, can be titled *multiple discrepancies theory.*

Michalos (1986) applied his theory in the context of two surveys. He found that, on average, three types of comparison variables (i.e., goal-achievement gap, comparisons with previous best, and social comparisons) accounted for 53% of the variance in satisfaction in 12 different areas of life. Michalos also undertook a comprehensive review of other gap theorists' work between 1979 and 1982 and discovered that in 37 of 41 studies, the gap-theoretic explanations were useful. This means that 90% of the time, when a researcher looked for an association between satisfaction and a perceived gap, the search was successful.

Gutek, Allen, Tyler, Lau, and Majchrzak (1983) made an important contribution to theory in this area with their assertion that "internal referents," such as one's comparison level and level of aspiration, are cognitive variables that mediate between objective and subjective indicators. In a random sample using a city telephone directory, they investigated people's satisfaction in four domains (families, jobs, experiences with government agencies, and neighborhoods). They found that the variables *comparison level* and *aspiration level* accounted for 29% of the variance (not a considerable amount) in quality of life.

Despite the logical appeal of the gap approach to quality of life assessments, it has been criticized by Day (1993) on the grounds that it is difficult to determine who the comparison referents are. It would seem that the number of different possibilities is endless and the probability is that many different ones come into play simultaneously.

Personality Variables

Recognizing the personal nature of quality of life assessments, some researchers have argued that personality must certainly play a role in how people view the quality of their lives. Some of the variables investigated are self-esteem (Kozma & Stones, 1978), locus of control (Brandt, 1979/1980), optimism (Scheier & Carver, 1985), and sociability (Emmons & Diener, 1985). For example, Kozma and Stones found a positive relationship between self-esteem and quality of life in an elderly population. Locus of control was found by Brandt to be positively related to quality of life in an institutionalized elderly sample. Emmons and Diener (1985) demonstrated a positive linkage between sociability and quality of life in undergraduate university students. In a study of undergraduate university students, Jankey (1992) also found that both perceived control and sense of *coherence* (a term popularized by Antonovsky, 1987, and defined as one's capacity to view his or her world in a comprehensible, manageable, and meaningful way) were positively related to quality of life. In fact, perceived control and sense of coherence jointly accounted for over half of the variance in quality of life.

But an obvious criticism of this approach is that the emphasis on personality factors in assessing quality of life is limited and could even be used as a justification for reactionary approaches to program planning. If an argument could be made that quality of life resides within the person and is not reflective of environmental conditions, programs designed to enhance it could be curtailed. The argument could be made that the individual is deficient in some way and programs to improve external conditions would be useless.

The Medical Approach

Historically, the overriding emphasis in the medical profession is on cure and survival. With the realization that many medical interventions have the potential to cause unpleasant side effects, however, it has become clear that the quality of life of the individual undergoing treatment is important, apart from cure and survival. This realization came as a result of the awareness by some medical practitioners that medical or surgical treatments, although extending life on the one hand, may, on the other, actually reduce its quality as a result of multiple or lengthy hospitalizations, intrusive and often painful procedures, or highly aversive side effects (Eiseman, 1981). This orientation is in keeping with the medical precept of *primum non nocere,* which means that the benefits of treatment must be greater than the suffering that may be entailed (Greer, 1984).

From a medical point of view, quality of life assessments have been used to justify or refute different forms of medical treatment, resolve disputes concerning different therapeutic approaches, and provide a basis for allocating resources to those treatments judged to be most effective (Goodinson & Singeton, 1989). But as Day (1993) points out, these assessments have often been used to justify the obvious, such as the fact that lifesaving heart surgery enhances a heart patient's quality of life. In fact, as Hollandsworth (1988) argues, so heavily biased are the studies in favor of showing higher quality of life as a result of the intervention, it is remarkable that there have been medical studies that failed to find positive results.

Scrutiny of the medical literature finds a marked absence of quality of life theory associated with medical research. A search of Medline—a comprehensive database of literature in medicine and related disciplines—indicates that for the years from 1989 to 1995, few researchers even used standardized quality of life scales, preferring to create study-specific, often nontransferable scales. Measures such as severity of pain, severity of symptoms, and exercise tolerance are accepted as measures of quality of life. These investigators suggest that a patient's quality of life has been enhanced if an improvement in these measures can be demonstrated. The absence of a theoretical conceptualization of quality of life is lacking in virtually all studies in this area, and rarely is quality of life even defined.

Another characteristic of quality of life studies in this area is the absence of reference to emotional and social factors (Cella & Tulsky, 1993). Although medical researchers acknowledge the importance of subjective assessments, their definition of *subjective* is asking patients personally about their physical condition, such as whether their symptoms had been alleviated by a specific treatment. They merely assume that their alleviation results in higher quality of life. It appears that the major argument offered by the medical profession for not assessing variables in the psychological domain is that the data obtained from these assessments are too "soft" (Hollandsworth, 1988). By contrast, it has been argued (Schipper, 1983) that indicators of aspects of a patient's physical condition, such as severity of pain, severity of symptoms, and exercise tolerance, are "harder" data and consequently more valid. Whether, in fact, these indicators point to harder and more meaningful data is questionable (Hollandsworth, 1988).

The Rehabilitation Approach

In the past few years, the goal of rehabilitation has shifted from the restoration of function and integration of persons with disabilities into society, to the notion that rehabilitation also involves enhancing their quality of life (e.g., Day, 1993; Schalock, Keith, Hoffman, & Karan, 1989; Wood-Dauphinée & Kuchler, 1992). This shift is expressed in the recent mission statement of Rehabilitation International (Seton, 1993), which states this goal: "To improve the quality of life of people with disabilities throughout the world" (p. 10).

Moreover, rehabilitation professionals concern themselves more with the welfare of the individual in a program rather than focusing primarily on how the group is being affected. In general, rehabilitation practitioners support the notion of the personal nature of quality of life (Goode, 1994e); however, measures that are used to assess it do not appear to reflect this approach.

It has been argued (Scherer, 1988) that quality of life is best assessed through a combination of both subjective and objective measures. Even when subjective reports are elicited, however, they commonly are only subjective assessments of a researcher-imposed view of life (Gutek et al., 1983). Individuals whose lives are being assessed have little input into the determination of which aspects of their lives will be considered relevant to the determination of the quality of their lives. Veenhoven (1984) pointed out the inherent weakness of a researcher-driven approach to the study of quality of life. When researchers impose the domains of life to be measured, they risk omitting important aspects that may have greater relevance to that person or imposing aspects that have little or no relevance. The results may, therefore, have little validity.

A goodness-of-fit model proposed by Murrell and Norris (1983) achieved popularity in the literature with respect to people with disabilities. This model grew out of research (e.g., Liu, 1976; Milbrath, 1979) that argued for quality of life research to identify unmet needs in different populations and use of this information to differently weight the importance of their needs. This approach could then be employed to influence the allocation of resources to these populations. According to this model, quality of life is the yardstick for determining the goodness of fit between a person and the environment. A central tenet of the model is that the quality of life of a person is a function of the discrepancy between resources and stressors. Akin to gap theory, quality of life is determined by assessing the size of this discrepancy. If the discrepancy is large, quality of life is low, whereas with a small discrepancy, quality of life is high.

As was characteristic of the medical approach, quality of life research in the field of rehabilitation also shows that relatively little work has been done on definitions and conceptualizations of quality of life compared to the number of instruments that have been devised to measure the construct (Woodill, Renwick, Brown, & Raphael, 1994).

In keeping with the goal of rehabilitation that places importance on the individual's subjective experience, rehabilitation practitioners have devised measures that reflect this subjectivity. Researchers would determine the areas of an individual's life they wished to sample, and information on various aspects of that person's life was obtained. Thus, more information was available about a person's quality of life than a single score as favored by some. Although it has been acknowledged by some rehabilitation researchers (e.g., Stensman, 1985) that people with disabilities put different weightings on various aspects of their life than people without disabilities, the measures in popular use tend not to reflect this. This could explain some of the contradictory research findings that are apparent when the quality of life of people with disabilities is compared with that of the general population. For example, Crewe (1980), in a study conducted with 128 people with spinal cord injuries, concluded that quality of life may be lower for people with a disability than for the general population. On the other hand, Cameron, Titus, Kostin, and Kostin (1973) compared questionnaires of 190 persons with physical disabilities and 195 without but failed to find differences between the groups in ratings of satisfaction. Another study by Ramund and Stensman (1988) examined 36 people with severe mobility disabilities and 36 nonhandicapped matched controls and found no differences in quality of life between the two groups. Day (1981), in a study of 151 people in vocational rehabilitation programs, found that quality of life was poorer than it was for a normative population but when participants were asked about the best life they expected to have, the difference disappeared completely.

These conflicting findings underscore the need for a reevaluation of our commonly accepted methods of conceptualizing and measuring quality of life. Rather than having researcher-defined criteria imposed on them, the people being assessed should be asked to directly evaluate their quality of life and state the basis for their evaluation. This would require taking into account the personal nature of quality of life. The data collected would be in an open-ended form and would allow us to learn about the issues of importance to the individual whose life is being assessed. This approach would also take into account the problems that arise when researchers determine what is important to the person being assessed (see Veenhoven, 1984).

A Holistic Model of Quality of Life

Day, Jankey, Alon, Clingbine, and Reznicek (1993) took a different approach to the manner in which quality of life has been historically assessed. Rather than employing researcher-defined criteria, they adopted a qualitative research approach in which 15 people were asked how they assessed their quality of life on a 10-point scale and the basis for their evaluation. This method avoided the fixed-format questionnaire that asks for objective information or subjective feelings about objective phenomena. However, it forces the respondent to fit into the schema that are created by the researcher and may disregard what may be of greater interest to the respondent.

Grounded-theory methodology, developed by Glaser and Strauss (1967), was adopted with the goal of clarifying the concept of quality of life and providing a model to direct its measurement. This approach appears to be most promising for phenomenological research (Rennie, Phillips, & Quartaro, 1988). It provides a systematic approach for analyzing qualitative data while at the same time placing less emphasis on the researcher's role in constructing the respondent's accounts. This aspect is particularly important, as it tends to reduce researcher bias when developing a model of the concept under investigation.

Three different groups of five people were interviewed in private sessions that took more than an hour each. These groups consisted of five people with disabilities, five with chronic illnesses, and five members of the population at large. Separate models were generated on the basis of the interviews. The models were then synthesized to form an overarching model, presented in Figure 4.1, that encompassed essential characteristics of the individual models.

It was impossible to construct a model at this stage to include every element of the concept. Rather, it was deemed preferable to create a simplified model that incorporates essential higher-order factors and allows for their elaboration in the future. For example, the nature of *personality* was presented as a single unit with the expectation that future research would detail its complexity.

It must be recognized that the elements of the four original models were not adopted naively but were influenced by the unique experiences and personal values of the team members. In fact, the models developed separately by each interviewer were similar yet unique. Moreover, the final model did not incorporate all the elements of the three models. Rather, it was a synthesis of those elements of the models that were found to be common.

Some elements, such as early experiences, comparisons with peers, and satisfaction or dissatisfaction with economic status, were incorporated into higher-order factors. Members of the team used different names for identical concepts and these had to be translated (after heated discussions) into accepted versions to allow their integration into the final overarching model.

The model takes the position that quality of life is a subjective condition that reflects the level of *life satisfaction.* The evaluation process that leads to the appraisal of life satisfaction is one in which one's *life circumstances* are examined and evaluated. One should note that external circumstances of life were not unimportant to the interviewees, but, they tended to talk about objective circumstances that reflected inner evaluations that had meaning to them. For example, one elderly interviewee referred to having adequate living accommodations and stated the following:

> We moved into one storey. . . . It's an excellent place, except they don't have any facilities right there, as far as groceries or the mail, so we're kind of debating whether to go back to a condominium or something like that. . . . The trouble is, if we both go down at the same time . . . then we need some outside help, and we haven't quite figured out how we'll get that yet. We already have planned to try and find out what's available, . . . where you can have your own

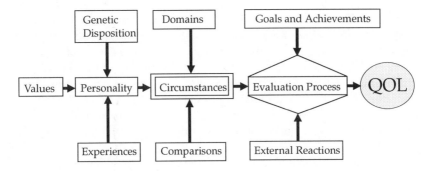

Figure 4.1. Model of Evaluation Process of Quality of Life (QOL)

apartment, but you can go to the dining room and there's assistance . . . and I can go out of the house and do the shopping.

It is clear from this excerpt that it is not so much the living conditions themselves that affected her quality of life but the personal meaning of the living conditions with respect to the effect they have on her independence.

At this point, the question of what constitutes quality of life becomes more relevant. Our study found that the determination of the constituents of one's life circumstances is unique. There is an infinite array of inputs into the determination of life circumstances, and we can venture to suggest that the composition of the array considered important to any individual changes from time to time. Attempting to identify interviewees as disabled or terminally ill or young, healthy adults was impossible because differences in responses were great.

One might speculate that interviewees with disabilities and terminal illnesses would reflect on their *achievements* and past *experiences* as compared with young, healthy adults who would evaluate their circumstances as a gap between their present circumstances and their future aspirations. But with qualitative research and a small, nonrandom sample of interviewees, we could not generalize and, in fact, we found that no two interviewees, even in the same group, responded similarly. Clearly, translation is entailed, and validity requires a great deal more investigation.

Some of the criteria that contributed to the self-assessment of many interviewees were in the *domains* of social relationships and control or power. *Values,* as a component of *personality,* also appeared in the protocols as expressions of the importance of goals, the interpretation of past experiences, and the choice of various domains, such as education and family relationships.

The importance of the foregoing discussion is to underscore that there is a tendency in quality of life research to develop a test for every occasion. Each test is designed to justify the researcher's theory, the therapist's intervention, or the engineer's new assistive device. And each test does what is asked of it because it is user-driven and biased. Such tests are not transferable to different situations or different groups of people. They have little reliability and validity (Wood-Dauphinée & Kuchler, 1992). Nor are they flexible so that respondents can impose their own structure and highlight their major concerns.

The model presented here highlights the complexity of the quality of life concept and argues that researchers must be cognizant of its complexity and must not perceive it in terms of moulds shaped by the researcher. Researchers can investigate aspects of the elements used by people in their evaluation of quality of life, but they must not presume to argue that they are measuring quality of life. For example, one of the researchers reported on various personality traits that contribute to quality of life, traits such as optimism and perceived control over one's life. But in a recent study, Jankey (1992) found that these accounted for only a small proportion of the total variance in quality of life.

To return to the fable of the elephant, we learn that perhaps the reason that there is so much disagreement among theorists in defining quality of life is because researchers have perceived it only from their narrow perspectives. Rehabilitation professionals choosing instruments to measure quality of life should begin their quality of life assessments by asking the respondents to identify the criteria they themselves deem most important in defining the circumstances of their lives. Only then can they continue assessing quality of life and do so by including and weighing the importance of each of these contributory criteria.

5

Exploring Current Conceptions of Quality of Life

A Model for People With and Without Disabilities

David Felce
Jonathan Perry

Quality of life has a central position in the evaluation of services for people with pervasive disabilities, due to the major role that support services play in contributing to or even determining individual lifestyles. Many indicators of service process and outcome have been developed to characterize the effect of services on the lives of people with developmental disabilities, chronic psychiatric morbidity, physical disabilities, or infirmity due to old age and to assess the effects of fundamental policy change. As service complexity has grown and the range of intended outcomes for service

AUTHORS' NOTE: This chapter arises from research on the quality of community residences for people with developmental disabilities in Wales, which was funded by the Welsh Office and the Department of Health.

users has become more ambitious, so, too, have the requirements for evaluation, resulting in a widespread call to reflect the full meaning of quality of life (e.g., Landesman, 1986). Research on societal or community well-being has also responded to the demands of quality of life assessment. Social and psychological indicators have been defined for use in surveys of the general public (e.g., Campbell, Converse, & Rodgers, 1976; Flax, 1972). However, operational definitions of quality of life are diverse in both the general field and in fields applied to defined populations. It is our contention that work aimed at convergence is merited. In addition, we propose that the conceptualization of quality of life should be generic as well as applicable across society as a whole and to particular subgroups within it.

Considerable attention has been given to the definition and operationalization of the quality of life concept within the fields of general social welfare (e.g., Andrews & Withey, 1976; Campbell et al., 1976), mental health (e.g., Baker & Intagliata, 1982; Bigelow, McFarland, & Olson, 1991; Franklin, Simmons, Solovitz, Clemons, & Miller, 1986), physical disabilities and rehabilitation (e.g., Parmenter, 1988), and developmental disabilities (e.g., Borthwick-Duffy, 1992; Schalock, 1990b). In investigating the degree of consensus that exists, we have drawn on these and other key conceptualizations to identify definitional themes and construct a model of quality of life based on common ground (Felce & Perry, 1995). Our formulation comprises a three-element model in which personal values, life conditions, and personal satisfaction interact to determine quality of life. It reflects conceptual development in work on societal welfare in general as well as quality of life models proposed for people with disabilities or problems with mental health. Figure 5.1 illustrates this model and provides details of the life domain areas that may be considered within it.

Overview of Quality of Life

As the contributions to this book show, there is broad agreement that quality of life is a multidimensional construct. The three-element model and the five-way categorization of life domains shown in Figure 5.1 are consistent with this. *Quality of life* is defined as an overall general well-being that is comprised of objective and subjective evaluations of physical, material, social, and emotional well-being together with the extent of personal development and purposeful activity, all weighted by a personal set of values. *Objective evaluation* refers to the description of the life conditions under which people live, such as health, income, housing quality, friendship network, activity, social roles, and so on. *Subjective evaluation* refers to personal

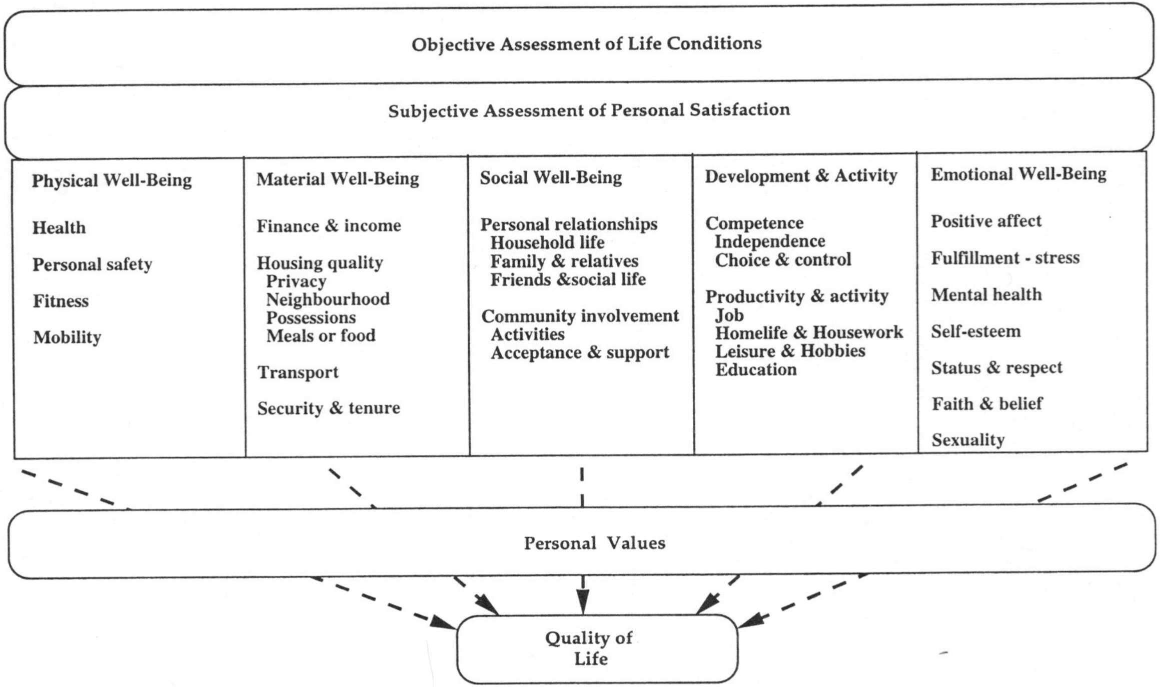

Objective Assessment of Life Conditions

Subjective Assessment of Personal Satisfaction

Physical Well-Being	Material Well-Being	Social Well-Being	Development & Activity	Emotional Well-Being
Health	Finance & income	Personal relationships	Competence	Positive affect
Personal safety	Housing quality	Household life	Independence	Fulfillment - stress
	Privacy	Family & relatives	Choice & control	
Fitness	Neighbourhood	Friends &social life		Mental health
	Possessions		Productivity & activity	
Mobility	Meals or food	Community involvement	Job	Self-esteem
		Activities	Homelife & Housework	Status & respect
	Transport	Acceptance & support	Leisure & Hobbies	
			Education	Faith & belief
	Security & tenure			Sexuality

Personal Values

Quality of Life

Figure 5.1. Conceptualization of Quality of Life

53

satisfaction with such life conditions. The significance of both is interpretable in relation to the value or importance the individual places on each area in question.

The categorization of life domains under the five headings shown was not empirically determined but was devised by us as a means of classifying the substantial agreement on the range of factors relevant to quality of life that the authors report in their analysis of the literature (Felce & Perry, 1995). Physical well-being subsumes health, personal safety, fitness, and mobility. Material well-being subsumes finance and income, various aspects of the quality of the living environment, transport, and security and tenure. Social well-being includes two major dimensions: (a) the quality and breadth of interpersonal relationships—within household life, with family and relatives, and with friends and acquaintances—and (b) community involvement—community activities undertaken and the level of acceptance or support given by the community. Development and activity is concerned with the acquisition and use of skills in relation to (a) competence and self-determination—independence and choice or control—and (b) the pursuit of functional activities—in different arenas, such as work, home, leisure, and education. Emotional well-being subsumes affect, fulfillment, stress and mental state, self-esteem, status and respect, religious faith, and sexuality.

The three-element model, incorporating personal values as well as assessment of life conditions and personal satisfaction, builds on the contributions of other commentators. Borthwick-Duffy (1992) presented three perspectives on quality of life defined in terms of (a) life conditions, (b) satisfaction with life conditions, and (c) a combination of life conditions and satisfaction. Equating quality of life with the assessment of life conditions is compatible with the argument that no citizen has the right to satisfaction with life but only the right to life and reasonable life conditions. Life conditions may well affect personal satisfaction but neither this potential relationship nor the subjective appraisal itself is germane to quality of life assessment. This will comprise a set of objective indicators capable of characterizing the salient life conditions of the population.

Many authors, however, caution against there being objective standards by which one can define a decent or reasonable quality of life (e.g., see Edgerton, 1990). Individuals differ in what they find important, and this has led to expressed satisfaction with life being seen as an ultimately more important criterion of individual welfare or quality of life. Individuals' personal autonomy to maintain or change their quality of life is a paramount consideration. Yet treating expressed satisfaction as a commentary on the acceptability of life conditions experienced is not without problems. First, reports of well-being may owe more to internal temperament than to external conditions (see discussion in Edgerton, 1990). Satisfaction may, therefore, prove to be an unresponsive quality of life indicator, sensitive only to gross and immediate changes in life conditions. Second, satisfaction is often a measure of comparison over time and across people, and therefore, it is impossible to divorce expressions of satisfaction from their context. Reports of satisfaction may adjust to habitual life conditions rather than reflect them, particularly if they are seen as typical of the individual's experience over time or of the people he or she sees as a main source of reference.

Moreover, quality of life defined as synonymous with personal satisfaction, without regard to widely different life conditions, is a less appealing formulation if reasonable independence and autonomy to change life conditions cannot be assumed. Many people with pervasive disabilities lack independence skills to some degree, a deficit that constrains their autonomy and frequently results in their inhabiting worlds of other people's construction. This may be seen as only an extension of a more general position applicable to a lesser or greater degree to many other societal groups disadvantaged economically, educationally, or by class or racial origin. The autonomy to maintain or change life conditions in accordance with subjective appraisal is constrained—for some groups, atypically so.

If satisfaction is a measure of comparison, one might expect that socially devalued people whose circumstances, status, and options to date may make them particularly prone to having low expectations may be the most likely to report satisfaction under adverse life conditions. Certainly, research concerning adults with moderate or mild developmental disabilities living relatively independently has provided a picture consistent with this expectation. Studies that have included the views of people with developmental disabilities have shown that individuals remain philosophical or satisfied about the present and remarkably optimistic about the future despite the adverse conditions under which they live, including poverty, poor housing, threats to health, threats to safety, victimization, social isolation, experience of loss, and failure to gain or retain employment (Close & Halpern, 1988; Edgerton, Bollinger, & Herr, 1984; Flynn, 1989). A definition of quality of life that ignores objective assessment of life conditions may, therefore, not adequately reflect societal division and stratification. It might also fail to provide the level of safeguard for vulnerable people that should be associated with a measure that is to be accepted as the criterion for the adequacy of social policy as well as the specific design and level of service support.

Nevertheless, most commentators would agree that satisfaction remains a relevant concept and that differences between individuals need to be reflected within a model of quality of life. Personal appraisal has a validity for which there is no substitute if one person's values are not to be imposed on another. In view of the weaknesses in defining quality of life in terms of either life conditions or satisfaction, it may be best seen as a combination of objective and subjective components, taking account of both. Such a formulation is commonly found (e.g., Bigelow et al., 1991; Brown, Bayer, & MacFarlane, 1989; Schalock, Keith, & Hoffman, 1990). Moreover, Cummins (1993) has suggested not only that quality of life should comprise objective and subjective assessments of a variety of life domains but also that the manner of combining expressions of satisfaction across life domains should take into account the relative importance the individual places on the various aspects considered.

This approach is consistent with the conceptualization that well-being stems from the degree of fit between an individual's perception of his or her objective situation and his or her needs, aspirations, or values (Andrews & Withey, 1976; Campbell et al., 1976). The principle of taking account of an individual's scale of values, however, can also be applied to the objective assessment of life conditions. The logic of this is strengthened by the fact that an individual may attach different relative weights to objective and subjective aspects of the same issue. For example, someone who is socially gregarious may give high weights to size of friendship network and frequency of friendship contact and to satisfaction with social affiliation. A person who is decidedly not gregarious, however, may give a low weight to extensiveness of social affiliation although still giving a high weight to satisfaction with friendships. Thus the model we propose broadens the application of the goodness-of-fit approach by using individual value structures to weight the importance of both objective and subjective components. In so doing, the concern that only individuals can decide the trade-off between competing aspects of their own personal welfare is met.

The Representation of Conceptual Themes in the Research Literature

The validity of a specific multidimensional formulation of quality of life clearly requires an empirical basis that has not been achieved here and remains to be tested in the context of future research. The importance of the themes embraced by the proposed model can, however, be illustrated by reference to evaluation practice. Objective assessment is well represented in many research literatures, but there has also been much recent attention given to satisfaction with lifestyle. Subjective appraisal has been a cornerstone of research on the quality of life of the general population. The two principal dimensions of our model can, therefore, be found in a range of evaluation literatures. As yet, how to take account of individual value structures is less well developed.

As to domain content, Emerson and Hatton (1994) show, for example, that two of the five domains we have described, social well-being and development and activity, have received particular attention in recent British research on the deinstitutionalization of people with developmental disabilities. Allied to this emphasis has been a smaller number of studies of material well-being and personal satisfaction with living arrangements or lifestyle. The relevance of such domain content is echoed in the suggestion of Bellamy, Newton, LeBaron, and Horner (1990) that the assessment of lifestyle quality should have a multidimensional scope and attend to five areas: (a) physical integration—the number of activities performed outside the home, (b) social integration—the number of activities performed with other community citizens, (c) variety—the diversity of activity, (d) independence—the range of activities performed autonomously and without assistance, and (e) security—tenure and continuity of relationship ties and other associations. Such scope is also found in some of the more comprehensive research studies of, for example, residential services for people with developmental disabilities (Burchard, Hasazi, Gordon, & Yoe, 1991; Conroy & Bradley, 1985; Felce, 1989; Felce, de Kock, Thomas, & Saxby, 1986; Lowe & de Paiva, 1991). One can conclude, therefore, that many researchers have seen social relationships, family and friendship contact, community integration, community acceptance and support, independence and skill development, degree of choice, and engagement in functional activity as important facets of quality of life (see also Allen, 1989; Lakin, Bruininks, & Larson, 1991).

Research has also examined physical well-being and level of income, other material circumstances, and the character of the neighborhood, although with less emphasis than might be expected given their general importance to most members of the population. Instruments exist to measure health status in the population generally, and screening tools applicable to people with disabilities have been developed (e.g., Wilson & Hare, 1990). Material well-being has been reflected in research studies by reference to disposable income, quality of housing, and the level of furnishings, equipment, and possessions.

Social well-being has, as indicated, received considerable attention. Direct observation of social interaction among householders or between individuals and their caregivers has explored the quantity, quality, and reciprocity of interaction within the home in the fields of mental health (Liberman, de Risi, King, Eckman, & Wood, 1974), developmental disabilities (Felce & Perry, 1995; Landesman-Dwyer, Berkson, & Romer, 1979), and aging (Blackman, Howe, & Pinkston, 1976). Rating scales have been developed to measure the social climate of a variety of settings serving different groups (Moos, 1974). The extensiveness and character of people's social networks and the frequency and nature of their social affiliation have been investigated using data from interviews or the direct recording of social events, again for a variety of client groups (Felce, 1988; Greenblatt, Becerra, & Serafetinides, 1982; Knapp et al., 1992; McConkey, Naughton, & Nugent, 1983).

Community presence has also been a common area of assessment (de Kock, Saxby, Thomas, & Felce, 1988; Shadish & Bootzin, 1984). The range and frequencies of community activities undertaken by people with disabilities supported by services have been measured through the use of questionnaires (Lowe & de Paiva, 1991), rating scales (Raynes, Pratt, & Roses, 1979), and direct recording and categorization of events (de Kock et al., 1988). Use of community amenities has been assessed by direct observation (Saxby, Thomas, Felce, & de Kock, 1986). Acceptance within the community has been explored in terms of community or neighbor attitudes to residential services (Lubin, Schwartz, Zigman, & Janicki, 1982; McConkey, Walsh, & Conneally, 1993; Pittock & Potts, 1988) and by gaining the views of business proprietors, managers, and staff of amenities frequented by people with developmental disabilities (Saxby et al., 1986). In addition, the direct experience of people with disabilities of the general public's reaction to them has also been described (Close & Halpern, 1988; Flynn, 1989).

The measurement of developmental progress reflects the importance of developing competence and independence and service goals such as "maximizing potential." Such outcomes have been seen as some of the most immediate consequences of service treatment or support arrangements, whether in health promotion, rehabilitation, mental health, or developmental or other disabilities. One aspect of independence is reflected by adaptive behavior for which a range of alternative measures exists (Reiss, 1988). Another is the degree of autonomy or opportunities for control over day-to-day living decisions. Various scales have been developed to address autonomy in this sense, including the social climate scales referred to earlier and the Characteristics of the Treatment Environment Scales (Jackson, 1969; Sutter & Mayeda, 1979), which have separate psychiatric and developmental disability versions.

The extent to which people participate in the range of activities typical of ordinary living is a direct measure of environmental opportunity and the use of skills. Direct observation of activity patterns has contributed to the assessment of the quality of services in several fields, including preschool and school (Risley & Cataldo, 1973), aging (Jenkins, Felce, Lunt, & Powell, 1977), mental health (Desmond Poole, Sanson-Fisher, & Thompson, 1981), and developmental disabilities (Felce, de Kock, & Repp, 1986). Research on activity patterns has also been conducted by interview (Knapp et al., 1992). In addition, large-scale surveys have described activity patterns among the general population (Robinson, 1977).

Evaluation of emotional well-being is represented in the general literature on quality of life (e.g., Andrews & Withey, 1976) but is relatively neglected in some of the disability literatures. For example, Emerson and Hatton (1994) identified no studies in the recent British developmental disabilities deinstitutionalization literature concerned with affect, mental well-being, or self-identity. The potential exists for using measures developed for general application. For example, Zautra, Beier, and Cappel (1977) used 16 items from the Perceived Quality of Life Scale (Andrews & Withey, 1976) to measure pleasure and contentment of a sample of the general population. They also used the Positive Affect Scale (Bradburn, 1969) to the same end and the Negative Affect Scale (Bradburn, 1969) and a psychiatric screening instrument to reflect problems in mental state. Scales of life stress are commonly used, and general measures may be adapted for use with people with particular disabilities (Bramston, 1994). Similarly, research on self-concept or self-identity may follow application of general approaches, such as repertory grid technique (Oliver, 1986). Cummins (1993) has included consideration of intimacy in both the general and disability versions of his quality of life scale. This may be considered as a quality of relationship issue or as an aspect of life that may be closely associated with self-esteem, understanding of sexuality, and general emotional well-being.

Assessment of inner states such as those considered within emotional well-being leads on to the issue of subjective appraisal and satisfaction. The multidimensional nature of the quality of life construct illustrated in Figure 5.1 implies that assessment of satisfaction will be equally broad ranging. This is an area of recognized importance. Despite the problems in understanding and communication inherent in developmental disabilities, the development of quality of life scales that reflect the users' perspective has been a growth area in recent years (Cummins, 1993; Heal & Chadsey-Rusch, 1985; Schalock et al., 1990). The satisfaction section of the Quality of Life Questionnaire (Schalock et al., 1990) invites respondents to rate 10 items, which include (a) an overall view on life, (b) how much enjoyment they derive from it, (c) how well off they are compared with others, (d) whether most events or activities are rewarding or not, (e) their satisfaction with their living arrangements, (f) how well they are treated by neighbors, (g) whether their education prepared them for what they are currently doing, (h) the extent of their problems, (i) whether they feel lonely, and (j) whether they feel out of place in social situations. The Lifestyle Satisfaction Scale (Heal & Chadsey-Rusch, 1985) contains 29 yes-no items and addresses satisfaction with residence and associated living arrangements; satisfaction with the neighborhood, friends, and the use of leisure time; and satisfaction with generic or professional services. Cummins (1993) gains subjective appraisals of material well-being, health, productivity, intimacy, safety, place in community, and emotional well-being.

Concluding Remarks

A fundamental consideration in the conceptualization of quality of life is that the resulting formulation should be equally applicable across disability groups, other special populations, and society as a whole. In accordance with our aim to look for common ground between models, content has been made to fit a pragmatically determined framework. Clearly, the social validity and domain structure of the proposed framework remains to be established. This will need to be achieved by reference to a population cross-section as well as to any defined groups of interest. The five domains suggested here to categorize the content areas relevant to quality of life are all of a general nature, which is desirable from the perspective of developing a quality of life measurement system that has broad utility. The content embodied has been shown to reflect many of the outcome indicators used in evaluation research across a number of related fields. This too testifies to its potential general relevance. As a consequence, the model may be seen as a framework by which to investigate the generalized effect of social policies and arrangements for any particular subgroup irrespective of its precise defining characteristics. The specific concerns of health promotion, rehabilitation, disability, mental health, and aging have common cause with respect to this conceptual framework.

Another issue is how best to conceive of the measurement task. There has been a tradition of scale development; that is, quality of life is measured by a quality of life scale. However, separate aspects of the domain content considered here could also be assessed using different measures, allowing variation of the method of data collection to the specific task in hand. The quality of life construct would, in this case, more clearly be seen as a composite attribute. As the foregoing selective review makes clear, many measures exist that are relevant to the assessment of the five domain areas. Measures have proliferated, and a key research task is now to compare different ways of measuring similar entities so that their relative properties can be established. In the same way that broad agreement on the definition of quality of life is required, it is also important to establish related measurement methodologies that can command broad support. An example, albeit a rather limited one, of the type of research that could be conducted is illustrated by one of our recent studies. To gain more information on the extent of agreement between different objective measures of material and social well-being, personal development, and activity of residents of supported housing services, we used several measurement methods for each of the aspects in which we were interested to explore the correlation in the rank order of settings that they generated (Perry & Felce, 1995). Replication of this type of research would establish the extent to which ostensibly similar measures do measure the same thing, and if they do not, precisely how they differ.

Relatively little mention has been made to the point about good practice in gaining subjective views. In particular, problems of understanding and communication can be encountered for a variety of reasons: traumatic brain damage, degenerative disease, psychiatric illness, dementia, sensory loss, and severity of developmental disability. What has been learned methodologically about how best to gain complex subjective opinion needs to be consolidated. So too do indications about where the limits of possibility lie. Lack of language ability will inevitably constrain the extent to which obtaining informed opinions can be universally achieved. For example, experience to date suggests that most people with severe, and all people with profound, developmental disabilities will be unable to express their satisfaction with global quality of life concepts. That is not to say that such people do not have preferences and cannot indicate them. Rather, it is to recognize that day-to-day choice making and reaching an encapsulated view of satisfaction differ, the latter being significantly more difficult.

Research is also required on how to gain information on the relative value structures of individuals. Ascertaining the relative importance of issues may call for even greater cognitive abilities than the expression of satisfaction as it involves the ranking of relative values. Exploration of the values that people with disabilities attach to various aspects of life has been limited, but the scale being developed by Cummins (1993) does this. Further work is required in this area but the qualification mentioned earlier about language and understanding limiting the universal feasibility of gaining subjective views is equally relevant. Where this can be done, a full assessment of quality of life can be obtained that matches the model in Figure 5.1. Where not, quality of life assessment may be limited to objective indicators.

Such considerations again emphasize the significance of developing a common approach to quality of life applicable not only to defined groups but also to society as a whole. This is vital if information regarding one section of society is to be interpreted with confidence. The quality of life concept originated in the concern to encapsulate the well-being of populations rather than individuals. Problems in inferring what alternative quality of life might be reasonable in the individual case are compounded by the fact that life conditions and satisfaction with life inevitably vary across individuals in all groups within society. Making judgments about an individual's quality of life is a separate issue from measuring quality of life: Translating quality of life data into prescriptive action requires a separate basis for reaching decisions. There is an obvious objection to an externally imposed quality of life framework replacing personal autonomy as a mechanism for making choices and determining personal circumstances, a prospect that Goode (1994c) has referred to as a "tyranny of quality" (p. 41). At the aggregate level though, quality of life data applied to the question of evaluating major policy or service provision movements (e.g., deinstitutionalization) may provide a better rubric than measures of more limited scope. Quality of life data for a defined group of interest may be compared with those for the total population to establish whether or not aspects of quality of life are similarly distributed. Social policy may then respond to conspicuous inequality.

6

Social Well-Being

A Framework for Quality of Life Research

Michael Bach
Marcia H. Rioux

We live in an age where technological development is guided by a logic of its own, independent of societal values and commitments (Franklin, 1990). The consequence of this discontinuity between development and values poses serious environmental, social, and economic risks for individuals and communities. This discontinuity is evident in a number of fields of technological development, including rehabilitation. In this particular field, the health promotion framework may help to recast the aims of rehabilitation, thus establishing parameters for the development and application of rehabilitation approaches and technologies.

Health promotion places an emphasis on individuals and communities exercising greater control over the conditions and decisions that affect their health and well-being (Epp, 1986; Health & Welfare Canada, 1988). Although health promotion provides an important philosophical direction for rehabilitation, the methodologies for measuring quality of life outcomes of rehabilitation are out of step with the conceptual advances the health promotion framework brings. The consequence has been that the standards by which to measure rehabilitation efforts and to guide rehabilitation programs have not promoted individual, community, and societal health and well-being to the extent they might.

This chapter argues for quality of life assessment in rehabilitation that is guided by a framework of social well-being. As discussed here, social well-being incorporates the principles of health promotion and can serve as a standard when designing quality of life research. Rather than pointing to a set of specific indicators for measuring quality of life, the framework of social well-being provides a conceptual and methodological direction. With this standard for quality of life research, the effect at the individual, community, or societal scale can be examined. It can also be used as a basis for cross-national studies of quality of life, although recognizing that specific indicators of social well-being have to respect community and societal differences. Beginning with a critique of conventional approaches to quality of life measurement, this chapter lays out an approach to conceptualizing social well-being as a standard for quality of life research.

Health Promotion and Quality of Life Research: Critique

Drawing on research literature primarily in the area of disability, three broad approaches to conventional quality of life research can be identified (Bach, 1994)—namely, client satisfaction, functionalist, and ecological. The primary distinguishing factor is the underlying assumption about what constitutes the standard of "quality" when it comes to measuring quality of life.

THE CLIENT SATISFACTION APPROACH

The *client satisfaction approach* is based on the assumption that the standard for understanding the quality of a person's life lies in that person's subjective sense of well-being (Diener, 1984). On the basis of this approach, a number of life satisfaction scales have been developed to measure people's sense of satisfaction using "feeling measures" that typically range from something such as "bad" to "happy." By itself, this approach is clearly inadequate for measuring the extent to which rehabilitation efforts promote health or greater control by a person over the conditions that affect his or her health. Nor is it able to assist in understanding the realities of exclusion of certain groups or individuals and victimization in people's lives. Further-more, research that has examined the relationship between subjective indi-cators of a person's environment and objective social indicators of the same environment has not found a positive relationship between them. This is not to suggest that, thereby, objective social indicators are the only valid indica-tors but simply that subjective assessments provide one among many per-spectives on quality of life.

THE FUNCTIONALIST APPROACH

The same limitation (i.e., the reduction to a single perspective) is inherent in *functionalist approaches* to quality of life that view the person from a so-called objective standpoint of "normal" social roles, "typical" behaviors, "basic" needs, or a combination of these (Braybrooke, 1987, 1991). Although this broad category encompasses many approaches to quality of life research, they are unified in the sense that there is assumed to be an objective set of standards that can be constructed by the research community to guide research. The concept of the person is radically different from the previous approach but just as limited. Whereas the client satisfaction ap-proach assumes that the person defines himself or herself by virtue of his or her feelings, the objective approach is based on an assumption that the person is defined entirely by socially established categories of role, behavior, and needs (Lewis & Lyon, 1986). This approach draws its logic and its justifica-tion from functionalist social theory in which valued social roles, behaviors, and needs are considered self-evident. Indicators of quality of life can then be objectively defined, not from the perspective of the individual whose quality of life is in question but from some other transcendent, "objective" standpoint.

The underlying limitation of this approach is that certain actors and processes are given the power to define the needs of others, as well as their appropriate place in society, in accordance with certain assumptions that are never made fully explicit. Conceptually, this approach makes some advance over the client satisfaction approach. It moves beyond indicators of quality of life that are based simply on subjective feeling measures. But it raises as many problems as it solves because it is not able to confront the issue of who is to have the power to define need. The idea that needs are not fixed and immutable entities, but, rather, the outcome of a social, political, and cultural process has been argued by social scientists and moral philosophers alike (Benhabib, 1986; Leiss, 1978).

THE ECOLOGICAL APPROACH

There is a substantial body of quality of life research in the field of disability that draws on what has been termed the *ecological approach* (Keith, Schalock, & Hoffman, 1986; Landesman-Dwyer, 1986; Murrell & Norris, 1983). The ecological approach seeks to address the dilemmas raised when either the subjective perspective of the person or the objective assessment of the environment is drawn on exclusively to investigate quality of life. Rather, an ecological standard of quality of life focuses on the degree of "fit" between a person and his or her environment, between a person's expectations in his or her environment and the resources that environment provides to that person. *Environment* in an ecological approach has been defined in a number of ways to include the social supports in a person's life, the settings in which he or she lives and works, and the broader policy environment that regulates the provision of supports and services.

In recognizing that a person cannot be separated from his or her environment, this approach makes substantial advances over the client satisfaction and functionalist approaches. It provides no way of judging what the relationship between a person and his or her environment or society *should* look like, however, or the extent of control a person should have over conditions in his or her environment. This is because this approach, like the others, lacks an ethical framework. It rests squarely on a naive positivism that assumes that degrees of positive and negative person-environment fit or environmental stressors can be measured and that this information will provide a basis for designing environments. There are ecological studies that do critically examine the residential and other environments in which adults with an intellectual disability are supported, from ethical standpoints such as that of self-determination (Bervovici, 1983). But the importation of ethics into the ecological approach is at odds with its exclusively positivist foundations.

Quality of Life Defined as Social Well-Being

The three approaches just discussed offer different answers to the question What standard should we use to know when a person has a high quality of life? The analysis suggests these approaches do not provide an adequate standard for measuring the outcomes of rehabilitation. We suggest here that a much more comprehensive standard for determining quality of life is the social well-being enjoyed by people, communities, and their society.

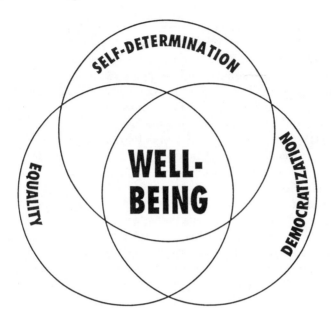

Figure 6.1. A Framework of Social Well-Being

Social well-being has three core elements, which appear in Figure 6.1. The choice of these elements reflects the empirical literature on well-being, the philosophical literature, and the fundamental commitments to the well-being of societies as expressed by governments through international human rights conventions, declarations, and national constitutions (Roeher Institute, 1993). These core elements are discussed in the next three subsections. The accompanying examples are drawn from Canadian society; however, they are similar to situations that exist in other democratic countries.

SELF-DETERMINATION

People attain well-being when they are able to achieve their aspirations for themselves, their communities, and their society (Herbert & Milsum, 1990). Self-determination is exercised when persons, communities, or governments articulate aspirations and make plans and decisions to achieve them (Beauchamp & Childress, 1983; Rawls, 1971). Self-determination means that choices are made autonomously and without coercion and that people consent in an informed way to their rule by others or by government. Self-determination is exercised both as "freedom from" resistance or repression by others and as a positive freedom, a "freedom to" do or enjoy something worth doing or enjoying (Green, 1964; Qualter, 1986). Positive freedom implies that, although governments may have legitimate reasons to restrict freedoms, they also have a role to play in ensuring the conditions necessary for people and communities to exercise their self-determination.

Self-determination also entails the development by people, communities, and society of the resources and capacities they need to achieve their aspirations (Doyal & Gough, 1991). Without nurturing and support from their families or other personal relationships, individuals do not develop the capacity to make life plans and to exercise self-determination throughout their lives. In addition, people often need other kinds of support to exercise self-determination. They may require assistance in making decisions about health care; about the community supports they will use; and about their education, training, and paid work. Many groups need resources and supports to participate effectively in decision-making processes in political and other institutions. Others require supports to participate in education, jobs, and community activities. Without this support, more powerful interests tend to monopolize the decision-making process.

People's sense that they are able to be self-determining plays a critical role in mediating the effect of stress on well-being. Those best able to deal with the increasing stresses associated with the workplace, family life, lack of income, and job loss in ways that do not result in ill health perceive that, despite the stresses, they have some control over themselves and their life situations (Kobasa, 1979).

A health promotion approach recognizes the importance of fostering the development of self-determination rather than assuming that it is an inherent and voluntary capacity. Health promotion asks how individuals, groups, and communities can be enabled to make choices that lead to health as well as the necessary strategies and resources for this (Hamburg, Elliot, & Parron, 1982; Herbert & Milsum, 1990). A constructive health promotion approach does not blame the victim for his or her lifestyle choices but recognizes that a whole range of environmental, income, workplace, and household factors may severely limit the capacity of people and communities to make choices that promote rather than diminish health.

A strong commitment to self-determination is an integral aspect of well-being for any society. The basis for such a commitment is articulated in most countries' constitutions and in the international human rights instruments to which most countries are signatories. Commitments to collective rights to self-determination are also often embedded in these documents.

DEMOCRATIZATION

The struggles through which people and groups seek to obtain recognition for themselves and for their aims and to exercise greater control over the conditions that affect them have been defined as *the politics of recognition* (Taylor, 1992).

Democratization makes a constructive politics of recognition possible. It goes beyond the conventional meaning of the term *democracy*. It is the process of enabling the democratic participation of individuals and diverse groups in a wide scope of decision-making processes that directly affect their lives and their well-being. It is based on an understanding that interdependence is inevitable and essential. Democratization points to the importance of recognizing, respecting, and drawing on diverse points of view in decision-making processes at all levels of society. Without democratization, diversity becomes a breeding ground for conflict rather than a basis for cooperation in achieving individual and group ends.

Can democratization provide the conditions for social well-being and result in sustainable economic development? In the current economic environment, this is an unavoidable question. If institutional arrangements allowed communities to measure the costs and the benefits of trading arrangements and allowed them to participate in investment and production decisions, it is entirely possible and probable that choices would be made to pursue directions for growth that would perhaps lower the gross national product but increase satisfaction and better secure environmental sustainability (Block, 1990; Bowles & Gintis, 1986; Mishra, 1990).

The underlying principle of such an economy and society would be participation in decision making (Albo, Langille, & Panitch, 1993; Heilbroner, 1992). The economy would not rest on global forces or market pressures. It would rest on the idea that economies should serve people and communities and that broader representation and participation in economic decision making is a means to secure that end (Heilbroner, 1992).

Social well-being is achieved in a society where democratization is an integrating force (Drover & Kerans, 1993). There are existing obligations and commitments in most countries and at the international level to provide the foundation for democratization. For instance in Canada, the right to vote, collective bargaining arrangements, and individual and collective rights entrenched in the *Charter of Human Rights and Freedoms* reflect this commitment. In addition, Canada's first constitution in 1867 provided a foundation for democratization and mutual recognition by granting status in institutions and decision-making processes to both French and English communities. The process of democratizing institutions to give greater representation to the communities that make up Canada has not stopped since.

EQUALITY

Equality is another element of social well-being when it is defined as the absence of barriers to mutual respect and recognition between people "who are equally free from political control, social pressure and economic deprivation and insecurity to engage in valued pursuits, and who have equal access to the means of self-development" (Lukes, 1980, p. 218).

To a large extent, society's institutions are not designed to enable this kind of equality to be practiced. The formal interpretation of equality that has predominated in public policy and court rulings requires treating similar cases in similar ways. This formal interpretation, however, no longer responds to the demands for equality now made by different groups. This is because the formal interpretation does not accord women and others who have been marginalized the basis of a claim to equality. It is difficult, if not impossible, to claim that women, for example, are situated in society in the same way as men or that people with disabilities are the same as or are similarly situated as people without disabilities (Rioux, 1994).

Challenges to this formal understanding of equality have been advanced in recent years (Smith, 1986). For example, since the introduction of the equality provisions of the *Canadian Charter of Right and Freedoms,* courts in Canada have begun to rewrite the standards of equality indicating that the principle of equality does not necessarily imply similar treatment: It may require treating people differently. In this view, differences (e.g., arising from nationality, gender, race and ethnicity, religious belief, or disability) are not a reason to deny people the supports they need to exercise their self-determination. If people are to exercise self-determination, institutions in society should be structured to recognize, respect, and support the presence of diverse languages, identities, and cultures (Kymlicka, 1989; Young, 1990).

Society's institutions enable equality among individual persons when they are organized to value differences, address disadvantages, and recognize that people have differing needs. When this happens, the well-being of some does not depend on denying well-being to others.

There are growing commitments in Canadian and other societies to an interpretation of equality that accounts for differences. The enactment of human rights laws and the establishment of human rights commissions have been one set of responses to demands for equality and freedom from dis-crimination on the basis of gender, race, disability, and other differences. A model of equality that takes account of differences is increasingly recognized to be a defining feature of well-being (Abella, 1985; Bayefsky & Eberts, 1985; Brodsky & Day, 1989; Cholewinski, 1990; Rioux, 1994).

Levels of Social Well-Being
in Quality of Life Research

The framework of social well-being as a standard for quality of life takes into account the interdependence of various levels within society. If a high quality of life is to be realized, then self-determination, democratization, and equality must be achieved at the individual, community, and societal levels. What does well-being mean at each of these levels? *Individual well-being* has been defined as the extent of the gap between a person's aspirations and the degree to which these aspirations are actually achieved (Herbert & Milsum, 1990). The narrower the gap, the greater a person's well-being. This notion means that well-being is a dynamic relationship between, on the one hand, an individual's developing capacities and sense of purpose and, on the other, the changing social, cultural, and economic conditions that affect the pursuit and achievement of a person's goals.

Individuals cannot attain well-being by themselves. They do so in the context of the communities they belong to—geographic communities as well as communities defined by common interest, language, culture, gender, and other characteristics. Through institutions associated with education, government, media, and culture, communities can transmit values and traditions to their members. They provide the language and ideas that people use to express what they want (Kymlicka, 1989) and the resources people need in order to participate and be included in society. When communities, supported by society at large, provide the social, economic, cultural, and environmental context for enabling the well-being of their diverse members, important steps have been taken to secure individual well-being. When the capacity to do this is equally enjoyed among the various communities in a society despite their diversity, then community well-being is in the process of being developed.

Like individuals, communities cannot achieve well-being on their own. Nor can they alone provide all the necessary conditions for individuals to achieve well-being. Larger institutional structures are required to enable the social, economic, and environmental sustainability of communities and to enable individual well-being to be achieved. Economic, social, and political institutions create a context for realizing community and personal well-being. They are also the means by which a society can pursue broad and collective goals. When individuals and communities express their aspirations and develop capacities to pursue and achieve them, their well-being is well on the way to being secured. When a society makes it possible for its members and communities to contribute to the well-being of that society, the society is closer to social well-being. Ultimately, when nations, as well as international institutions, provide the conditions for this to happen in a context of mutual recognition and equality among nations, it can be truly said that they have achieved well-being.

Applying the Standard of Social Well-Being to Quality of Life Research

Using the social well-being framework to design standards for quality of life research results in a reconceptualization of both dependent and independent variables. Quality of life, measured by the extent of social well-being achieved (i.e., self-determination, opportunities for participation in decision making, and equality), is an approach consistent with a health promotion focus in rehabilitation. These elements provide a new direction for measuring the dependent or outcome variable in rehabilitation and quality of life research. They go beyond the measures of adaptation, functional development, and satisfaction that have traditionally been used to measure rehabilitation outcomes, in the absence of the health promotion framework.

The social well-being standard also reorients conceptualization of the independent variables. This is because any rehabilitation service or program is shaped by a wide range of funding and policy parameters established at the societal level and because its delivery interacts in a particular way with a mixture of services and supports depending on the agencies, communities, and recipients involved. To examine how a rehabilitation program affects the quality of life of a person, factors at all of these levels need to be taken into account. In this way, the rehabilitation program is contextualized within a broader set of institutional arrangements. The specific outcomes for a person may be due to the way a rehabilitation service is provided or to the eligibility, funding, and other requirements that are established as a matter of policy, statutory law, or fiscal arrangements of governments. Thus research in health promotion and rehabilitation may point to the limitations of existing policies and funding arrangements in enabling individuals who require rehabilitation services to exercise greater control over the conditions affecting their health, which constitutes the very essence of health promotion.

Examining rehabilitation efforts from the social well-being standard of quality of life can bring new perspectives and questions to the field of rehabilitation research. First, given its source not only in empirical and philosophical literature but also in the commitments that governments make, it can be used to critically analyze the aims of public policy. In applying this standard, policies worth pursuing are those that contribute to social well-being. A wide variety of policies and institutional arrangements for rehabilitation, which affect rehabilitation outcomes, could be evaluated against the social well-being framework.

Second, the social well-being standard encourages a focus on sustainability. It leads to questions about how to facilitate the social, economic, and environmental sustainability and security of the communities in which people who require rehabilitation live. These are different questions from ones usually asked in quality of life research in rehabilitation. We need to begin asking them because the communities that people currently depend on for their long-term support and rehabilitation are often under serious economic and environmental threat. Successful rehabilitation in a disintegrating community is difficult to imagine.

Third, the social well-being standard of quality of life stresses the importance of decision-making structures in managing the differences in society and the conflicts that arise in allocating limited resources fairly. By stressing democratization of decision making, the social well-being framework recognizes that society, the economy, the environment, and government are not isolated entities but, rather, all necessary parts of a whole. If rehabilitation efforts are to promote health, then decisions about how such services are to be funded and delivered need to be made in concert with other decisions about the economy, labor markets, social supports, and the environment. In addition, this needs to be done so that relevant interests are adequately represented. Democratization, as an element of social well-being, does not provide a formula for resolving the conflicts that arise or for making decisions. It can provide a measure to assess how decisions are made about rehabilitation funding and delivery. It also offers a means of examining the relationship of these decisions to other policy and program decisions that affect the promotion of health and may engender or resolve social conflict.

Conclusion

The conventional methodologies for measuring quality of life outcomes of rehabilitation are not able to measure the reorientation that the framework of health promotion brings to the field of rehabilitation. Nor can the standards of quality of life that have been traditionally used take into account the wider set of institutional arrangements and policies that constitute the delivery and practice of rehabilitation. It is these arrangements and policies that shape the outcomes of rehabilitation in people's daily lives. This chapter has pointed to an alternative standard for quality of life, namely, social well-being, which incorporates the principles of health promotion and emphasizes the interdependence of individuals, communities, and society.

Application of a standard of social well-being to quality of life research can underscore the many factors that shape people's lives and the extent to which they can exercise control. It can also illuminate the influence that funding as well as delivery and decision-making processes associated with rehabilitation services have on individuals, communities, and society as a whole.

7

The Centre for Health Promotion's Conceptual Approach to Quality of Life

Being, Belonging, and Becoming

Rebecca Renwick
Ivan Brown

This chapter presents a conceptual approach to quality of life that was developed by a multidisciplinary research team from the Quality of Life Research Unit at the Centre for Health Promotion (CHP), University of Toronto (Renwick, Brown, & Raphael, 1994; Rootman, Raphael, Shewchuk, Renwick, Friefeld, Garber, Talbot, & Woodill, 1992a, 1992b). Its development was influenced, in part, by earlier theoretical work on quality of life, some of which has been discussed in previous chapters in this section. This chapter presents an overview of the process of developing the CHP framework and

AUTHORS' NOTE: The CHP framework was developed during Phase 1 of the Quality of Life Project that was funded under contract with the Ministry of Community and Social Services (Ontario, Canada). However, the views expressed here do not necessarily represent the views of the Ministry or the Government of Ontario. The CHP approach was developed by the chapter authors in collaboration with G. Woodill, I. Rootman, S. Friefeld, D. Raphael, and M. Garber. The figures presented were developed by the chapter authors in collaboration with D. Shewchuk.

outlines this conceptual approach, including the assumptions that underpin it and the definition of quality of life on which it is based. Finally, existing and potential contributions of the CHP conceptual approach to theory, research, health and social policy, and service provision are considered.

Development of the CHP Approach

The CHP approach was formulated as the conceptual foundation of an ongoing (1991 to 1998) three-phase research project that examines the quality of life (and related issues) of persons with developmental disabilities living in Ontario, Canada's most populous province. Although the quality of life project focused on one particular population, the research team realized in the early days of the research that the CHP approach to quality of life has broader relevance. That is, it is a useful way to conceptualize quality of life of people in general, whether or not they have disabilities (see Raphael, Brown, Renwick, & Rootman, 1994a). The research team also recognized that quality of life assessment for any subgroup of persons needs to be based on a broader, more comprehensive conceptualization of quality of life that is relevant to the general population. Thus, the approach developed was intended for a general population. Within this broader conceptualization, however, allowances were made for tailoring assessment methods based on this approach to persons with developmental disabilities (Raphael, Renwick, & Brown, 1993) as well as to other groups, such as older adults, adolescents, and persons with physical and sensory disabilities (see Raphael et al., 1994a).

The conceptual framework and the definition on which it is based were developed as the result of three inquiry processes that were carried out concurrently. One process consisted of a critical evaluation of the existing literature on quality of life of persons with and without disabilities. Literature in the areas of health, rehabilitation, medicine, disability, psychology, sociology, and philosophy was reviewed. Some of the major themes that influenced the formulation of the CHP model are outlined in a subsequent section.

A second process involved detailed consultation with prominent researchers and theorists on issues related to quality of life, health, and disability. They discussed current and visionary issues in quality of life with the research team and provided feedback on the emerging CHP model in its various developmental stages. The major themes that emerged from this process were the contribution of personal empowerment and choice to quality of life and the primary importance of individuals' perspectives on their own quality of life.

The third process consisted of collection of detailed information from persons with disabilities, their families, and service providers about their perspectives on quality of life (see Rootman et al., 1992a). This information was gathered in the context of focus groups and in-depth personal interviews with the informants. At various stages of its development, the conceptual framework was tested against the lives of real people, with and without disabilities, by means of personal interviews and case studies that combined interview and observational methods (Rootman, Raphael, Shewchuk, Renwick, Friefeld, Garber, Talbot, & Woodill, 1992). Some particularly significant themes that emerged from this process were individuals' needs for personal control in many areas of life and for opportunities that foster quality of life.

Influencing Themes From the Literature

The CHP conceptual approach was broadly influenced by the humanistic-existential tradition (e.g., Bakan, 1964; Becker, 1971; Merleau-Ponty, 1968; Sullivan, 1984; Zaner, 1981). A detailed discussion of these philosophical foundations of the CHP approach appears in Woodill, Renwick, Brown, and Raphael (1994). By way of summary, however, this literature recognizes that individuals have physical, psychological, and spiritual dimensions. It also acknowledges people's needs to belong, in both physical and social senses (i.e., to places and social groups), as well as to distinguish themselves as individuals by pursuing their own goals and making their own choices and decisions. In the context of the CHP framework, these themes are incorporated in three major domains of quality of life—namely, *being, belonging,* and *becoming.* These are discussed in a subsequent section.

The other body of literature that most informed the development of the CHP approach is focused on quality of life of persons with disabilities, especially the work on developmental disabilities. Several conceptual frameworks and analyses were particularly influential. Taylor and Bogdan (1990) argue convincingly for focusing attention on how individuals view their own quality of life and that taking such an approach is necessary in order to really understand their lives. Goode's (1990b) concept of "goodness of fit" between the person and the environment encouraged the CHP research team to further develop the idea that the nature of the interaction between the person and the environment and the ongoing outcomes of this interaction are the basis for individuals' perceptions about their quality of life.

The Brown, Bayer, and MacFarlane (1989) quality of life framework emphasizes life satisfaction and well-being as well as growth and mastery by individuals as critical factors (among others) in their quality of life. The satisfaction dimension is also incorporated in the conceptual model developed by Schalock, Keith, Hoffman, and Karan (1989). Halpern, Nave, Close, and Wilson (1986) include the notions of social networks and social support as critical features in their quality of life framework. Constructs similar to the ones offered by these authors are encompassed, although in a broader fashion, by the CHP approach. In addition, the CHP framework offers a unique conceptualization of the interrelationships among these elements that is discussed in detail in the next section.

Distinctive Attributes
of the CHP Approach

Diversity in interpretations of the quality of life construct has led to diversity in representing it at both the conceptual and operational levels. This has presented challenges and problems for both conceptualization and measurement, many of which are addressed in other chapters of this volume. It is puzzling, however, that the commonalities among the approaches that have already been developed have received scant attention. The CHP approach attempts to address this issue by drawing on and integrating broader, common themes underlying other conceptualizations of quality of life. The CHP approach builds on the valuable principles inherent in other approaches (as summarized in the foregoing section) and draws on their strengths. Although it incorporates similar concepts, it deals with these comprehensively and at a much broader level. For instance, the CHP framework centers around three broad areas of life (i.e., being, belonging, and becoming) that are common to all human beings and that are essential to human experience. As such, these are the natural arenas in which to explore the lives and activities of human beings.

These natural arenas are the general areas of life that all people share and in which they strive for quality. Thus it is commonly believed and commonly understood by all people that quality living is important and desirable within these broad areas. The specific ways that quality is represented within these broad areas, however, vary from person to person, from group to group, and from culture to culture. For example, the importance of having a home within one's physical environment is universally valued, but that home may be an igloo, a tent, a bungalow, or a palace, depending on life circumstances. The uniqueness of the CHP approach is that it clearly sets out nine broad areas in which to explore quality of life but allows for the wide variety of ways that quality can be realized within these areas.

The CHP approach also organizes and interweaves some common themes from other recent conceptualizations of quality of life with new constructs in ways that go beyond existing frameworks. The CHP approach takes into account individuals' perceptions of what are relatively important and unimportant areas in their lives. It also emphasizes the central role that personal choice and available opportunities in each of the major areas of life play in the attainment and enjoyment of a good quality of life.

A review of the current literature indicates that few instruments that measure quality of life are explicitly tied to comprehensive, coherent conceptual frameworks (for many examples of this, see Bowling, 1991; McDowell & Newell, 1987). Furthermore, conceptual models of this construct do not seem to have been formulated with a view to developing instrumentation based on them. The CHP model is notable in this respect because it was developed with the explicit intention that it would serve as the foundation for both qualitative (Rootman et al., 1992a) and quantitative measures (Raphael et al., 1994a; Renwick, Rudman, Brown, & Raphael, 1994; Rudman, Renwick, Raphael, & Brown, 1995). Thus its development included considerable attention to clear conceptualization that would readily lend itself to translation into more concrete operational terms.

The CHP Conceptual Approach

UNDERLYING ASSUMPTIONS

Several assumptions underpin the CHP approach to conceptualizing quality of life, the most significant of which are presented here (for a more detailed and expanded discussion of some of these, see Woodill et al., 1994). It should be noted that some of these assumptions were shaped by the literature noted in the foregoing section.

First, equal respect for persons, whether or not they have disabilities, is inherent in the CHP conceptualization of quality of life. Thus, the fundamental constituents and determinants of quality of life are viewed as the same for all persons, with and without disabilities. Second, any meaningful view of quality of life must take into account the holistic nature of individuals. That is, it will recognize their physical, psychological, spiritual, and social aspects and the major human needs associated with these. Third, quality of life is seen as a multidimensional phenomenon. Fourth, it is a dynamic, complex constellation of interacting components. Thus, it can change for individuals over their lifetimes in terms of some or all of its components or dimensions. Fifth, the quality of life experienced by individuals arises out of their ongoing interactions with their environments. Sixth, although its components are the same for all people, the quality of life experienced by individuals will vary from one person to another. For instance, there will be differences in degree of quality of life across its various dimensions because no two individuals will have the same life circumstances. Furthermore, individuals evaluate their quality of life within the framework of their own personal system of cognitions, beliefs, values, and interests. Seventh, quality of life takes account of the health of the individual as broadly defined (e.g., World Health Organization [WHO], 1986) as well as the social determinants of health (for details, see Evans & Stoddart, 1990). Finally, the perspectives of individuals are most important in understanding their quality of life.

DEFINITION OF QUALITY OF LIFE

As is already evident from the foregoing chapters, quality of life has been frequently measured but seldom explicitly defined. Those definitions offered in the literature emphasize various aspects of the construct. For instance, some emphasize physical or psychological or social functioning (or some combination of these), life satisfaction, or psychological well-being (Bowling, 1991; McDowell & Newell, 1987; Schalock et al., 1989). Others highlight "the discrepancy between a person's achieved and unmet needs and desires" (Brown, Brown, & Bayer, 1994, p. 41).

The definition developed as part of the CHP conceptual approach is distinct from these earlier definitions. It views quality of life as "the degree to which the person enjoys the important possibilities of his or her life" (Rootman et al., 1992a, p. 23). Possibilities refer to the opportunities and constraints in people's lives as well as the balance between these. They result from the ongoing interaction between persons and their environments and thus depend on characteristics of both persons and environments. There are two types of possibilities that operate in concert. These appear in the top portion of Figure 7.1. Some possibilities occur "by chance," in that they are not primarily under a person's own control. An individual's gender, genetic endowment (including inherited physical disorders), historical time of birth, and socioeconomic status of the person's birth parents are exemplars of this kind of possibility. Other possibilities occur "by choice"; that is, they are, to a great extent, amenable to much more control by individuals. Individuals' decisions and choices about a whole range of life events exemplify this second kind of possibility. These include decisions about how to spend one's discretionary savings, selection of friends, joining groups and organizations, and choice of occupation. Although there has been some scholarly debate

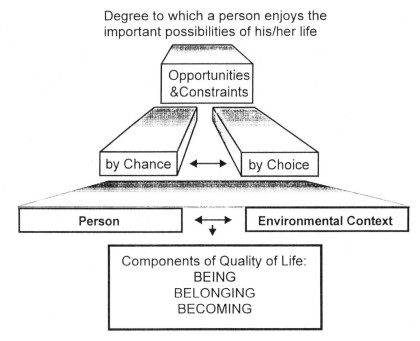

Figure 7.1. Relationship of Definition to Conceptual Framework

about the actual locus of control of the events that occur in people's lives, that is not a central issue in this context. Rather, the CHP framework emphasizes that opportunities and constraints occurring by chance and by choice interact to produce the things that are possible in a person's life.

Many possibilities occur over a person's lifespan and, of course, at any point in a person's life. Therefore, an individual can deal with only some of these possibilities. Furthermore, not all possibilities are equally important to all people and their lives. Quality of life results from those possibilities that have become important to people and the way they live their lives. For instance, personal hygiene and grooming are common activities of daily living, but for some people these assume special significance (e.g., for reasons related to their occupation, age, health, culture, or religion).

The term *enjoyment* implies two interrelated ideas. One refers to the pleasure or satisfaction a person experiences. The second refers to possession or attainment as embodied in the expressions, "they enjoy a good standard of living" and "they enjoy the ability to get along well with others." These aspects of enjoyment are closely connected. Anticipated fulfillment of a need often motivates a person toward possession or attainment of some goal and in turn pleasure often results from such possession or attainment. In essence, enjoyment of important life possibilities includes both the attainment of meaningful things or goals (e.g., personal skills, relationships with others, achievements, and accomplishments) that are possible in people's lives and the pleasure associated with this.

COMPONENTS OF QUALITY OF LIFE

The CHP conceptual framework focuses on the person's possibilities in three fundamental areas of life that are common to the human condition and are essential dimensions of human experience. They are referred to here as being, belonging, and becoming. These possibilities arise out of the ongoing interaction between persons and environments as described in the foregoing section. Figure 7.1 represents the relationship between the CHP definition and conceptual framework and presents the three broad areas of life in which these life possibilities occur.

Being encompasses the most basic aspects of who people are as individuals. *Belonging* is concerned with the fit between individuals and their various environments. *Becoming* focuses on the purposeful activities in which individuals engage in an attempt to realize their goals, aspirations, and hopes. Each of these three components of quality of life has three subcomponents. These nine subcomponents are summarized in Figure 7.2.

Being

Physical being encompasses physical health, including nutrition and fitness. It is also concerned with physical mobility and agility as well as personal hygiene and grooming. *Psychological being* embodies individuals' feelings, cognitions, and evaluations concerning themselves. It focuses on self-confidence, self-control, coping with anxiety, and the initiation of positive behaviors. *Spiritual being* consists of personal values and standards to live by, spiritual beliefs (which may or may not be religious in nature), transcending daily life experiences (e.g., through nature, music), and celebration of special life events (e.g., birthdays, Thanksgiving, and other cultural or religious holidays).

Belonging

Physical belonging refers to the links that people have with their physical environments (i.e., home, neighborhood, workplace, and the larger commu-

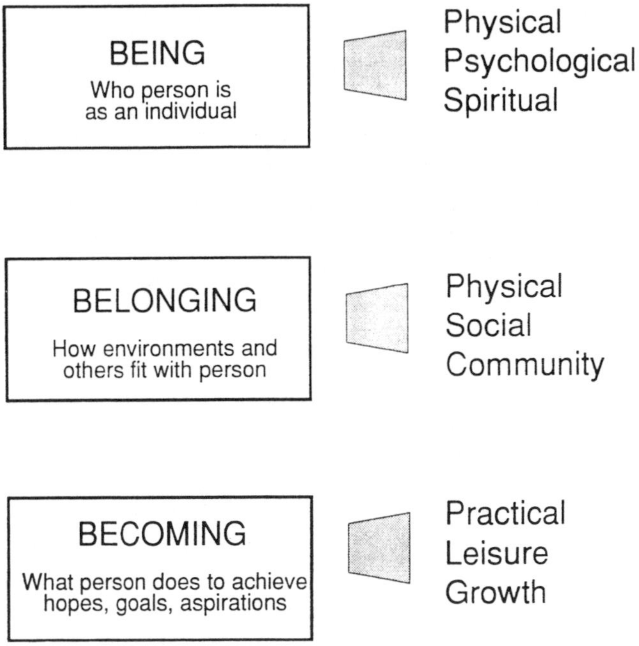

Figure 7.2. Quality of Life: Essential Components and Subcomponents

nity). This subcomponent includes their feelings of being at home in these environments. This subcomponent also encompasses the freedom to display one's personal possessions as well as having privacy and safety in these environments. *Social belonging* consists of the links people have with their social environments. It focuses on meaningful relationships with others (i.e., a partner, friends, family, coworkers, neighbors, and members of cultural or ethnic groups). *Community belonging* embodies the connections people have with resources typically available to members of their community and society. This includes information about and access to sources of adequate income, employment, educational and recreational programs, health and social services, and community events and activities.

Becoming

Practical becoming consists of practical, purposeful activities that are typically done on a daily or regular basis. These activities include household chores, paid or voluntary work, participation in school or educational programs, self-care, and seeking out helpful services (e.g., health or social services). *Leisure becoming* refers to leisure and recreational activities that do not necessarily have an obvious instrumental value. These activities promote relaxation, stress reduction, and "recreation" of people's balance of work and play in their lives. It includes activities of relatively short duration (e.g., socializing with friends, a stroll in the park, or a game of tennis) as well as clusters of activities of longer duration (e.g., taking a vacation). *Growth becoming* encompasses activities that promote the development of individuals' own skills and knowledge, whether this involves formal or informal education and learning. These include learning new information, improving existing skills or learning new ones, and adapting to changes in their lives.

DETERMINING AND
INFLUENCING FACTORS

The CHP approach considers *importance* and *enjoyment* to be the factors determining quality of life for individuals. Thus, quality of life in each of the nine areas (discussed in the previous section) is determined by both the relative importance or meaning attached to each dimension and the extent of individuals' enjoyment in each area.

Basic quality of life is the product of perceived importance and enjoyment; however, quality of life is moderated (i.e., increased or decreased) by two other factors. These are *control* and *potential opportunities*. The former refers to individuals' perceptions concerning how much control they can exert with respect to the important possibilities of their lives in each of the nine areas subsumed by being, belonging, and becoming. The latter refers to individuals' perceptions about the extent of their potential opportunities in each of the nine areas. In essence, opportunities are the perceived chances for change or enhancement in each area of life. Potential opportunities include those currently perceived to be available as well as those that are seen as likely to be available to the person in the future. Examples of potential opportunities are perceived (present) chances to make new acquaintances at a social gathering or perceived (future) chances to obtain better living accommodations or a new position at a company that will begin operation in 3 months' time.

Implications and Future Directions

The CHP framework makes a significant contribution to the theoretical knowledge about quality of life. It offers a broadly grounded perspective that integrates important elements of earlier conceptualizations in an innovative way as well as emphasizing new aspects of quality of life. Such theoretical work is important because there is a remarkable dearth of comprehensive detailed conceptualizations in the literature on quality of life, particularly in the areas of health promotion and rehabilitation. This framework has already served as the theoretical foundation for development of several instruments designed to measure quality of life of persons with and without disabilities. This is important given that most measures purporting to tap quality of life are not grounded in a clear, explicit conceptual base (see Bowling, 1991, for various examples of this). Thus, these instruments have the potential to make a significant contribution to the research on quality of life within health promotion and rehabilitation. They also offer a meaningful way to test the relationships among the proposed elements of the CHP model. In fact, some preliminary testing is currently being conducted in the context of several projects of the Quality of Life Research Unit at the Centre for Health Promotion, University of Toronto.

One set of these instruments was designed for use with adults who have developmental disabilities (Rootman et al., 1995). After preliminary validation, these have been demonstrated to have adequate psychometric properties (Rootman et al., 1995). This instrument package will be validated further in the context of the third phase of the quality of life project referred to at the beginning of this chapter. Another measurement tool based on the CHP model has been constructed for older adults (Raphael, Brown, & Renwick, 1993). The Raphael chapter on older persons provides some details about this instrumentation and its validation to date. An instrument for the general adult population (Brown, Raphael, & Renwick, 1993) is currently being validated. Another instrument for persons with physical and sensory disabilities (Renwick, Rudman, et al., 1994) has also been developed and has demonstrated adequate psychometric properties following preliminary validation (Rudman et al., 1995). All of these instruments tap the same components of quality of life as well as the determining and moderating factors (all described earlier). However, specific items associated with each have been tailored to the particular population after detailed input from and rigorous review by members of that population. These instruments are useful for assessments of individuals' quality of life as well as for the collection of data from groups of individuals.

The CHP theoretical framework can also be employed in the context of both health promotion and rehabilitation to analyze, plan, and evaluate. Specifically, it can be used in conjunction with input from potential users of particular settings (e.g., classrooms; the workplace; and residential settings, such as group homes) as a guide for designing and developing environments that promote quality of life, which includes health, as discussed in the *Ottawa Charter for Health Promotion* (WHO, 1986). At the community level, the framework can be used to elicit citizens' input about the quality of life they experience in their immediate neighborhoods or in their larger communities and can help identify areas that need enhancement. For instance, the CHP framework could be employed in the context of social diagnosis (Green & Kreuter, 1991). The subcomponents of belonging as well as the concepts of importance, enjoyment, control, and opportunities would be particularly useful in this regard. Such environments could be planned to foster quality living for persons with and without disabilities. The CHP approach also provides the basis for instrumentation to evaluate the efficacy and acceptability of such quality-promoting environments. In the area of rehabilitation, this is particularly significant because currently used quality of life measures typically focus on narrower dimensions of individuals' functional performance and do not accord adequate attention to the environments with which they interact.

Because quality of life has been a major issue for many governments in Canada and other countries, it would be useful to consider the value of the CHP approach as a framework for integrating health and social policy for citizens with and without disabilities. It has the advantage of incorporating elements that are consistent with the concerns of both health and social policy makers (e.g., control, opportunities, being, belonging, and becoming). Many other approaches tend to focus on either health (Bowling, 1991) or social issues (Dennis, Williams, Giangreco, & Cloninger, 1993). Further, this framework is inclusive, having been repeatedly tested for relevance with people with and without disabilities.

The CHP approach is a versatile framework for conceptualizing and thinking about quality of life in the context of health promotion and rehabilitation. It has considerable potential value for stimulating new research in that it provides a guiding framework for studying quality of life of persons with and without disabilities and the basis for instrumentation (e.g., Brown et al., 1993; Renwick, Rudman, et al., 1994) to measure this construct. Because it is a systematic and detailed model, it can also be practically applied in health promotion and rehabilitation (Renwick, Brown, et al., 1994), as some of the preceding discussion illustrates. Finally, the conceptual model has great potential for guiding health and social policy and for integrating these around the construct of quality of life.

PART

III

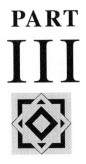

SOME CRITICAL ISSUES

8

The Use of Quality of Life as a Construct for Social and Health Policy Development

Trevor R. Parmenter

In his discussion of the state of Oregon's attempts to extend the coverage of health services by prioritizing services on the basis of their cost-effectiveness, John Kitzhaber (1994), then president of the Oregon State Senate, presented graphic examples of the dilemmas faced by legislators and the public at large when faced with decisions to contain escalating health care costs. Kitzhaber outlined one such example in which a 2-year-old boy who suffered irreversible brain damage after a near-drowning accident was placed on sophisticated life support systems that cost hundreds of thousands of dollars. All prognoses indicated the boy would remain in a permanent vegetative state or at best be severely impaired.

Kitzhaber pointed out that all parties to the procedures, including government officials and policy makers, claimed credit for being able to at least save the boy's life. What they implicitly ignored, however, was that approximately 40,000 children in the United States die before their first birthday because of their being unable to access basic health care. These deaths cause little public consternation. One can readily understand the difficult decision. The community at large and the families of persons with acute life-threatening traumas immediately demand that all steps be taken to save a life at risk, especially if the case is well publicized. Seldom is there a public uproar if the same situations are occurring but are not well publicized.

A second example of the dilemma facing developed countries is portrayed in a lead article in an Australian newspaper ("Counting the Cost of the Good Life," 1991) that asked readers to play the role of a doctor, politician, or bureaucrat by rating in order of priority the spending of the health dollar on a number of scenarios (see Table 8.1).

The article also referred to a discussion paper commissioned by the New South Wales Department of Health in which the author, Niki Ellis (1991), suggested that changes would have to occur in the way decisions are made about how health funds are used if we are to get better health outcomes for the money spent. She posed these questions:

- Should more be spent on health at the expense of roads, education, and welfare?
- If significant funding for roads were transferred to health, what would then be the effect on health?
- Would worse roads lead to more serious road accident injuries?

Ellis pointed out that one of the major factors in the perceived "blow-outs" in health spending is the dramatic increase in medical technology, from the discovery of penicillin in the 1940s to the more recent developments in heart, lung, and liver transplants. With each new advance in medicine, the general public has come to expect it will be available immediately on demand.

These examples illustrate the highly emotive questions surrounding any attempts to address issues of equity and ethics in social and health policies. Nowhere is this better illustrated than in the disproportionately high amount of funds countries allocate to acute medical procedures in contrast to preventative health programs. Given changes in demographic patterns, the increasing sophistication of medical technology, and the subsequent demands for lifesaving and life-prolonging treatments, ever-increasing demands are being made on health care and rehabilitation budgets. This situation has led to a close examination of the nature of health services provided and the manner in which they are delivered, with governments applying fiscal pressures to contain the burgeoning costs of health care. In many Western industrialized countries, there are increasing numbers of examples of rationing medical procedures according to predetermined schedules, the Oregon case being one. The use of cost utility analysis (CUA), including quality of adjusted life

TABLE 8.1 Examples of the Costs of Medical Interventions

Patient	Age	Medical Condition	Prognosis	Cost of Treatment
Michael	Newborn	Premature birth (27 weeks); birth weight, 900 g; survival at 2 days old rated > 90%	Chances of long-term medical problems < 10%	$48,000
Margaret	32 years	Contracted HIV from blood transfusion; has symptoms of AIDS	Will not live beyond 30 months; treatment with AZT may prolong her life	$50,000/ year
Geoff	35 years	Detached retina— loss of vision	Operation will restore full vision	$3,000
Doris	68 years	Deteriorating hip joint— extreme pain	Requires hip replacement, 2.5 to 3 years waiting time; pain will cease after operation	$7,000
Janet	46 years	Cancer of larynx (possibly related to history of smoking)	After throat surgery and follow-up radiotherapy, 75% chance of living to old age	$14,000
Fred	42 years	Final stage of renal failure due to glomerulonephritis	Requires thrice-weekly hemodialysis	$45,000

SOURCE: Adapted from *Counting the Cost of the Good Life* (1991) with permission.

years (QALYs), has become a popular procedure by which to estimate the relative value of health-related procedures in economic terms.

Each of these attempts to impose a purely economic approach to health services, however, basically looks at the quantity of life rather than quality of life, or in Aristotelian terms, *eudaimonian*—the good life (Nordenfelt, 1994). People discharged from services prematurely to meet fiscal criteria may ultimately cost the community more if their illnesses recur or worsen. The social costs for caregivers (e.g., family) are seldom taken into account in these approaches to health care cost containment. This chapter will critically review the literature concerning the CUA and similar approaches, outlining their advantages and disadvantages with a view to evaluating their ability to inform social and health policy development. In particular, the use of the quality of life construct as a dependent variable in the evaluation of health and rehabilitation services will be examined.

There is not an easy relationship between the quantitative approaches to estimating quality of life (i.e., via CUA and QALYs) and qualitative measures that emphasize client-patient satisfaction and are more amenable for use in program monitoring or as process measures. Clinical judgments that address program effectiveness during the process of intervention and that involve people such as medical patients or persons with disabilities in program planning are obviously as important for policy development as are data that address outcome measures in terms of cost-effectiveness. An examination of the social measurement and social indicators movements will serve as a useful framework in which to examine these issues.

Social Measurement and Social Indicators

Carley (1981) has emphasized that there are two important characteristics of social indicators, namely, *surrogates* and *measures.* As surrogates, social indicators do not stand by themselves. They take quite abstract and intrinsically unmeasurable concepts and translate them into operational terms. Thus a social indicator is a proxy for an unmeasurable concept. On the other hand, as measures, social indicators seek to deal with information that is quantifiable. A good example is the notion of *well-being.* Because we cannot measure well-being directly, we have to resort to indicators that may be either objective or subjective. For example, objective indicators may appraise the status of a person's health in physiological terms, whereas a subjective index may consist of data derived from people's expressed feelings concerning their health.

An early but widely publicized definition of social indicators was contained in a U.S. Department of Health, Education, and Welfare (HEW) (1969) publication *Toward a Social Report.* The thrust of this document was that indicators would be useful for social policy development and the evaluation of programs. The essence of the definition was that a social indicator is

> a statistic of direct normative interest which facilitates concise, comprehensive and balanced judgment about the condition of major aspects of a society. It is, in all cases, a direct measure of welfare and is subject to the interpretation that if it changes in the right direction, while other things remain equal, things have become better, or people are better off. (p. 971)

The HEW definition heralded a significant departure from earlier input-based approaches to the assessment of health and welfare programs in its emphasis on output measures. Under the input approach, it was assumed that there was some direct causal effect, for instance, between the number of empty hospital bed spaces and improvements in public health. The HEW approach denied that the volume of resources allocated to health problems was a suitable proxy for the concept of "good health." A second important feature of the HEW definition was its emphasis on the normative nature of indicators. The salient point here was that the measure could be used to show that things are getting better (or worse) and by how much. But this requires a judgment that is not value free. Someone has to decide what "getting better" is. This is a crucial issue germane to the study of the concept of quality of life, for in the search for indicators that are most representative of the quality of life, one has to question on whose values quality is to be judged.

Carley (1981) has indicated a number of the early problems faced by the social indicator movement. One, identified as early as 1975, was that in focusing strongly on attempts to quantify aspects of human existence and in adhering almost blindly to statistical procedures and models, researchers lost sight of the complex political reality of policy issues. Another difficulty was the possibility that specific political agendas might be advanced on the basis of specious or poorly provided data. Such data can be used to camouflage problems or to make past policies look successful. If accurate data are provided, they may acutely embarrass politicians or bureaucrats whose policies may be proven to be flawed.

A further problem concerns methodology. Carley pointed out that if indicators are quantified surrogates for unmeasurable phenomena, it can be rather difficult to demonstrate a correlation between what is measured and what is unmeasured. This difficulty is especially relevant to subjective judgments on quality of life. It was suggested that these indicators might help establish validity for other objective indicators. It soon became established, however, that there was not a significant correlation between these two indicators (Lewis & Lyon, 1986; Muthny, Koch, & Stump, 1990).

If subjective indicators alone were to be used to make policy, it is prudent to ask whose judgments are to be used and by what method those judgments are to be made. Although subjective indicators may demonstrate quite significant social problems, they are prone to measurement errors, which makes it quite difficult to allocate scarce resources in an equitable manner. To accommodate this problem, a combination of subjective and objective measures is called for, but a basic flaw in this procedure has been the relative ad hoc way in which the social indicators movement has grown. Generally, politicians and bureaucracies have called for specific answers to immediate problems that are seldom located in "any systematic framework based on social theories and established cause-and-effect relationships" (Carley, 1981,

p. 13). Therefore, much of the approach of the social indicator movement has been unsystematic and atheoretical—a phenomenon particularly evident in the context of much of the work on quality of life.

To be useful, social indicator research must be policy relevant or related to social goals. To achieve this, such research needs to be undertaken in a policy context where political value judgments are explicitly acknowledged. This also raises the question of whether social indicators sit within a social system. Land (1975) has argued that a social indicator should be a component in a sociological model of a social system or some part of a social system. However, in attempting to derive models of a social system, social indicators have not had conspicuous success in detecting causal relationships between variables that may contribute to a specific social problem. Lineberry, Mandel, and Shoemaker (1974), who explored the use of social indicators by town councils, attributed this failure to the general lack of a coherent social theory.

The New South Wales Office on Social Policy (1994), in its discussion paper *Quality of Life: A Social Policy Approach,* suggested the following:

> Policy informed primarily by social theory is concerned with the functioning of society as a whole. . . . [It] recognizes that the multi-dimensional nature of social life and well-being is too complex to be represented by a single measure . . . as such quality of life is often monitored through a range of social indicators. (p. 12)

But this raises the question of the nature and validity of the social theory being used (Weiss & Bucuvalis, 1977).

An example cited by Lineberry et al. (1974) concerned juvenile crime. Indicators that show the incidence of juvenile crime in a city seldom point to the variety of psychological and environmental determinants of the crime. These are factors that need to be considered when deciding whether to provide increased recreational facilities or increased law enforcement. Bunge (1975) has suggested that social indicators, by their very nature, imply a causal relationship between the indicator and well-being. He argued, however, that this would be acceptable if there were a model or theory of well-being. He then pointed out that

> since no such theory has been constructed so far, we are forced to use our treacherous common sense to an extent that is uncommon in science. Which is a polite way of saying that, so far, the study of the quality of life has not been thoroughly scientific. (p. 75)

Disappointingly, two decades later, the same observation may be made.

Need for a Sound
Theoretical Framework

Carley (1981) has outlined a number of essential factors for the development of social indicators within a sound theoretical framework. First, because one of the essential elements of a theory is an attempt to explain why or how something has happened, or in other words, to provide a set of propositions that are interrelated, its choice of a unit of analysis is critical. Such units of analysis include the individual; a particular group of people; or an act, division, or policy. Second, a theory must generate hypotheses that are amenable to empirical testing. Hence Carley draws on Merton's (1967) distinction between *unified social theory,* or a total system theory, and theories of the *middle range,* which deal with limited or micro aspects of social phenomena. However, as the social system is so complex, Carley has argued that an aggregation of microlevel hypothesis testing may lead to the attainment of a knowledge threshold at which a paradigm shift or change may occur. It is suggested that such a change has occurred in the way quality of life research has developed, for major sociopolitical changes, such as the rise of a consumer advocacy movement and the view that disability is as much a social construct as it is a result of an impairment, have made a complementary contribution to the development of a social theory in which quality of life may be embedded (Schalock, 1991).

It is here that another major problem is raised: Once a hypothesis is formulated that one variable is validly related to one or more other variables, it is necessary to quantify the variables and their subsequent relationships. Here is the nub of the problem, for the rather nebulous concept of quality of life has to be defined and operationalized in quantitative terms. For several decades, research into quality of life has been pursued without any agreement on those social indicators that can reliably claim to measure it. From a social theory perspective, it is the testing of the theory per se that will lead to a justification for the selection of one social indicator rather than another. Much of the instrumentation that has been developed to measure quality of life has not been located within a coherent theoretical base (Parmenter, 1992, 1994).

Here it is useful to explore the relationship between the terms *social indicator model* and *social theory.* In its simplest terms, suggested Carley, "a model is a likeness of something" (1981, p. 71). An alternative definition put forward by Forcese and Richer (1973) is that a model is "an imitator or abstraction from reality while still capturing its essential characteristics" (quoted in Carley, 1981, p. 71). Forcese and Richer (1973) have made a distinction between *descriptive* models, which contain only descriptive state-ments in which the concepts are not operationalized, and *explanatory* models, which contain explicit explanatory hypotheses in which the con-cepts are operationalized. At the level of theory, all the concepts of a model have been operationalized and the relationships between them have been validated. Thus there is a logical continuum from descriptive model to tested theory.

Land (1975) suggested that sound indicators should demonstrate a histori-cal pattern of timing and covariation with social change. The need for valid, reliable results that require extensive periods of research, however, can be in conflict with the equally urgent need to obtain results quickly and at minimum costs. There are competing claims for research funding between research that requires a longitudinal approach, such as the long-term effects that education or family assistance may have on an individual's life cycle, and research into the effectiveness of innovative government poli-cies to solve acute problems, such as poor schools or deprived inner city residents.

It is imperative, therefore, that data should be kept by governments that are amenable to the needs of predictive and causal research via a time series approach. Measurement systems must ensure that such data are constant and sufficiently rigorous to allow analyses that may validate social indicators as effective components of social policy models. It is obvious that there are competing forces between academic research and policy analysis. Academic research is usually motivated by a desire to establish quality research and the pursuit of the intrinsic value of knowledge. In this context, the researcher is often remote from the decision-making processes. On the other hand, Coleman (1972) has identified characteristics of policy analysis that include (a) an audience of political actors, (b) short-term satisfaction of information needs, and (c) an ultimate product that is designed to influence policy rather than contribute to existing knowledge.

Rather than perceiving a dichotomy between academic research and policy analysis, Carley (1981) has argued that there should be a symbiotic relation-ship between the two, wherein "good policy analysis is predicated on a theoretical base provided by academic researchers, which in turn justifies itself by its relevance to policy analysis and ultimately the process of government" (p. 103). Nowhere is this issue of complementarity more needed than in the use of quality of life as a construct for social and health policy development. As indicated in the introduction, health economists, in tackling the escalating costs of health care, have sought to ration medical services according to a metric that involves relative judgments about a person's quality of life.

Quest for a Generic Measurement of
Health Status and Health Service Outcomes

In the North American context, it has been suggested that the collection of data on health indicators gained strength through their association with the social indicators movement, which emerged as a critique of the exclusive use of economic indicators in the making of national policy (Larson, 1991). Thus social indicators supported the notion that health is more than absence of disease but includes a number of positive elements as well. However, Land (1975) pointed out that in its attempt to supplement economic indicators with information on the quality of life, the term itself has since become virtually identified as *the* rationale for social indicators. He further suggested that

> this excessive use of the term quality of life and the resulting confusion of meaning leads to the conclusion that it serves more as a political slogan for social indicator advocates than as a convincing rationale for their development. Thus, like other political slogans, the phrase benefits from a nebulous meaning, in that this facilitates the use of the slogan for many different purposes. (p. 12)

Before proceeding to analyze further the utility of quality of life as a metric for health services outcomes, it is useful to clarify the concept of health. Ware (1991) has suggested that we should begin by looking at the two dimensions of life, namely, its quantity and its quality. Quantity can be indicated in terms of the length of one's life, life expectancy, and mortality rates, but Ellinson (1979) has pointed out that these indicators have little value in capturing the quality of years lived in developed countries. It is important to note also that the definition of health is significantly dependent on the historical period in question and the culture in which it is defined (Larson, 1991). Hadley's (1982) definition of health as a multidimensional concept that encompasses not only the absence of disease and disability but also the ability to carry out normal tasks and activities and to maintain an overall sense of well-being reflects the broad contemporary approach.

Larson (1991) has classified five general approaches to defining health: the medical model, the holistic model, the wellness model, the environmental model, and the eclectic model. The medical model is predicated on the perspectives of illness, disease, and proper functioning. The holistic model is a broader concept encompassing physical, mental, and social health of the whole person. This approach is best identified with the definition of health advanced by the World Health Organization (WHO), which defined health as a state of complete physical, mental, and social well-being and not merely the absence of disease or infirmity (WHO, 1980a). The wellness model encompasses "better than normal" states as well as subjective feelings of health. It is often criticized as being too subjective, with attendant measurement difficulties, especially as it includes happiness, quality of life, and other global factors. From the medical model perspective, one can be healthy but not feel happy or experience a high quality of life. If happiness and quality of life can be accurately measured, it is a moot point whether they ought to be included in the definition of health or seen as separate concepts.

The environmental model focuses on the relationship of the individual with his or her environment. A person's state of health is related to adaptability to the environment and therefore can vary with environments. This approach is consistent with quality of life concepts developed in the disability field, especially the "goodness of fit" model (Schalock, 1990b). The environmental model of health finds support from a number of researchers. For instance, Hunt, McEwan, and McKenna (1985) found that changes in socioeconomic, environmental, and education conditions have effected greater advances in health status than medical interventions. Being embedded in systems theory, the environmental model has been criticized as being difficult to operationalize, thus presenting measurement problems (Larson, 1991). As this model views health as a relative concept, the environment is perceived as the proper standard against which to measure it. This can lead to a situation where an individual may be seen to be healthy in one environment but unhealthy in another. Again, there are parallels in the disability field. The WHO distinction between impairment, disability, and handicap views "handicap" as the extent to which a disability reduces one's ability to function in a specific environment that may or may not provide necessary support.

The eclectic model is typified by approaches that emerge from sociopolitical views of society, especially those that reflect economic determinism and the Marxist perspective of capitalism. For instance, Dolitel (quoted in Navarro, 1977) suggested that "health is institutionally defined as the capacity to help produce the very surplus the owners of the means of production appropriate" (p. 14). The conflict, social justice, and social control perspectives on viewing social policy and disability described by writers such as Oliver (1989) are in sympathy with this approach. Although the eclectic model appears to contain rather atypical definitions, it nevertheless points to an increase in the politicization of the health debate and the conflicting economic paradigms in which the debates are located, all of which are having profound effects on the way health policies are being developed.

As indicated in the discussion of the emergence of social indicators, policy analysts in the health field have moved from evaluating health services from an input perspective to an assessment of outcomes. This has led to a search for an elusive gold standard by which to make this assessment. In an attempt to move closer to a generic measure, Dowie (1991) made a distinction between *health status* and *health services outcome*. He pointed out that health care services are only one of the variables that may bring about a change in the overall health status of an individual or a population, and he was particularly unimpressed by health service outcomes being tackled as a separate exercise from health status measurement. There is a need for comparability, as it has a significant bearing on the total resources devoted to health services.

Applications of the Quality of Life Concept in the Domain of Health Care

Although much of the controversy surrounding the quality of life concept in health care is concerned with resource allocation, the concept has been used in a diverse range of other health settings, including health needs assessment, clinical trials, evaluation research, and clinical care (Fitzpatrick & Albrecht, 1994; Parmenter, 1994). In the context of health needs assessment, quality of life measures have been used to obtain more patient-focused, nonmedicinalized data concerning the total effect of health problems on individuals' lives (Wilkin, Hallam, & Dogett, 1992).

In the *clinical trials* context, quality of life measures that reflect patients' views are increasingly being used to supplement the traditional physiological indicators (Deyo, 1991; Parmenter, 1994; Schumacher, Olschewski, & Schulgen, 1991). Perhaps, as the questions addressed in this context are domain specific, the case of the quality of life concept has its most relevance for the health field. There is also a high degree of optimism for the use of quality of life measures in the evaluation of health and disability services (Emerson, 1985; Goode, 1990b; Greenfield, 1989; Landesman, 1986; Parmenter, 1992). In the case of individual patient care, there is little evidence of any widespread use of quality of life measures, possibly because the instruments are too complex and time-consuming to be routinely used in clinical settings. The development of shorter, more specific instruments may encourage their use by physicians, particularly as patients regard the information in such questionnaires important for their doctor to know (Nelson & Berwick, 1989).

It is in the area of resource allocation, however, that the most controversy has been generated. Calls for a rational system for the allocation of health services resources have led to the use of cost utility analyses associated with measures of quality of life. The approach associated with quality of life measures uses information concerning the costs of particular health service interventions in association with their respective benefits to health expressed in terms of survival, adjusted for what it terms QALYs. The debates concerning the use of CUAs essentially center on two areas. The first concerns the attempt to assign interval-level quantification to all states of health-related quality of life. The second concerns the use of such global measures, especially the moral and ethical acceptability of utilitarian approaches to resource allocation. QALYs have been used in two separate contexts: first, where choices have to be made among different possible forms of treatment for the same individual and, second, where a choice must be made among alternative ways of allocating resources for a diverse range of health interventions.

The North American approach to QALY measurement, based on economic decision analytic techniques formalized by Von Neumann and Morgenstern (1944), was pioneered by Torrance (1976). This approach was initially directed toward making intervention decisions for an individual. Here, the basic idea behind the QALY concept is that a person who is faced with the prospect of living Y years at less than full health may be able to equate this with the prospect of living X years (where $X < Y$) at full health. In explicating this approach, Loomes and McKenzie (1990) pointed out the following:

> The idea then is that any number of profiles of survival duration in a whole range of health states can be converted to their respective "full health life years" equivalents. Such QALY measures may be used as a decision aid in cases where different therapeutic options may produce quite diverse combinations of lengths and quality of life. (p. 85)

There are a number of problems associated with this approach to clinical judgment. One is the assumption of a consistent proportional trade-off between length of life and health status. This proposes that people are prepared to sacrifice some constant proportion of their remaining years of life to achieve a given improvement in their health status, despite the number of years that remain. This interval scale approach assumes, for instance, that a person might regard 12 years in excellent health as equivalent to 15 years in a reduced health state.

There is clear evidence, however, that people place different values on various health states according to the duration of the state (Pliskin, Shepard, & Weinstein, 1980; Sackett & Torrance, 1978). Also, this model makes no explicit allowance for time preference—that is, the varying value a person places on an event according to the timing of the event. For instance, people usually prefer present consumption of a commodity to the future consumption of the same commodity. Likewise, immediate periods in a specific health state may be valued more highly than distant periods in a similar state. Young adults may place lower weight on present good health than on good health later, when they may be raising a family. It may be different again in middle age when the family has left home and different yet again in the years following retirement. Support for these variations comes from a study by Williams (1988), who suggested that many people value certain stages of life more highly than some earlier stages, thus casting further reservations about the validity of a constant proportional time trade-off assumption.

The QALY utility model also requires that a person's risk attitude toward uncertain duration of survival should be independent of health state and should exhibit a constant proportional risk attitude. Loomes and McKenzie (1990) have pointed out that there is substantial evidence that "clearly undermine[s] the QALY assumption of constant proportional risk attitude" (p. 90), especially that which shows that the same individual may systematically exhibit both risk aversion and risk seeking.

There are also methodological problems associated with the way alternatives are framed. For instance, McNeil, Weichselbaum, and Parker (1982) showed that the method of describing the outcomes of a treatment affected the patients' preferences for surgical or nonsurgical options, especially where the outcomes were described in terms of probabilities of living or probabilities of dying.

Possibly the most serious reservation concerning individual utility-based QALYs is the rather uncritical way in which they are used to provide measures of cost-effectiveness to guide the setting of community-based health care priorities. Implicit in this approach is the view that the "values to be used in social decision making should be some aggregate of individuals' values" (Loomes & McKenzie, 1990, p. 94). In practice, though, it is not the individuals' values that are obtained but, rather, a political system may delegate government officials to make decisions on society's behalf. Their views on values may not necessarily reflect an aggregate of individuals' values. In the United Kingdom context, Williams's (1988) work on QALYs is possibly the best known and most frequently criticized, especially for his providing a basis for health care rationing (Brahams, 1991).

In a recent commentary on the usefulness of quality of life measures to social policy, Clemenster (cited in Hopkins, 1992) argued for open explicit criteria to be available and used in quality of life measurement in the rationing of services. He suggested that the more important quality of life is to the final decision, the less the rationing should be in the hands of professionals or government officials. In the United States, intense debate has followed the state of Oregon's plans to prioritize health care services, with most of the criticism focusing on the validity of the rankings of different health services determined by benefits to survival and quality of life (Dixon & Welch, 1991).

The rationing of health services raises important equity and ethical issues in the minds of many. Significant groups that oppose the QALY concept on these issues are those advocating for elderly and disabled persons. A typical antagonist in this field is Wolfensberger (1994), who has trenchantly criticized the use of the term *quality of life,* especially because it now carries so much "baggage" as to render it useless for scientific examination. For issues of life and death, particularly for the unborn or the economically and intellectually disadvantaged, quality of life is often blurred with the concept of sanctity of life, which raises the highly emotive issues of abortion and euthanasia. In this context, the question of who defines quality of life is again raised, for the motivation of the observer affects the definition. The economist focuses on issues of cost in dollars, whereas individual definitions tend to be oriented toward daily function, often extending beyond basic health factors to include social health, including social support and social interaction.

Despite acknowledgment of the inherent weaknesses in the current approach to QALYs, health economists are adamant that until more precise instruments or concepts are available, it is best to pursue the QALY line (Dowie, 1991; Richardson, 1992). Loomes and McKenzie (1990), however, have warned that it may be better to scuttle the approach and seek a new direction, especially if we arrive at the conclusion that there are too many limitations involved, limitations that are too fundamental to be overcome by applying more sophisticated measurement techniques.

Conclusions and Recommendations

It is enticing to dismiss the use of the quality of life construct in the context of social and health policy development and to omit it from economic appraisal because of difficulties in its measurement and evaluation, its attendant complex ethical problems, and its lack of a sound theoretical base in much of its formulation. In addition, the analysis of social indicators showed that there are several methodological problems in their development and validation. Generally, an atheoretical approach has been taken in establishing quality of life indicators and insufficient use has been made of the philosophical and epistemological underpinnings of the "good life." All of these factors have weakened the validity of current quality of life indicators as factors contributing to social and health policy development. This is not to deny their potential use, however.

To redress the problems raised, the following issues adapted from Nordenfelt (1994) need to be addressed:

What is the basic purpose of assessing or measuring quality of life? For instance, is it to inform global policies, to evaluate an intervention for a person in a clinical context, or a basis for the rational distribution of health care funds?

Having decided the purpose, one needs to determine the specific aspects of the person's life to be assessed. In this context, it may be asked who should determine the relevant evaluative dimension—the person or someone else? In a paternalistic mode, "experts" or politicians may decide the dimensions. A more liberal and individualistic approach generally leads to a situation where people's quality of life becomes identical with their own evaluation of their quality of life and there is no necessity for a general assessment instrument.

Once the purpose of the assessment and specific aspects of people's lives have been established, the particular scale or measurement device has to be selected or developed.

A plausible way forward, it is suggested, is to use Sen's (1980) construction of a plurality of independent vectors, each of which may be seen as an independent component of a full assessment of an individual's quality of life. Each of these components may be weighted by the person according to his or her view of its importance to having the good life. The *Comprehensive Quality of Life Scale* developed by Cummins (1993) is a good example of this approach. The artificial boundaries posed between objective and subjective indicators and those between qualitative and quantitative research methodologies need to be removed. There is also an urgent need for researchers coming from differing philosophies and discipline bases to join together in a common search for a deeper understanding of the complexities of the concept. Quality of life, from a subjective perspective, is an amalgam of cognitive and emotional factors that influence and are influenced by more objective external factors. The search for an elusive gold standard by which we may capture the full richness of the concept may be as productive as was the search for the Holy Grail.

9

Quality of Life and
Quality Assurance

Robert L. Schalock

◈ The concepts of quality of life, quality enhancement, and quality assurance are currently significantly affecting rehabilitation and community health programs. Their effect stems from at least the following three sources: (a) The current paradigm shift, with its emphasis on inclusion, equity, empowerment, and community-based supports, has forced service providers to focus on person-referenced services and outcomes (McFadden & Burke, 1991; Schalock, 1990b); (b) the quality revolution, with its emphasis on total quality, quality leadership, and total quality management, has resulted in habilitation services managing for quality (Albin, 1992; Schalock, in press); and (c) documentation has indicated that persons can be more independent, productive, community integrated, and satisfied when habilitation services are based on quality enhancement and integration principles (McGrew & Bruininks, 1992; Schalock, Keith, Hoffman, & Karan, 1989).

The term *quality of life* denotes a person's desired conditions of being as related to home and community living, school or work, and health and wellness (Schalock, 1994c). An enhanced quality of life represents both the purpose for and the desired outcomes from rehabilitation programs (Dossa, 1989). Throughout this volume, critical issues regarding the emerging concept of quality of life and its application have been addressed. The purpose of this chapter is to continue that dialogue by discussing the relationship between quality of life and quality assurance on rehabilitation and community health programs.

The chapter is based on a quality of life model that attempts to integrate major factors in one's perceived quality of life. Throughout the chapter, four fundamental points are made. First, quality of life is a subjective phenomenon based on a person's interpretation of various aspects of life experiences, including personal characteristics, objective life conditions, and the perception of significant others. Second, quality of life can be measured adequately by using subjective and objective measures (Schalock, 1990a). Third, a person's perceived quality of life can be influenced positively by education, health promotion, and rehabilitation programs. Fourth, quality assurance should be person referenced and involves a shared process of internal program evaluation and external validation. The chapter is divided into three sections that include the description of a quality of life model, a discussion of quality assurance "then and now," and the characteristics of a person-referenced quality assurance system.

A Quality of Life Model

Recent quality of life models have focused on process (Goode, 1991), community adjustment (Halpern et al., 1986), programmatic intervention (Brown, Bayer, & MacFarlane, 1989), person-environment interactions (Parmenter, 1988, 1992), or program improvement and outcome evaluation (Schalock, in press; Schalock & Keith, 1993). A recent review (Schalock, 1994c) of these models and the assessment instruments that accompany them indicated that a person's perceived quality of life is related significantly to factors within three major life domains that include home and community living, school or work, and health and wellness. These three factors are depicted in Figure 9.1. In the model, *satisfaction* serves as an intervening variable between each of the domains and a person's perceived quality of life.

The importance of models is that they help guide our thinking and assist in bringing about systems change. To that end, the model depicted in Figure 9.1 provides a framework for implementing a person-centered approach to quality assurance. Before describing what such a system would look like, however, it is important to review briefly quality assurance from a historical and current perspective.

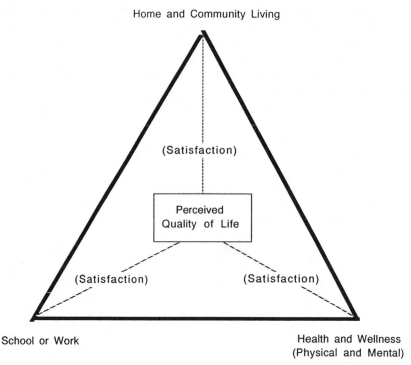

Figure 9.1. Quality of Life Model

Quality Assurance, Then and Now

Historically, quality assurance methods have involved certification, licensure, accreditation, citizen monitoring, or a combination of these (Bradley & Bersani, 1990; Gardner & Chapman, 1993). These approaches were based on the belief (that is still valid) that through its standards, monitoring, and response processes, an effective quality assurance system ensures high quality services. In addition, the conceptual framework for quality assurance proposed that a comprehensive assessment should address the three programmatic dimensions: program structure, process, and outcomes (Donabedian, 1966).

In actuality, however, quality assurance has focused primarily on program process, with minimum attention given to program structure and outcomes (Zeithaml, Parasuraman, & Berry, 1990). This overreliance on program process (sometimes called "the paper chase") has been further complicated by the views that service quality is more difficult to evaluate than product quality, that people do not evaluate services on outcomes alone, and that the only considerations that matter in determining service quality are set by the user of the service (Gardner & Chapman, 1993).

Because of these problems and the fact that we need to change systems faster (Shea, 1976), we have begun to rethink the purpose and process of quality assurance in light of the quality revolution. At least three phenomena are significantly affecting this reevaluation:

A focus on quality enhancement rather than quality assurance (Albin, 1992; Gardner & Chapman, 1993)

A paradigm shift that places the focus of best practices on the strengths and capacities of the person, normalized environments, integrated services with supports, and the empowerment of persons served (Bradley, Ashbaugh, & Blaney, 1993; Schalock & Kiernan, 1990)

A person-centered planning and supports model that focuses on developing partnerships with families, professionals, and communities (Smull & Danehey, 1993)

These three phenomena have resulted in a significant reformulation of how quality assurance should be viewed and implemented. In addressing this reformulation, I would like to suggest that we consider the concept of a person-referenced quality assurance system. What would such a system look like? In the remainder of the chapter, I discuss its five characteristics:

1. It is based on a comprehensive framework.
2. It begins with the end (that is, person-referenced outcomes) in mind.
3. It considers quality assurance as a form of internal program evaluation.
4. It is a shared process involving consumers, providers, and regulatory bodies.
5. It results in quantitative information that can be aggregated for multiple uses.

Characteristics of a Person-Referenced Quality Assurance System

COMPREHENSIVE FRAMEWORK

A comprehensive client-referenced quality assurance system should focus on three major program-related factors: desired person-referenced outcomes, program structure, and program process. This framework is shown in Figure 9.2.

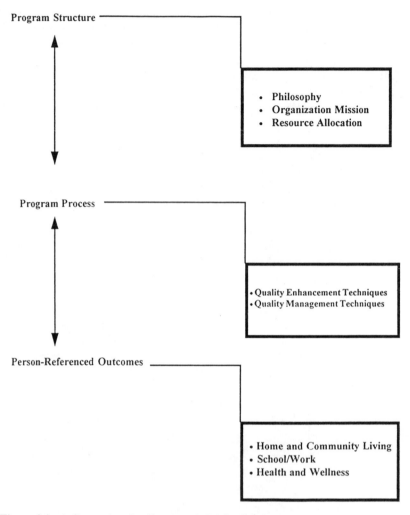

Program Structure

- Philosophy
- Organization Mission
- Resource Allocation

Program Process

- Quality Enhancement Techniques
- Quality Management Techniques

Person-Referenced Outcomes

- Home and Community Living
- School/Work
- Health and Wellness

Figure 9.2. A Comprehensive Framework for Quality Assurance

In a recent summary of the quality revolution in management, Albin (1992) discussed five basic principles that summarize how human service management has responded to the quality of life movement and has enabled the management-programmatic structure to affect, in a significant way, the objective life conditions of persons and thereby enhance their quality of life. These five principles include (a) establishing a mission to lead quality improvement, (b) developing an obsession with quality, (c) creating a unity of purpose, (d) empowering employees to work to achieve the mission, and (e) using a systematic approach to find opportunities and to improve performance. Operationally, a comprehensive framework is seen in a program's structure, process, and outcomes. Each area is described briefly.

Program Structure

The focus here is primarily on the program's mission statement and conversion activities. In reference to the need for a strong mission statement, Albin (1992) stated the following:

> Whatever your business happens to be, your mission must be able to lead quality improvement efforts. Establishing such a mission provides the context to support efforts toward quality [and] must guide continuous improvement of the quality of services. To do that, an organization's mission must be defined in a way that will assist its members in recognizing quality, in determining how well the organization is achieving that quality, and in taking any steps needed to improve its performance. (p. 14)

Currently, we are seeing tremendous efforts toward program conversion. Critical components of this process include moving toward supported living, supported employment, and recreation and leisure from a wellness perspective (Schalock & Kiernan, 1990).

Program Process

The focus of looking at (and evaluating) program process is to continue emphasizing the critical nature of the quality enhancement and quality management techniques discussed in a later section on data use.

Program Outcomes

Although quality enhancement and management techniques use different words, the desired result is enhanced quality outcomes. How these outcomes are defined varies but frequently involves the monitoring and evaluation of critical quality indicators that reflect enhanced independence, productivity, community integration, and health and wellness.

BEGIN WITH THE END IN MIND

As shown in Figure 9.2, quality assurance involves delineating significant person-referenced outcomes. Consistent with the current paradigm shift toward person-centered planning and service delivery, the selection of these desired outcomes is made primarily by consumers and their advocates. A number of possible quality of life indicators, aggregated according to the three factors depicted in the quality of life model (Figure 9.1), are listed in Table 9.1. This list is not exhaustive but hopefully will give the reader some suggestions.

Internal Program Evaluation

Quality assurance can be considered a type of internal program evaluation that uses a decision-making model and focuses on self-monitoring and self-evaluation (Mathison, 1991). According to Clifford and Sherman (1983),

> Internal evaluation is a tool of management science as much or more than it is either a product or tool of social science. The internal evaluator has a long-term commitment to change through enhancement of the quality of decision making in the organization. (p. 23)

The attractiveness of an internal program evaluation approach to quality assurance includes the following: (a) It is part of the organization's information processing system and thus does not require duplicative evaluation-monitoring efforts and data; (b) the decision-making model draws heavily from the systems perspective, which is consistent with the need to relate a program's mission statement to processes and quality outcomes; (c) it focuses on self-monitoring and self-improvement; (d) it attempts to be comprehensive, correct, complete, and credible to partisans on all sides; and (e) it allows for a better understanding of the contextual variables of the organization and the perspectives of the various stakeholders (Torres, 1992).

A Shared Process

Consumer empowerment and equity represent the essence of the paradigm shift currently affecting rehabilitation and health promotion services. Thus a reformulation of quality assurance should incorporate this change as shown in Figure 9.3, which graphically summarizes the key aspects of the shared process.

> There is a parallel set of activities completed by the provider (internal evaluation) and the consumer-advocate-regulatory body (external validation).
> Internal evaluation is a data-based process built around the desired person-referenced outcomes (summarized previously in Table 1) and monitored jointly by the service provider and external validator(s).

TABLE 9.1 Exemplary Person-Referenced Quality of Life Indicators

Domain	*Potential Indicators*	
Home and community living	Ownership of home	
	Private telephone	
	Name on mail box or rental lease	
	Possessions	
	Family-social relationships	
	Use of generic services	
	Safety and security	
	Integrated recreation and leisure activities	
	Activities of daily living, such as meal preparation, housekeeping, transportation, taking medicine, money management, and telephone use	
Work-school	Work	School
	Integrated employment	Age-appropriate materials
	Fair salary	Age-appropriate tasks
	Employment benefits	Functional skills
	Safe work environment	Integrated classrooms
	Feedback	Integrated recreation-
	Meaningful avocational activities	leisure activities
Health and wellness	Activities of daily living	Wellness indicators
	Eating	Number of days sick
	Transfer	Number of days of missed work
	Toileting	Number of doctor appointments
	Dressing	Medication level
	Bathing	Time out of bed or chair
	Good nutritional status	Number of hospitalizations
	Health care access	Physical fitness indicators
	Mobility	Strength
	Minimum medication	Flexibility
		Agility
		Balance
		Cardiorespiratory endurance
		Activity indicators
		Number of activities (full)
		Number of activities (partial)

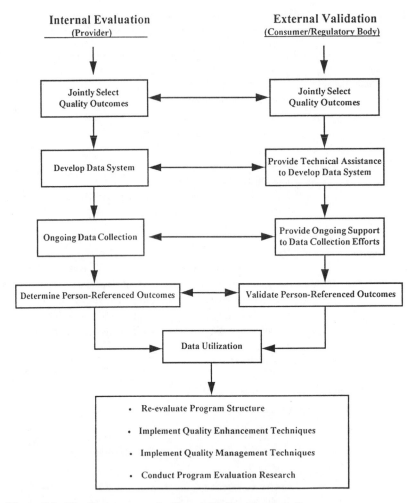

Figure 9.3. The Components of a Shared Quality Assurance Process

External validation involves agreeing on the quality outcomes to monitor, providing technical assistance and support to the development and maintenance
of the data system, and validating the critical quality outcomes.

Data from the quality assurance process are used for a variety of purposes,
including reevaluating program structure, implementing quality enhancement and management techniques, and conducting program evaluation
research.

Using the Data

This section suggests four uses for data from the quality assurance process. As will be seen, the specific use will depend on a number of factors, such as whether or not the outcomes meet the needs and expectations of the consumers and the capacity of the program to change.

Reevaluating Program Structure. Figure 9.2 indicated that evaluating program structure is a key aspect of quality assurance. If person-referenced outcomes are lacking, then one needs to evaluate the program's philosophy, mission, and resource allocation. Change must begin at the top. The current efforts at rehabilitation program conversion stress the critical need to align a program's philosophy and mission statement to its ongoing service delivery system.

For example, the author has recently been involved in providing training to 60 vocational rehabilitation agencies who want to convert their sheltered employment programs to ones based on the principle of integrated employment with supports. Part of the training has involved evaluating their current programs across nine conversion factors using *The Program Capacity Checklist and Manual* (Calkins, Schalock, Griggs, Kiernan, & Gibson, 1990). The results of pre- and post-training comparisons are presented in Table 9.2.

Although it is apparent from these data that there was considerable change (that is, a change ratio of .20 or better) in these programs' philosophies and missions, there is still considerable work to do to bring program practices into alignment with the changed philosophy and mission. Part of the necessary conversion activities will involve resource allocation but part will also involve implementing quality enhancement and management techniques.

Implementing Quality Enhancement Techniques. If the person-referenced outcomes are less than optimal, the key players can sit down and problem solve as to how specific quality enhancement techniques can be implemented. A number of approaches are currently being used to enhance person-referenced outcomes. Goode (1990a), as one example, uses group discussion, including persons with disabilities, parents, and staff. During the discussion, various topics are explored, beginning with the question, "What is a good life?" Other topics include important needs and ways to fulfill them in different settings. The results of these sessions can be analyzed using a number of need-goal matrices consisting of dimensions such as work, housing, leisure time, friendships, self-image, security, and integration. The goal of this approach to

TABLE 9.2 Changes in Overall Organizational Functions

Function	Average Evaluation		Change Ratio[a]
	Pre-Training	Post-Training	
Philosophy	2.1	2.6	.24
Program and resources	2.4	2.7	.13
Program practices	2.3	2.5	.09
Program evaluation	2.0	2.4	.20
Person-job match	2.5	2.8	.12
Employer expectations	2.4	2.7	.13
Systems interface	2.1	2.4	.14
Natural environment- supports	2.2	2.6	.18
Quality of work life	2.5	2.8	.12
		Average =	.15

a. Change ratio = $\dfrac{\text{Postevaluation} - \text{Preevaluation}}{\text{Preevaluation}}$

quality enhancement is to test the capacity of the service system to satisfy the expressed needs of its consumers.

A second quality enhancement technique focuses more on what program personnel and program services can do to enhance the person's perceived quality of life. For example, Table 9.3 summarizes a number of quality enhancement techniques that are related to home and community living, school or work, and health and wellness. The goal of this second approach is to encourage programs to implement quality enhancement techniques that can have a significant effect on person-referenced outcomes.

Implementing Quality Management Techniques. Probably the best example of how quality management principles have brought about quality improvement is reflected in the Malcolm Baldrige Award for Excellence. This award is based on a number of fundamental principles (American Society for Quality Control, 1992; Deming, 1986; Rosander, 1991; Wood & Steere, 1992), including the following:

- Quality defined by the customer
- Services continuously improved based on feedback about their quality
- Employee participation and development
- Management by data
- Partnership development

TABLE 9.3 Quality Enhancement Techniques

Domain[a]	Exemplary Enhancement Techniques
Home and community living	Allow for choices, decision making, and environmental control
	Interface with person's social support systems
	Maximize use of natural supports such as family, friends, and neighbors
	Stress normalized and integrated environments, social interactions, and community activities
	Emphasize family-professional partnerships
	Promote positive role functions and lifestyles
School-work	**School**
	Use age-appropriate materials and tasks
	Teach functional skills
	Promote critical and interactional activities
	Teach across settings and in the natural environments
	Work
	Facilitate integrated employment, work status, avocational activities, and nonemployment volunteerism
	Use job accommodation and job restructuring
	Foster coworkers as natural supports
	Develop supported employment alternatives
Health and wellness	Promote wellness by emphasizing physical fitness, nutrition, healthy lifestyles, and stress management
	Maximize health care coverage and access
	Maximize use of prosthetics that facilitate mobility, communication, and self-help
	Maintain as low a psychotropic medication level as possible
	Promote stable, safe environments that lessen stress and increase predictability, control, and positive behaviors

a. Domains are based on the quality of life model shown in Figure 9.1.

- Constant monitoring of future trends that will influence customer needs
- Well-designed and executed service delivery systems

Conducting Program Evaluation Research. Once a quantitative quality assurance system is in place, then systematic program evaluation studies are possible. For example, recently we (Schalock, Lemanowicz, Conroy, & Feinstein, 1994) used the model in Figure 9.1 and the Quality of Life Questionnaire (Schalock & Keith, 1993) to determine empirically a number of model-related correlates to measure quality of life. The study involved 989 persons with mental retardation who were administered a number of measures reflecting their personal characteristics, objective life conditions, and significant others' perceptions. In the analysis, the total quality of life score was used as the dependent measure. A hierarchical regression analysis was conducted in which predictor variables were entered in three blocks: personal characteristics, objective life conditions, and perceptions of significant others. The results, as shown in Table 9.4, show clearly that personal characteristics explained the most variance, followed by objective life conditions and the perception of significant others.

Conclusion

The concepts of quality of life and quality assurance are having significant effects on program planning and evaluation efforts within rehabilitation and health promotion. An example of these effects is seen clearly in the author's longitudinal studies of the community placement outcomes of persons with mental retardation.

In our first studies (Schalock & Harper, 1978; Schalock, Harper, & Carver, 1981), we were interested primarily in the "placement success" of individuals whom we had placed 5 years previously into independent living and competitive employment environments. The dichotomized dependent variable was whether or not the individual remained in the placement environment or returned to the habilitation program. During that period, the organization's primary goal and staffing patterns were directed at placing individuals with mental retardation into community environments that increased their independence and productivity.

Five years later (10 years after the initial placement), we reevaluated the status of these individuals, expanding our data sets to include a measure of the persons' quality of life (Schalock & Lilley, 1986). This addition reflected the organization's commitment not only to place persons into the community but also to assist them to become better integrated and satisfied with their community placements. Although the organization's mission statement reflected an enhanced quality of life for its clientele, program structure during the 5-year period had not changed significantly in terms of the quality

TABLE 9.4 Results of Hierarchical Regression

Block-Predictor Variable	R^2 Adjusted	R^2 Change	F for Block	Beta Coefficients
Personal characteristics	.426		89.34*	
Age				−.08
Gender				.04
Adaptive behavior index				.40
Challenging behavior index				.21
Health index				−.01
Need for medication				−.06
Objective life conditions	.506	.08	53.17*	
Earnings				.17
Integrated activities				.12
Physical environment				−.03
Social presence				−.01
Living unit size				.01
Residential supervision				−.05
Home type				.16
Employment status				.07
Perceptions of significant others	.519	.01	43.75*	
Client progress				.03
Environmental control				−.03
Job satisfaction				.07
Working with person				.07

* $p < .0000$.

enhancement techniques summarized in Table 9.3. What we found in the 1986 study was that, essentially, the organization had fulfilled its goal of placing people into community-living and employment environments but had overlooked the multifaceted quality of their lives.

Based on that finding, the processes outlined in Figure 9.2 were implemented. Specifically, program structure (staffing patterns and resource allocation) was aligned with the mission statement, focusing on enhanced quality of life outcomes; quality management principles were implemented that empowered employees to find community-based opportunities and supports that would enhance the person's independence, productivity, community integration, and satisfaction; and quality enhancement techniques related to increased use of natural supports and the permanence of one's home were integrated into staff training.

The net result was to change significantly the evaluation paradigm used in the 15-year follow-up of the original group. In that study (Schalock & Genung, 1993), personal interviews and observational data were used to evaluate the person's social and support networks, lifestyles and role functions, activity patterns, measured quality of life, and expressed satisfaction. Currently, the quality assurance process is being changed significantly as reflected in Figure 9.3 to evaluate, during a person's annual individual program review, mutually agreed-on person-referenced quality of life indicators to ensure that the program's mission statement is being fulfilled on an ongoing basis as seen by the heterogeneous constituency.

In summary, what I have attempted to do in this chapter is to suggest that the concept of quality of life is the overriding principle of the 1990s and will continue to influence significantly rehabilitation and community health programs. If this is true, then it is essential that (re)habilitation and community health programs be guided by quality of life models that provide a framework for service provision, quality assurance, and program evaluation. Furthermore, we should embrace a quality assurance system that is consumer-referenced and results in quantitative data that can be used to enhance quality, including one's quality of life.

10

Overcoming the Social Construction of Inequality as a Prerequisite to Quality of Life

Marcia H. Rioux

There have been a number of major shifts in the framing and justification of state obligations in Canada toward persons with disabilities (Drover & Kerans, 1993; Roeher Institute, 1993; Yalnizian, 1993). These suggest that the culture of justice and the public ownership of private disadvantage is too often lacking in the organization of our social and legal institutions. What is needed is not a culture that sees poverty as a problem just for the poor and homeless but one that celebrates diversity and sees each people's place in the world as integrally related to that of others in other nations.

This chapter explores the process of the social and legal construction of inequality and, more specifically, the way in which those with disabilities have been distinguished from other citizens to permit differential treatment and to justify fewer rights although purporting to uphold the central democratic tenet of equality. It also examines the implications of that process of differentiation for both the conceptualization and measurement of quality of life and its application in health promotion and rehabilitation.

The social and legal construction of inequality, although having some elements particularized to nation-states, also has some elements that are common across nations. In other words, there are some ways in which we construct the inequality of people on notions that are thought to be universal. It is clear that in nearly every nation of the world, women hold a status that is less valued than that of men. That lesser status varies from nations where women cannot vote, cannot drive a car, and cannot go out in public without their husbands to nations where they are accorded full social and legal rights but their employment opportunities and child care responsibilities result in an overall lower socioeconomic status. Likewise in virtually every nation in the world, people with disabilities hold a lesser status than other people.

Particular policies, programs, and services established in different countries are often legitimated by obligations that are circumscribed or limited by assumptions of inequality based on ability to contribute economically. The social, legal, and economic policies in place at any given time in history reflect the ways that principles of justice have legitimated differential treatment. This chapter will trace the development of some prevalent general understandings of disability. It will also trace the shift in the conceptualization of equality. Assumptions arising from both these developments, which form the basis for many state policies, programs, and services, have made the differential treatment of people with disabilities seem both just and fair. They have been the foundation for keeping people with disabilities in the status of second-class citizens both within nation states and as world citizens. They have also influenced the meaning and parameters of the assumptions about quality of life and have arguably limited the goals of rehabilitation to fit particular political and professional views of disability and equality.

Disability as an Example of
the Social Construction of Inequality

We are seeing within the disability movements in many nations a resurgence of a discussion of some fundamental principles of how all people should be treated. Questions are being asked about the quality of the care being provided (or lack of it) and whether it meets even minimum notions of what is fair and just. People with disabilities and their advocates are recognizing the need to put these questions within the broader context of principles of justice, fairness, and equality as they recognize that the way people are treated and the share of the national funding allocations they receive reflect much more fundamental inequalities in society (Barton, 1993; Leal Ocampo, 1995; Oliver, 1990; "Pathway to Integration," 1993; Riddington, 1989). It is these inequalities that will have to be addressed if people with disabilities are to be full participants in their societies. To study the case of disability, therefore, is to reflect on the struggle for social justice and the parameters of political obligation to relieve inequality. I am not suggesting that this particular case is unique. A similar analysis of other disadvantaged groups would be equally enlightening. The case of disability, however, provides insight into the interplay between notions of quality of life and, in particular, rehabilitation based on enhancing quality of life directed toward those with disabilities and how these have contributed to and result in differential treatment. The case of disability enables us to tease out the way in which the conceptualization and measurement of quality of life supports and reinforces both state and professional obligations to people with disabilities. It finds its roots in particular theoretical and scientific constructs of disability and equality.

The examination of these constructs is thus important to an understanding of the issues associated with conceptualizing, measuring, and applying information about quality of life.

Stages in the Legal and Social Construction of Inequality

There are a number of identifiable stages in the social construction of inequality and in determining standards of equality. First, a person is labeled or distinguished from others in such a way that he or she is considered socially inferior. Second, care and treatment, including professional standards and practice, law, policy, and political rights, are developed and legitimated on the basis of this label of social inferiority. Third, a paternalistic denial of liberties and self-determination is imposed, premised on the social obligation that attaches to the status.

In the case of disability, these have been fundamentally influenced by the interaction of two major trends. On the one hand, there has been a paradigm shift in the social and scientific characterization of disability and, coincidentally, there has been a legal and philosophical reconceptualization of the meaning of equality and its implications.

Social and Scientific Change in How Disability Is Perceived, Diagnosed, and Treated

The social and scientific change in how disability is perceived, diagnosed, and treated is reflected in assumptions about the social responsibility toward people with disabilities as a group. The assumptions or postulates about

disability are not mutually exclusive nor have they been temporally chrono-
logical. Some disciplines have clung tenaciously to the historical characterization of disability solely as a medical condition or as a personal deficit,
whereas others have adopted the framework of disability as either a social
or a political condition or have adopted some hybrid of these two major
schools of thought. Consequently, policy and programming, both within the
professional sphere and coming from government, reflect attempts to accommodate these shifting understandings of disability as a status.

The most widespread way of dealing with disability has been to portray it
as a biological condition. The perception of disability as biologically determined replaced the earlier understanding of its source in demonic possession. This switch from religious to scientific doctrine was accompanied by
the belief that disability was a sign of inferiority that, once diagnosed, could
be eradicated or treated. Biological determinism has played a significant role
as a basis for classifying and labeling people since the early part of the 20th
century. This has been particularly evident for people with intellectual disabilities with the development, scientific endorsement, and use of intelligence
tests. A principal theme within biological determinism is that worth can be
assigned to individuals and groups on the basis of their heredity, and that the
nature of their heredity is reflected in the nature of their intelligence. By
measuring intellectual potential or intelligence as a single quantity, heredity
and therefore social worth was argued to be identifiable. Society, and its
economic and social distributions, was then argued to be a reflection of
biological order. It followed that political inequality could justifiably be
attributed to biological characteristics. Similar arguments have been used to
justify the political and social inequalities of women and people of color.
The use of intelligence testing and arguments drawn from biological determinism has, in other words, rendered the social fact of discrimination, a
scientifically justified "fact."

Given the medicalization of disability, many instruments have been developed for the purpose of diagnosis. These include the *International Classification of Impairment, Disability, and Handicap* (*ICIDH*); the *Diagnostic and
Statistical Manual* (*DSM-IV*); the *International Classification of Disease*
(*ICD* 10); and various intelligence tests.

Labeling or diagnosing the physiological or psychological state has been
important as a means of determining the individual pathology or functional
disabilities and as a basis for undertaking curative or remedial treatment. On
the basis of such diagnoses, medical or rehabilitation therapy is initiated to
address the diagnosed problem, which if cured medically or remediated will
enable a person to function as independently as possible—within the social

and economic environments designed and used by able-bodied persons. Where environmental modifications are made, these have tended to be limited to the personal or immediate sphere rather than the macro or systems level of social and economic organization.

This therapeutic or remediative care has sometimes been taken to extremes. For example, there is a huge literature on the effectiveness of one therapy or another in changing the behavior or adaptive skills of individuals. For many people, such as people with an intellectual disability, learning how to cook is referred to as "culinary therapy," learning how to speak becomes "speech therapy," listening to music for enjoyment becomes "music appreciation therapy," and learning how to make friends becomes "social network therapy." The result of all this therapy can be an extremely "clinical" lifestyle; but more important, characterizing everyday activities in this way has important implications for individual status and for the interpretation of quality of life. Notwithstanding the American Association on Mental Retardation's fairly recent recognition of the interplay between environment and individual impairment, the professional field remains generally focused on diagnosis-assessment, prevention, and amelioration of individual skill deficits and building individual competencies (American Association on Mental Retardation, 1992).

The social obligation attached to such characterizations of disability is limited to medical-biological diagnosis and medical or technological treatment, including medically directed therapeutic interventions. For those who cannot be cured or rehabilitated, institutions and other segregated housing and all-encompassing service provision centers have been the conventional model of care. Until quite recently, people with disabilities were expected to make little or no contribution to society and, in many cases, were considered a danger to society (Cohen, 1985; Cohen & Scull, 1983; Law Reform Commission of Canada, 1979; Sutherland, 1976). As a result, families were encouraged to place their children in institutions. The alternative was to keep them at home with few services or supports. Quality of life within this framework was then measured within a set of parameters limited to basic needs.

Scientific study contributed to the rationale for putting people in large institutions that have housed up to 3,000 people at various times in this century in Canada. The rationale was that society had to be protected from the effect that such people might have. There were fears they might reproduce and fears that society would be overridden by people who could not work and would not be able to take care of themselves (Brynelson, 1990). Chappell (1992) suggested that the emergence of wage labor contributed to the perception of disability as an individual pathology and that institutionalization was used as a form of social engineering.

The medical model has matured to encompass the characterization of disability as a service or social problem rather than solely as a biological problem. Using this formulation, the hypothesis is that the deficit lies within the individual, but the concept of treatment is broadened to include both ameliorating the condition and developing ways to enable people to develop the potential they have. From this perspective, there has been no attempt to reframe the notion that the problems experienced by people with disabilities are a result of their individual impairment.

Within this model, services are developed and provided to enable the individual with a disability to be as socially functional or as normal as possible (Meyer, Peck, & Brown, 1990; Wolfensberger, 1972). The social responsibility in dealing with disability is to develop systems of assessment, habilitation, and measures to improve self-care and social skills. This responsibility derives principally from a sense of charity and benevolence (and reducing social cost). Concentration is on issues of importance to professionals and on a professional service paradigm commonly based on the best interests of the individual as the ethical criteria for professional practice. Success in meeting the social and professional obligation (to ensure quality of life) is measured by how closely people with disabilities who use services can approximate so-called normal people.

A third identifiable way of dealing with disability is to understand it as a problem that is not a result of the individual deficit but is a consequence of social organization and the relationship of the individual with the society (Beresford & Campbell, 1994; Canadian Society for ICIDH, 1991; Oliver, 1990; Rioux & Bach, 1994; Roeher Institute, 1992; Roth, 1983). From this perspective, disability is regarded as a predetermined and inevitable part of the population, not as an anomaly. The treatment is to identify the barriers in society that restrict the participation of people with impairments or disabilities in economic and social life. Structural barriers to independent living or community living become the site of therapy (Canadian Association of Independent Living Centres, 1994; Goundry, Peters, & Currie, 1994; Roeher Institute, 1988). The indicator of quality of life from this perspective is the degree to which there has been a reduction of civic inequalities—that is, the degree to which social and economic disadvantage has been addressed. Recognition of social and political entitlements is based on people's humanity rather than on their ability to contribute economically, and rights are equated with all others in society. The social obligation is to provide supports, aids, and devices to enable social and economic integration, self-determination, and legal and social rights.

Changes in Understanding
the Concept of Equality

Whereas there have been changes in how disability is perceived, there has been a concurrent shift in the theoretical constructs of equality. They fit generally into three categories. One is the formal theory of equality—that is, the equal-treatment model (Aristotle, 1980; Nozick, 1974). The second is the liberal theory of equality (Dworkin, 1977; Rawls, 1971; Williams, 1962), incorporating the ideals of both equality of opportunity and special treatment. The third is the equality of well-being or equality of resources model (Baker, 1983; Dworkin, 1981a, 1981b; Rawls, 1971; Veatch, 1986). Each of these models claims that different elements compose equality. This has importance for people with disabilities, particularly in light of the ways in which disability has been perceived. If the status quo (the social, economic, and political organization) is assumed to be necessary for society to function and if differences are defined as intrinsic to the individual and in conflict with the status quo, then those who might make a claim for greater equality (that is, those with differences) have no grounds on which to challenge the label of difference and its consequences, which include unequal status and benefits.

If equality depends on sameness (the equal treatment model) and on being *similarly situate* (in the same circumstances), the concept of equality requires that like people be treated alike and presumes the impartial enforcement of legal and social rights. It makes no difference to attempt to clarify what makes people equal—that is, alike in particular circumstances or for particular purposes. There is no prescriptive element to the principle on which governments might base their decisions about which people are to be accorded the unequal treatment. The principle simply establishes the generally accepted rule of law (Tarnopolsky, 1982; Tarnopolsky & Pentney, 1985) that procedural fairness must be applied for law to be legitimate. Neutrality in the application of the law and the absence of different treatment are presumed to result in equality. The differential effect of the law or the treatment is of no consequence to whether equality has been achieved. Individual difference justifies limiting claims to entitlement and still meeting the standard of equality.

This standard of equality can be relatively easily met, even where the social and economic entitlements and outcomes are significantly different, if the social and scientific perception of disability results from and rests in an individual deficit (as when it is characterized as a medical, therapeutic, or service problem). Failure to provide education or the same standard of education for people with disabilities has been justified on this basis. The restriction of immigration of people with disabilities has also been justified on this basis. Therapeutic interventions, such as prevocational training, sheltered workshops, and others, have met this standard of equality.

This standard of equality justifies many of the predominantly used measures of quality of life that are based on notions of diminished capacity, competence, and exercise of social life as determined by some objective standard. For example, there are a number of cases where babies with serious physical and mental disabilities have been denied medical interventions because professionals have predicted that their quality of life will be considerably limited (Endicott, 1988; *Superintendent of Family & Child Service v. R. D. & S. D. et al.,* 1983).

Much recent discourse on equality has addressed the inherent problems of such a limited notion of equality. It draws attention to the substantive inequality between disadvantaged groups and advantaged groups in society. Equality of opportunity addresses some of the limitations of formal equality by taking into account and redressing historical conditions of inequality. It removes the necessity for disadvantaged groups to prove that they are the same as others with the same skills and abilities. Equality of opportunity recognizes that there may be prejudices and barriers to participation (for example, in education or the labor market) that have led some groups of people to be disadvantaged unfairly. They, therefore, have a legitimate claim to compensation—in such forms as affirmative action, employment equity, and so on—to enable them to start in a position relatively similar to that of others.

The dilemma for enabling equality for people with disabilities with this model is that their differences are not solely the result of historic circumstances, and there is no compelling obligation for social institutions to address such disadvantage when this model is used. As Smith (1986) argued, the equal opportunity model fits well in such cases as race, where physical differences can be legitimately argued to be legally irrelevant. However, it is not always so clear for other groups of people:

> There are physical differences between the sexes in relation to child-bearing and breast feeding which make identical treatment of the sexes unequal in some contexts. Running the race from the same starting line does not solve the problem of maternity along the way. Classifications based on sex may be legally relevant. Similarly there are differences between the able-bodied and the disabled and between young, middle-aged, and old people which can make identical treatment unequal. Simple equality of opportunity cannot conceivably produce equality of results in many of these situations. Such issues do not arise as squarely with respect to racial discrimination. (Smith, 1986, p. 365)

In most cases, people with disabilities cannot overcome natural characteristics and become like the norm, even with equality of opportunity,
because it is based on the assumption that the aim of equal opportunity is to
provide access to the competitive, individualistic market, not to such non-
comparable goods as minimal nutrition and medical support. The basis for
their claim to equality can be made only on their citizenship or on their
humanness or on a general egalitarian value assumption—for example, that
all people should be accorded equal respect by their government because
they are persons (Greenawalt, 1983), not because of their ability to compete.
Their claim on resources is to enable participation, even though in some cases
it will be unlikely in the long term that they will be competitive (within the
existing social and economic climate) without some degree of ongoing
support. Their claim is not a claim for support to redress past discrimination
or to overcome particular barriers to participation (equality of opportunity).
Instead, the claim of people with disabilities is for redistribution of state
resources and for ongoing systemic support to be able to exercise the same
rights as others. This claim is not premised on the measurable social benefits
(economic efficiency and effectiveness) foreseen to be achievable in exchange for additional state costs or support.

The unarticulated premises of the equality of opportunity model are
homogeneity and interchangeability. Combined with a perception of disability as an individual deficit rather than a structural or systemic problem, the
implications are obvious. The individual will be expected to integrate within
social and economic structures that are based on substantively male nonhandicapped standards and that make no long-term allowances for the
individual's inherent differences. The organization of society around people
with disabilities is based on an implied assumption that disability is an
intrinsic inequality. The differentiation between intrinsic and extrinsic inequality is not made. As a result, inequalities arising from such extrinsic
factors as the way income, employment, housing, and services are organized
are presumed to arise because of factors intrinsic to the individual. Simply
establishing that a class of individuals possess a specific characteristic does
not address such a problem. The weakness of this approach is that it can even
make disadvantage invisible (Brodsky & Day, 1989) because it is difficult
to identify anything but the most obvious intrinsic distinctions and easy to
ignore subtle but pervasive issues of power in society that create disadvantage. It is true that the equality of opportunity model can recognize and
address blatant prejudice. It is questionable, however, whether people with
disabilities are disadvantaged by inequalities arising from overt prejudice
rather than from the much more extensive inequalities arising from how
society is organized.

   A model of equality based on well-being as an outcome incorporates the premise that all humans—despite their differences—are entitled to be considered and respected as equals and have the right to participate in the social and economic life of society. Unlike the other models of equality, it would take into account that the conditions and means of participation may vary for each individual, entailing special accommodation to make this possible. Whereas the outcome—equality of well-being—would be universal, the programs or means to ensure equality could justifiably be targeted to enable those least able to achieve well-being to be supported on a temporary or long-term basis. Difference would be both acknowledged and accommodated in ensuring the outcome. Political and legal decisions would have to take into account differences in the achievement of well-being in the distributive paradigm of social justice.

   Well-being has a number of components, including equal achievement of self-determination, participation and inclusion in social life (through democratization), and the exercise of fundamental citizenship rights (Roeher Institute, 1993). Equality itself would be an end rather than a means to meeting other social goals. Alternatively, equal treatment and equal opportunity, in most of their formulations, treat equality as a means to ensure fairness in achieving some other ends. Thus in the latter case, people of equal need and ability should have equal opportunity to obtain desired scarce resources. Equality of well-being would recognize that although people are not equal in talent, social usefulness, or willingness to serve the community, they are entitled to make choices about how they want to live and what constitutes the good life for them, as long as it operates within the framework of the mutual recognition of others' self-determination. Quality of life is measured neither by an exclusively objectivist standard nor by an exclusively subjectivist one. It becomes the interpretation of generally accepted social values and goals and the personal and collective realization of such values and goals.

   Equality defined as the inclusion and participation of all groups in institutions and positions makes clear the onus to include even those people who cannot meet the standards of economic self-sufficiency. Young (1990) proposed this as a characteristic of a model of equality based on outcome and argued that it allows affirmative action to be seen as consistent with the principle of nondiscrimination and as a policy instrumental in undermining oppression. Equality as inclusion and participation shifts the basis for distributive justice away from economic contribution as the primary factor of entitlement and recognizes other forms of participation as valuable. The reproduction of the material and ideological conditions that benefit only one segment of the population would no longer be the primary rationale of social institutions, law, and policy. Rather, the rationale of social institutions, law, and policy would be to support the outcome of equality of well-being for all citizens.

Quality of life measures from this perspective are then not unidimensional and individualistic. They take into account the limitations of the perspectives on disability that see social and economic participation primarily as a product of individual ability and initiative rather than systemic condition and social organization.

In Practice

In practice, what we have seen with these various ways of perceiving, diagnosing, and treating disability, combined with the varying models of equality, are some identifiable legal, clinical, and service treatment modalities and differing standards and measures of quality of life. We can find evidence of these in our present policies and programs. They are reflected in entitlements based on the status of civil disability, in the charitable-privilege approach to disability, and in entitlement based on civil rights and equality.

Legal and clinical treatment of individuals, from the perspective of civil disability, guarantees or ensures protection and security for people with disabilities. The presence of disability in itself connotes a civil status that limits the rights of individuals. Treatment that includes institutionalization, the imposition of involuntary sterilization (or the differential prescription of drugs such as Depo-Provera®), prohibitions on immigration resulting from disability, the use of nonconsensual aversive therapies and drug regimes as therapeutic protocols, legal definitions of capacity and competency, and the refusal of medical treatment to newborns with disabilities are all examples of a civil status of disability. Such status maintains the need to protect society and the individual from the ill effects of disability. Quality of life can then justifiably be measured by the extent to which people are protected from harm to themselves and others. In such contexts, the measurement of self-determination as a standard of quality of life can be a parody of the principle of equality because people are confined to settings and lifestyles qualitatively more limited than those available for the general population.

There is a long history of providing care and treatment to people with disabilities as a charitable act. The charitable privilege that can be claimed is based on benevolence and compassion and on forms of paternalism. In this modality, people with disabilities generally trade rights for charity (Rioux, 1991). Involuntary treatment, imposition of *parens patriae,* denial of the right to own property, the structure of welfare programs (in which one trades employability for higher financial benefit), and segregated services (special education, sheltered workshops) have all been argued to be in the best interests of the individual. All of these are examples of care decided by third parties, in most cases professional gatekeepers, as being of benefit to the person with a disability.

In other words, we find reflected in clinical and service practice and law means of control exercised through medical decision-making and expert judgment with services provided through local authority and charity. The means of dealing with dependency is to provide compassionate care for those with disabilities under the direction of the experts in the field. Political obligation toward people with disabilities derives from the notion of "desert," or deserving, based on a presumption of intrinsic dependency and an assumption that others will have the knowledge to determine that person's best interests where there is any question. Again, where measures of quality of life do not question this context but accept it as a given, quality of life measurement has no place to go but to analyses of individual situations based on externally imposed criteria (measuring either subjective or objective factors).

An emerging modality is treatment and care based on entitlement to rights and equal outcome for people with disabilities. For example, in Canada, under the Canadian Charter of Rights and Freedoms, individuals are protected both before and under the law and are entitled to the equal protection and equal benefit of the law. A recent decision by the Supreme Court of Canada has suggested how extensively this is likely to be interpreted (*Andrews v. Law Society of British Columbia,* 1989). Although the legal decision did not concern an individual with a disability, it will have a significant effect because of the interpretation of the meaning of equality under the charter. The Supreme Court in this case extended the concept of equality beyond the formal notion that similarly situate should be similarly treated, and it recognized instead that "every difference in treatment between individuals under the law will not necessarily result in inequality and, as well, that identical treatment may frequently reproduce serious inequality." The court further held, "In fact, the interests of true equality may well require differentiation in treatment." If you understand equality to imply an even distribution of and access to justice, then the accommodation of differences is a substantial part of the essence of equality. The Court also held in that case that "distinctions based on personal characteristics attributed to an individual solely on the basis of association with a group will rarely escape the charge of discrimination, whereas those based on an individual's merits and capacities will rarely be so classed." If quality of life for people with disabilities were monitored according to this broad standard of equality, then the structural and systemic context of people with disabilities would come into view and the following would fall within the analysis of quality of life: the equitable access to social and economic opportunities that are open to citizens in general and the structural conditions that facilitate or inhibit access to those opportunities (including legal, financial, and service opportunities). In other words, quality of life would have to be measured according to the equitability of access and would have to question the legally and socially constructed barriers individuals face in access.

Conclusion

If we recognize how the inequality of people with disabilities has been constructed and has provided a basis for a social policy of exclusion, where do we go in quality of life research? Do we continue to confine the measurement of quality of life to individualistic criteria of the situation of those with disabilities? Or do we begin to recognize the inequalities inherent in our institutional structures, put the onus on the state to begin to develop policy based on principles that include supports for all people to participate and adjust our measures of quality of life accordingly?

Within a new framework for measuring quality of life, professional control of disability and the lives of people with disabilities will need to be re-examined so that people with disabilities themselves find their voices and dictate how they view the way they want to live their lives (Zola, 1994). This shift in measuring quality of life will involve redefining the so-called problem of disability as one of inequality rooted in the persisting social and economic structure rather than in the people with disabilities (Rioux & Crawford, 1994).

If we wish to work toward societies that are distinguished by a culture of justice and the public ownership of private disadvantage, we have to find a framework that takes into account and makes policy that includes all people, including those who do not fit conventional norms. This deconstruction of inequality will have to be addressed by concerted, coherent action.

Recognizing and tracing the social and legal construction of inequality is a step in moving toward a new framework and strategy for achieving social well-being. It permits the development of a conceptual model and indicators of quality of life that incorporate both structural and individual properties.

The recognition of quality of life as greater than simply the individualistic indicators inherent in the deficit model of disability and in equal treatment frameworks of equality places an accountability on the social, political, and economic structure to be organized in a manner that enables individuals to make appropriate life choices. Quality of life not only is a state for individuals to achieve but is inseparable from the underlying social and economic conditions without which individual and collective states of well-being cannot be achieved.

11

Measurement and Practice

Power Issues in Quality of Life,
Health Promotion, and Empowerment

Ronald Labonté

Quality of life, health promotion, and empowerment are different concepts claiming similar territory. This territory might be defined as posing and answering the question, What is it to be well? or as Raphael, Brown, Renwick, and Rootman (1994b) phrased it, "What is the good life?" When most people think about these questions, they probably use colloquial ideas such as happiness, contentment, a sense of meaning or purpose, control over important matters, and the like. Quality of life, health promotion, and empowerment are terms of primary interest to health and social service practitioners, the bureaucracies in which they work, and the research and academic disciplines that support them. Guba and Lincoln (1989) argued that all "disciplined inquiry," a term they use to encompass research, evaluation, and policy study, is purpose driven. Accepting that, our purposes in theorizing and researching quality of life, health promotion, and empowerment pertain to developing, implementing, and evaluating policies, programs, and professional practices that improve people's quality of life, health, and empowerment.

This process involves complex power relations between professionals and those with whom they work. This chapter will examine the concept of power and discuss some of its implications for concept development, research, and measurement and the "caring" professional practices informed by the three concepts in question.

Three Different Canvases
and a Few Common Brushstrokes

A striking feature in the literature on these three concepts is the degree to which they attempt to distinguish themselves from one another. Raphael et al. (1994b) claimed that quality of life is a determinant of health. The World Health Organization (WHO) (1984) defined health as a resource for everyday living, which renders it more a determinant of quality of life than the reverse. Similarly, Green and Kreuter (1991) claimed that health promotion has quality of life as its outcome. Schalock (1990a) argued that quality of life is enhanced by empowering persons to participate in decisions that affect their lives, identifying empowerment as a process integral to but distinct from quality of life. Writers such as Rappaport (1987) and Friedmann (1992) use empowerment as the outcome of many practices that others might claim as health promotion or quality of life. Those writing more exclusively in the health promotion field (e.g., Labonté, 1993; Wallerstein, 1992) either elide empowerment with health promotion or argue that empowerment is an important personal and social process that promotes health.

There may be good research reasons to keep some separation between these concepts. The approach that holds that "everything is connected to everything else" is not helpful for evaluation or theory building. In practice, however, the three terms overlap considerably and are often used interchangeably. They are different canvases on which discontented professionals and those with whom they work are painting their way free of rigidly reductionist theories and practices in the domains from which they arose. Quality of life emerged partly in response to patient-client challenges surrounding sophisticated but invasive medical treatments and patronizing approaches to the care of older adults or persons with disabilities (Raphael et al., 1994b). Subjective experiences of well-being began to supplement objective measures of disease or functional ability in decision making about treatment and service. Health promotion arose, in part, as a critique of the political conservatism and victim blaming inherent in biomedically defined and behaviorally individualistic health education programs (Labonté, 1986; Wallerstein & Bernstein, 1988). More broadly stated socioenvironmental models of health determination and health workers' practice were sub-sequently developed (e.g., Epp, 1986; Labonté, 1993; WHO, 1986). Health promotion became the process of enabling people to increase their control over and to improve their health, the prerequisites for which expanded to include peace, shelter, education, food, income, a stable ecosystem, sustain-able resources, social justice, and equity (WHO, 1986). Empowerment, despite more diverse roots in feminism, international development, educa-tion, social work, and mental health reform, generally summoned a stance against professional "others" defining the experience of the "self" in objec-tified terms. It emphasized a latent power-from-within (Starhawk, 1987) that we all possess and, in most uses, sought to locate that self-experience within larger social structures and belief systems (e.g., Freire, 1968; Freire & Macedo, 1987; Friedmann, 1992; Mondros & Wilson, 1994).

In brief, these concepts-as-canvases have painted health in different hues from pathology, sketched power's sociological meaning as "the ability to affect the actions or ideas of others despite resistance" (Weber, quoted in Olsen & Marger, 1993, p. 1) as merely one facet, and the "good life" as something far richer and more complex than a steady growth in the gross national product. They have expanded the frames in which health and social policies and professional practices might be analyzed and recast and so have stretched the canvas of future action. But there is a common heart uniting the artists who wield these new brushes, a latent or explicit concern with relations of power as they structure people's choices in their lives.

The Different Facets of Power

We see this concern with power in many of the definitions commonly encountered for these terms. Quality of life, as Schalock (1990a) tells us, increases as people are more capable (powerful) in making decisions that affect their lives. The model put forward by Renwick and Brown (this volume) has described quality of life as a "flexible and dynamic construct" in which "the individual evaluates . . . the importance or meaning of [new life] possibilities" (Raphael et al., 1994b, p. 33). But this evaluation is also subject to social influences in which power is central, for "humans have a remarkable ability to lower their aspirations and levels of dissatisfaction in the absence of any hope of realizing specific goals or attainments" (Campbell, Converse, & Rodgers, quoted in Raphael et al., 1994b, p. 26). The absence of hope presumably derives from a lack of power. Health promotion's concern with power is explicit in its notion of "control over" health's basic prerequisites, whereas power lies at the very root of empowerment.

Wallerstein (1992) provides a map of the relationship between empowerment and health that is instructive for persons working in quality of life and health promotion fields. Incorporating research using a variety of psychological and sociological constructs, she argued that certain objective social experiences (living in poverty, being low in hierarchy, having little or no decision-making authority, lacking material resources, lacking social support) coexist and interact with certain psychological or subjective experiences (learned helplessness, external locus of control, chronic stress). These experiences generalize to a more pervasive state of powerlessness and a lack of control over one's destiny, which in turn increase the risk of disease. Several other empowerment and health researchers and practitioners have constructed similar models and arguments (e.g., Eng & Parker, 1994; Evans & Stoddart, 1990; Israel, Checkoway, Schulz, & Zimmerman, 1994; Labonté, 1993). Empowerment reverses these relations, exhibiting changes at intrapersonal and interpersonal levels as well as changes in sociopolitical practices (community empowerment).

Following from Wallerstein's (1992) model, we might argue that quality of life and health (the root of health promotion) similarly manifest intrapersonal, interpersonal, and sociopolitical levels of power. It is at this point that some explicit analysis of social power relations needs to enter the research and practice discourses on quality of life and health promotion, which tend to emphasize intra- and interpersonal levels of empowerment over the sociopolitical level (Labonté, 1993).

This is not the same as saying that empowerment is, or should be, primarily concerned with people gaining power over others, an argument frequently encountered in the social work-community development literature. For example, in their study of community organizations, Mondros and Wilson (1994) argued that empowerment is a psychological state, "a sense of competence, control and entitlement—that allows one to pursue concrete activities aimed at becoming powerful" (p. 5). This resonates with quality of life and health promotion definitions cited earlier. But being powerful, they went on to argue, is "measured by the extent to which *another's* [italics added] activities conform to one's preferences" (p. 5). They are not alone in this argument, which tends to eschew a self-empowerment conceptualization as a false consciousness veiling objective forms of social oppression (Kilian, 1988) or, at best, a necessary step in the more important work of collective actions by the less powerful to have more powerful others heed their preferences.

Yet many powerless persons are more concerned with making their lives rather than with making history, as Minkler (1990) expressed in her study of poor senior roomers in San Francisco's Tenderloin district. From the practitioner's vantage point, the empowerment concern (for which one could easily substitute the quality of life or health promotion concern) becomes one of nurturing a trusting and mentoring relationship (Lord, 1992).

The significant qualities of the professional in this relationship are described as being a good listener, an equal, a guide, and a person who really cares (Lord & Farlow, 1990). One's quality of life is improved to the extent that mutuality and reciprocity are developed in the professional-client relationship and not necessarily in the client becoming dominant within it.

Feminist theories and experiences in consciousness-raising groups similarly challenged the notion that the only real power one has is that which is exercised over others. Kuyek (Kuyek & Labonté, 1994), a feminist community organizer, recounts an experience working with low-income women in a support group:

> Most women didn't want to discuss power. They said they didn't want to become more powerful. Power, to them, was so associated with dominance over others—the way they experienced it—that they didn't want any part of it. This way of viewing power, that it is only dominance or exploitation or "capricious authority," helps to keep many people powerless. (p. 22)

Other health promotion and empowerment conceptualizers have embraced this feminist recasting of power, arguing that psychological empowerment should be the end rather than the means of objective power struggles (Bernstein et al., 1994; Israel et al., 1994). Privileging objective over subjective power experiences defines power as *zero sum,* reifying it as a finite thing over which powerful and powerless groups conflict to possess (Boucher, 1992). Zero-sum models social relations of power such that for A to exercise X power over B, B must lack the equivalent amount of power. The sum of A's and B's power is zero. The counter position is that empowerment is nonzero-sum, "emphasiz[ing] participation, caring, sharing, responsibility to others, and [which] conceives of power as an expanding commodity" (Israel et al., 1994, p. 154). Nonzero-sum models of power emphasize their nonmaterial, communicative bases. Because nonzero-sum models lack a material base, their expansion is limitless. It is some variation on this construct of empowerment that one encounters most frequently in the quality of life and health promotion literatures.

Both claims are useful, presenting two coexisting facets of power (Pitkin cited in Wartenberg, 1990). Power in both cases ceases to be a thing. It exists only in, and expresses an aspect of, social relations. Starhawk (1987), a feminist writer, expanded the number of power's different faces to include *power-with,* the collective side of power from within. Power-with describes social practices in which the power (of some) over (others), an unavoidable characteristic of our social systems, is used to increase people's experiences of power from within, rather than to dominate or exploit them (Kuyek & Labonté, 1994). This conceptualization of power allows practitioners and researchers to approach quality of life, health promotion, and empowerment as social relations that simultaneously embody both zero-sum and nonzero-sum forms of power (see Table 11.1).

An empowered and healthy quality of life simultaneously challenges the zero-sum power-over practices of others (otherwise are we only accommodating ourselves to oppressive situations?) from an ethic of (a moral commitment to) nonzero-sum relations with others.

The remainder of this chapter examines how power-over relations inhere in our conceptualization, research, and practices related to quality of life, health promotion, and empowerment and discusses some of the steps that can be taken to transform them.

Power Issues in Conceptualization and Measurement

The first point to be made is that these concepts concern a process rather than an outcome, at least in the sense that an outcome is an objectively demonstrated thing. There is no objective state of quality of life, health, or empowerment. These concepts embody subjective evaluations shaped, in part, by social and cultural forces. Epistemologically, concepts such as quality of life, health, and empowerment are double hermeneutics, or interpretations (Sayer, 1984). A single hermeneutic occurs when what is named and studied exists in the realm of largely material or nonsocial phenomena, such as serum cholesterol. The choice and framing of the research question and the discussion of findings remain social (interpretive) acts, but the substance named *cholesterol* remains the same regardless of how it is labeled, studied, or measured. The same is not the case for *quality of life, health,* or *empowerment,* which are terms that become meaningful only in their particular usages. Thus, even when quality of life or empowerment surveys are initially constructed from interviews and when interviewees are actively engaged in naming the items of importance, there are problems with generalizing the items to other groups and with not recognizing that items of importance, even for those interviewed, change with time. Unless those persons initially interviewed are also involved in interpretation of the survey findings, the shifting importance or meanings people give to them will not be represented.

TABLE 11.1 Nonzero-Sum and Zero-Sum Forms of Power

Nonzero-sum power-from-within or power-with

  Respect for individuals and their autonomy

  Generosity to others

  Service and responsibility to others

  Experience of commonality-community ("sharing and caring")

Zero-sum power-over

  Control over (possession of) income, wealth, material resources, land, goods

  Control over capital or employment opportunities

  Control over decision making (authority)

  Control over ideology reproduction (dominant beliefs, values) via media, school,
    other forms of socialization

  Social status (privilege)

These epistemological concerns become power issues in a number of ways. The discussion that follows, though built primarily from experiences in the health promotion area, should be read as cautions by those eager to treat quality of life as some objectively discernible fact, particularly when that fact is used evaluatively to determine the usefulness of government programs and resources.

Power-over, in research practice, exists first in how some claims on knowledge are accepted as legitimate or scientific and others dismissed as special interest or opinion (Labonté & Roberston, in press; Rabinow, 1984). Usually, such claims to science are those built on positivist methodologies that rely on making causal statements between discrete variables in which the messiness of social context (historical and interpretive) is controlled for using statistical techniques. The concern is not with positivist methodology (as one approach to understanding) as much as with its underlying claim that its research can be value free and factual, generating causal laws that can (or should) be generalizable for all people in all situations at all times. The notion of science's detached objectivity tends to hide, rather than to reveal, practices of power-over (Tesh, 1988). It also risks reboxing practitioners within the narrow behavioral or disease-based approaches against which quality of life, health promotion, and empowerment critically positioned themselves. There is much call for, though little agreement on, indicators for positive health. Yet health, as a double hermeneutic whose contingent meanings are "free to vary across divergent contexts" (Gergen, 1986, p. 140), defies such indication, and the positivist imperative to define it in measurable terms tends to reduce health to disease prevention or, at best, the prevention of disease-related health behaviors (e.g., Evans & Stoddart, 1990; O'Donnell, 1986).

The noncontingent epistemology of positivism reinforces rather than transforms the technical rationality of the state (Adorno, 1976; White, 1988). This rationality holds that program or policy goals, objectives, and implementation strategies should be set at a given point in time (usually in annual cycles), administered by experts or authorities residing within the state structure, and accounted for strictly in terms of their stated objectives. It was this rigid rationality that was originally challenged by quality of life, health promotion, and empowerment concepts. It becomes disempowering to the extent that it "colonizes" the meanings people make of their "life-world" experiences (Habermas, 1984). Health workers on a chronic disease prevention program in a poor neighborhood became discouraged that local leaders were more concerned with poverty, unemployment, violence, racism, and housing (Shea, Basch, Lantigua, & Wechsler, 1992). Their response was to recommend a social marketing and community education strategy to convince these leaders that cancer and heart disease were objectively the most important problems. They wanted heart health higher on the community's agenda; there was no talk of placing the community's concerns higher on the health department's agenda. Indeed, a growing evaluation literature indicates how community concerns with issues such as racism and poor housing, which certainly bear on quality of life, have been derailed by epidemiological risk factor surveys that "prove" that heart disease and smoking are "objectively" the major health problems (Goodman, Steckler, Hoover, & Schwartz, 1993).

How Can the Power-Over of Our Conceptualizations and Measures Be Transformed?

We might answer this question recognizing the contingent usefulness of noncontingent measures. There remains a practical need for seeking more generalizable quality of life, health promotion, or empowerment measures— that is, measures that might be applied to more than one set of contexts. The radical relativism that emphasizes the nonreducible uniqueness of each person's experience of quality of life (or health or empowerment) does not account for the possibility that one's experience reflects dominant and disempowering ideologies nor does it equip groups with useful insights about how to challenge social practices of power-over. This practical need for new measures was recognized in the social indicators movement of the 1970s and 1980s, whose architects believed that narrow economic growth indicators were failing to capture more important human development or quality of life concerns. But from the earlier argument, this task should be undertaken only with an explicit awareness of the impossibility of succeeding in its accomplishment. Or as Morgan (1991) commented on positivism's claim to objectivity in research, "[science] can only claim any kind of objectivity by assuming otherwise" (p. 224). The difference lies in approaching the notion of generalizability as a practical (practice-based) need rather than as a means of determining what is "real." It also lies in acknowledging that practice-based needs are purpose driven: We are seeking some generalizable measures for a reason. In the case of social indicators, it was to challenge a narrow economic determinism. In the case of quality of life, the reasons could relate to political struggles over program resources, reviews of professional practice, establishment of better services, and so on. The same applies to health promotion and empowerment.

Rather than debate the generalizability of the measures, then, we need to debate the purposes for which the generalizability is thought useful or necessary. We also need to approach their use as taking on meaning only in their interpretation and not in their abstract statistical representation. For example, two recent articles describe quantitative measures of empowerment and community competence, both of which have some usefulness for researchers and practitioners interested in the sociopolitical levels of quality of life (Eng & Parker, 1994; Israel et al., 1994). Both of the measures identified their usefulness in assessment and evaluation. But neither of the articles discussing these measures claimed that the community empowerment maps created by their measurement tools actually represent some unique and universal characteristic called "community empowerment." Instead, the authors emphasized that without a qualitative dialogue, their quantitative measures would lack any meaning or relevance to the groups engaged in the empowerment project.

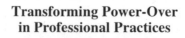

Transforming Power-Over in Professional Practices

So far, this chapter has focused primarily on power issues in the conceptualization, research, and measurement of quality of life, health promotion, and empowerment. It has described an empowering professional practice as one that mentors, cares, and listens. This sounds simple but it is often difficult to achieve. Perhaps the most pervasive power-over in professional practice inheres in the notion of professionalism itself and its presumption of specialized knowledge and authority (Freidson, 1972; McKnight, 1987). Most professionals are trained to give advice. Often this advice is desired and perceived as useful by the client-community. But often, it comes in the form of judgment (assessment) in which the professional fails to hear the client except through the rigid frames of his or her discipline expertise, an expertise enhanced by the use of objective assessment criteria (Kuyek & Labonté, 1994). This is still commonly encountered in the public-community health areas that provide many of the programs and services thought to enhance people's quality of life. Community nutritionists recently examined the means by which they had been taught to assess prenatal clients (see Table 11.2). They considered this a disempowering assessment. It presents an overwhelming burden of difficulties, which are actually professional power-over judgments. "No apparent substance abuse" implies that Marian could still be a substance abuser; she's simply clever enough to hide it.

Marian as a person is completely absent. There is no evidence of her own capacity or power, no reflexivity indicating whether the way the professional assesses Marian resembles the way Marian sees herself. In a second assessment (see Table 11.3), a completely different way of viewing Marian emerges. Here we see her abilities, many more opportunities for actual change, and the professional's role in helping that change.

The specialized jargon that accompanies professionalism also frequently serves a hegemonizing power-over in the professional-client relationship. Scambler (1987) cites an interesting example of the veiled power relations the argot of technical rationality entails. Transcripts of a consultation between a pregnant woman and her physician showed that the latter began his discussions in lay terms. When the former questioned his advice, however, he immediately switched to a technical-rational discourse that intimidated the woman and brought her into compliance with the physician's wishes without actually ordering her to do so. Even more intriguing is the possibility that the physician was also unaware of the veiled power he was exercising.

In subtle ways, professional-client relations are structured by such power-over domains as social status, authority, and influence. Professionals' education or training, higher incomes, and types of jobs often infer a higher social status. The positions professionals occupy in institutions often give them some decision-making authority over resources. Their social status and authority, in turn, can give them considerable power to influence or persuade, setting different political agendas around quality of life, health promotion, or empowerment. This status and authority can be used to dominate; it can also be used to transform. A few years ago, a group of poor women complained of conditions in a state-run rooming house. The group asked a public health nurse to represent their complaints to the authorities because of the legitimacy of her expert voice. Afterward, the nurse supported these women

TABLE 11.2 Judgmental Assessment

Marian

    Low-income, single mother

    Inadequate protein, calcium, and overall caloric intake

    One-bedroom basement apartment

    First child, low birth weight

    Insufficient weight gain

    Fears labor and delivery

    Does not speak or read English well

    No apparent substance abuse

to become their own advocates, while she served as mentor. She used her professional influence to persuade these women to act on their own when they were ready to do so. That is, an improved quality of life for these women was partially bound up in their relations with this health professional and her ability to use her professional power-over transformatively.

    Power or capacity also shifts from situation to situation. If power is an important element in quality of life, as has been argued, it is neither static nor absolute. A person might have decision-making authority in one situation but not in another. He may be a parent at home and a frontline worker at the office. She may be somebody's client coping with physical disabilities on Tuesdays and Thursdays but an esteemed leader in her church's social justice

TABLE 11.3 Empowering Assessment

Poor appetite due to stress and isolation; child's father is a political prisoner in Guatemala

Enjoys preparing traditional vegetable soups, bean dishes, and corn bread; would like more milk and meat but finds these too expensive

Healthy 3-year-old daughter born with low birth weight, no complications

Worried about income and child care when child comes; refugee status claim still pending

Has cousins locally who can help financially but not enough

Quilts and paints as hobbies; would like to sell her work

Spanish literacy, schoolteacher in Guatemala; concerned that poor English skills will be interpreted as stupidity

Small, tidy apartment

Wants refrigerator; afraid to ask landlord because she can't afford to be evicted committee on Fridays and Sundays. Recognizing this elasticity of power can remind professionals caring for those with specific problems (e.g., disabilities, physical illness, emotional distress) or in specific social disadvantages (e.g., poverty, unemployment) not to generalize this relative powerlessness to all facets of that person's life.

As with the definition of health promotion, there is also often an assumption that control over all aspects of one's life equates with a better quality of life. Yet there may be instances when the professional's or researcher's positive valuing of control over certain aspects of one's life may be experienced by clients-communities as disempowering. The significance of the experience of empowerment can be grasped only through interpretations of that experience that include the people (the clients-subjects) themselves.

Related to the fluidity of power experiences are the intentional efforts professionals can make to value individuals' and groups' differing capacities. In a group project involving immigrant and refugee Latin American women and their families, social work and health professionals who established the group sought to identify the different skills that individual members brought to the collective and its activities. Women who were skilled in writing prepared the grants applications and taught other interested women in the process. Women who were skilled in cooking took a leadership role in the collective kitchen and passed skills on to other interested women. The same process unfolded for women skilled in budgeting or in sewing. In the outside world, budgeting and grant-writing skills may be highly valued, and those who have them may be given more social status, experience more power, and be more satisfied with their quality of life. But in this particular collective, influenced by feminist principles, budgeting and grant writing became merely sets of social skills no more or less important than those involved in cooking, menu planning, or sewing. In other words, through their interaction with individuals and groups, professionals can shift the very frames of social status or authority, the socially dominant ways of valuing people, that constitute the backdrop against which individuals perceive or assess their own quality of life.

Of course, there are still real social practices of power-over that, although subverted through processes such as the one described, constrain the ability of persons to experience a good life. Health and social service professionals are often in a position to assist persons in organizing to challenge such practices. A few years ago, plans to implement welfare reforms in a Canadian province were stalled due to their costs, sparking the creation of a massive coalition of welfare advocates, organizations, professionals, church, and labor groups (Labonté, 1994). A local community health center became involved in the lobbying process. The center served a poorer neighborhood.

Many of the single mothers went to the center for medical care precisely because of the respectful, caring, and competent services provided by the primary care teams. But teams knew that these women's health problems (their quality of life or lack of it) were less rooted in their bodies, and even in their health behaviors, than in the structured inadequacies of the welfare system and the isolation of poverty it often created. These teams, with the center's health educator, created small groups on health exploration for these women that offered a supportive learning experience, breaking through some of the learned helplessness often engendered by poverty (Seligman, 1975). Such groups, Brazilian educator Paulo Freire (1968) argued, are important places where people can surface and question the dominant assumptions by which they live their lives, assumptions that often create a surplus power-lessness (Lerner, 1986) in which objective power-over practices are internalized as normal and unchangeable. The center's health promoter also helped some of the women organize a community action group, which on its own and in coalitions lobbied for reform. As they got stronger, the health promoter was able to reduce the initial support and mentoring role she had played in the group. The primary care teams also took case stories of these women's lives. These stories wove a tapestry with the studies collected by the health administrators in a powerful policy statement advocated by the board. Center staff, through their professional associations, lobbied senior government bodies, issued press releases, and joined with coalitions advocating reform, helping to legitimate the claims made by less powerful groups. An interesting aside to this story, pertinent to quality of life, is that for a brief period of time, much of the internal squabbling that often characterizes agencies and institutions disappeared in a focused endeavor, in which every staff person and citizen volunteer could see his or her role and its relation to other roles (Labonté, 1994).

Conclusion

Research is a practice that claims to enhance knowledge and understanding. Evaluation is a practice that claims to examine whether people's actions lead them toward what they value. The helping professions are practices that claim to improve people's quality of life, health, and empowerment. This chapter has argued that these relations are all structured, in part, by power. Moreover, the concepts of quality of life, health promotion, and empowerment all share a concern with the transformation of social power relations that are inimical to being well or living the good life.

All of these relations begin with the researcher, evaluator, and practitioner possessing more of at least some types of power than the client-community. Transforming this power-over to power-with does not mean negating the specialized knowledge or skills possessed by researchers and practitioners. It does require a stance on their part in which their knowledge and skills are seen as contributing to rather than determining the best decisions that might be reached by the client-community in relation with the researcher-practitioner. The essence of reaching these best decisions resides in a dialogue for shared meaning in which life-world (lay, subjective, traditional) knowledge is seen as complementary with, rather than subordinate to, "technical-rational" (professional, objective, scientific) knowledge.

There is one basic axiom in this sharing relationship and its attempt to transform structured forms of power-over to collective forms of power-with. It is the intention or purpose with which people, in this case researchers and professionals, act (Wartenberg, 1990). What allows a researcher's or caring professional's actions to be transformative (and in being transformative, to enhance health, empowerment, and quality of life) is the individual professional's commitment to create more equity in the relationship by nurturing more power-from-within in those with whom they work. This is, however, a difficult thing for human beings to accustom themselves to; there is a temptation for the dominant agent to seek to keep the subordinate agent from growing and developing in a way that transcends the initial power inequalities (Wartenberg, 1990).

For those of us in the caring professions, whether at the coal face of direct service or the supportive ranks of research and evaluation, the challenge of this transformative ethic to overcome the temptation of retaining power-over is perhaps best summed up in the evocative words of Lilla Watson, an aboriginal community organizer: "If you come here to help me, you are wasting your time. But if you come here because your liberation is bound up in mine, let us begin" (quoted in Wadsworth, 1991, p. 11).

12

Defining Quality of Life

Eleven Debates Concerning
Its Measurement

Dennis Raphael

It is not surprising that the idea of quality of life has spawned a multitude of conceptual models and measurement approaches in diverse disciplines such as gerontology, health promotion, medicine, psychology, rehabilitation, sociology, and social welfare (Parmenter, 1994; Raphael, Brown, Renwick, & Rootman, 1994b). What is surprising, however, is the limited effect that current debates concerning the nature of inquiry have had on the development of measurement approaches and the development of applications based on these approaches. These debates on the nature of inquiry are essentially debates on the nature of reality and have important implications for the conduct of quality of life research and the health promotion and rehabilitation applications arising from such research. Such implications are especially important when issues of disability or illness, marginalization, or unequal power relations are present. In this chapter, I examine the implications for quality of life measurement of 11 current debates on the nature of inquiry. Table 12.1 presents these debates.

TABLE 12.1 Eleven Debates Concerning Measuring Quality of Life

Debate 1	Sociological versus psychological perspectives
Debate 2	Positivist, idealist, and realist approaches
Debate 3	Naturalistic versus positivist methodologies
Debate 4	Quantitative versus qualitative methods
Debate 5	Values-based versus values-free approaches
Debate 6	Social policy versus basic research orientations
Debate 7	System versus individual data collections
Debate 8	Objective versus subjective measurements
Debate 9	Self-reports versus reports by others
Debate 10	Traditional versus participatory approaches
Debate 11	Critical approaches

These debates provide an 11-point framework for researchers and others to use for deciding on, and later describing, their quality of life measurement approach. The framework should also prove useful for interpreting the existing literature on quality of life because, in many cases, researchers do not explicitly state the assumptions underlying their measurement approaches.

The Eleven Debates: Some Signposts

My WordPerfect® 5.1 thesaurus provides the following synonyms for debate: *argument, controversy, disputation, contest, dialectic, discussion, match,* and *polemic.* None of these terms implies finality but, rather, ambiguity and uncertainty. The issues to be presented, in addition to not being resolvable, must by necessity be analyzed as simple dichotomies, even though all debates ultimately involve gradients of gray between black and white polarities. Even with such simplifications, illustrations from the quality of life literature clearly demonstrate the essence of these debates.

Each of the 11 debates exists within its own plane of discourse. I have placed the debates in the order in which I usually consider them, though others may disagree. At the highest levels, the nature of social reality and the appropriate means of investigating it are considered. At intermediate levels, debates concern use of either quantitative or qualitative approaches to methods and instrumentation. At the lowest levels, issues arise concerning objective versus subjective measures, self-report versus reports from others, and the methods by which the research is conceived and data are gathered and then applied. Although each level of debate is related to higher and lower levels, positions do not totally map across planes. Examples from existing quality of life conceptualizations will illustrate the implications of each debate.

DEBATE 1: SOCIOLOGICAL VERSUS PSYCHOLOGICAL PERSPECTIVES

For the sociologically inclined (and one need not be a sociologist to share this view), reality is ultimately social: "The sociological perspective enables us to look beyond individual psychology and unique events to the predictable broad patterns and regular occurrences of social life that influence individual destinies" (Wilson, 1983, p. ix). For the sociologist, the focus of inquiry is the individual in relations with others. The social milieu does not provide the context for understanding reality; it is the reality. The sociologist may study individual perceptions and behaviors but is not bound to do so.

For the psychologically inclined (and again, one need not be a psychologist to share this view), reality is ultimately individual: "Psychology is the scientific study of behavior and mental processes and how they are affected by an organism's physical state, mental state, and external environment" (Wade & Travis, 1990, p. 7). In this view, the focus of inquiry is the individual. The social milieu may provide a context for understanding individual behavior, but the psychologist is not required to include the social milieu in the inquiry.

The implications of this divergence for quality of life research are broad. Sociologically oriented quality of life researchers will usually choose to focus on the structure and content of societies, communities, and groups. The data of interest may include system-level indicators (e.g., structure of the health care system, number of senior centers per 100,000 seniors, percentage of individuals with disabilities employed, and number of public facilities with wheelchair access) or aggregated individual data (e.g., contacts with nurses and doctors, income and wealth, and contacts with friends and neighbors).

The psychologically oriented researcher will choose to focus on the structure and content of individual's well-being, mental health, personal adjustment, future time perspective, physical functioning, or any of a welter of other individual-based characteristics. Data collected may be objective (e.g., professionals' reports of mobility, quality of diet, number of activities, and number of social contacts) or subjective (individuals' satisfaction with mobility, diet, daily activities, or social contacts). Just as sociologically oriented researchers may choose to study individuals' perceptions of these societal and environmental factors, psychologists may choose to study environmental determinants of quality of life. In both of these cases of extradisciplinary inquiry, measures may be either objective or subjective. The main distinction remains: Within the sociologically oriented approach, the one certainty is focus on societal and group structures, whereas within the psychological approach, the one certainty is focus on the individual.

A few examples will illustrate these differing approaches. Health-related quality of life is usually seen as an individual (or psychological) construct. "Basically, quality of life is recognized as a concept representing individual responses to the physical, mental, and social effects of illness on daily living that influence the extent to which personal satisfaction with life circumstances can be achieved" (Bowling, 1991, p. 9). Besides dominating health-related quality of life research, the psychological approach is especially common in the gerontological (Birren, Lubben, Rowe, & Deutchman, 1991), medical (Spilker, 1990), rehabilitation (Livneh, 1988), and nursing literatures (Ferrans & Powers, 1992).

In contrast, some quality of life work focuses on the individual in relation with society. The volume *The Quality of Urban Life* (Frick, 1986) considers issues of measuring the quality of urban life, social networks within neighborhoods, physical aspects of urban environments, and the effect of these factors on psychological functioning and mental health. Lindstrom's (1994) work on the quality of life of children considers a range of important issues that move well beyond an individual perspective identifying issues of resource allocation and economic equity. Recent quality of life conceptualizations in the developmental disabilities area are also increasingly likely to be sociologically oriented: "Quality of life is the outcome of individuals meeting basic needs and fulfilling basic responsibilities in community settings (family, recreational, school, and work)" (Schalock, 1990c, p. x). Still, even when societal structures are included in particular models of quality of life, these structures are not necessarily the focus of inquiry. Most actual quality of life measurement efforts, including those from the developmental disabilities area, have a strong individual focus (Raphael et al., 1994b).

The focus that one chooses to emphasize when measuring quality of life will determine the parameters of the specific quality of life inquiry. When construed as an individual-level issue, potential assessments and subsequent interventions related to quality of life will be individually based, with the potential for ignoring important group, community, or society dynamics. Similarly, sole reliance on sociological analyses may lose the individual and ignore specific issues and needs that may occur among a study group.

DEBATE 2: POSITIVIST, IDEALIST,
AND REALIST APPROACHES

The second debate concerns what Wilson (1983) terms *world pictures* or *metatheories*. Wilson, a sociologist, presents no fewer than seven approaches to social theory categorized into three metatheories: positivism, idealism, and realism. Whereas the specific social theories Wilson examines are from the sociological tradition (e.g., exchange theory, structural sociology, functional analysis, and others), the mapping of the three metatheories are remarkably consistent with current thinking in psychological, educational, health, and disability research.

Positivist Approaches

Positivist approaches are well known and dominate quality of life research. Put simply, the positivist viewpoint has four assumptions (Wilson, 1983). First, there are no fundamental differences between natural and social science inquiry. The methods of natural science, such as hypothesis testing, operationalizing of concepts, empirical observations, and the carrying out of experiments and quasi-experiments are the preferred means of exploring reality. Second, the purpose of inquiry is to develop general principles and laws to explain social events and individual behavior. This assumption is an extension of the natural science approach. Third, social reality will be understood through the development of concepts based on what is observable and measurable; that is, there is a basic belief in empirical observation and data collection. The fourth assumption is that there is a distinction between facts and values, that scientific activity is value free.

Idealist Approaches

Idealist or interpretive approaches reject the assumption that social reality mirrors natural reality. Flowing from the sociological traditions of Max Weber, George Mead, and others, social reality is ultimately understood through the meanings that individuals place on events and objects. In additional, in contrast to the positivist model, the individual is seen as an active creator of the social world. Society results from the actions of individuals within social structures. Because social acts result from the intentions of individuals, understanding social reality is ultimately an attempt to understand the meanings that individuals place on their dealings within the world.

Realist Approaches

The realist approach is less frequently considered but differs in many ways from both positivist and idealist approaches. Similar to positivists, realists believe that there are objects and events that exist in the world independent of their meanings created by individuals. Also similar to idealists, realists believe that human beings are capable of creating and modifying the realities within which they are embedded. The unique defining characteristic of social realists is their quest to identify the societal mechanisms by which social behavior is regulated. Unlike positivists who create models and theories based on observables, the realists use models to serve as a means of understanding as well as investigating society and behavior. The realist search is for the underlying mechanisms that determine social realities.

The positivist focuses inquiry on the observable to create generalizable concepts and laws. Emphasis is on the creation of concepts and operationalizing the means of measuring these concepts (Bryman, 1988). Observations lead to generalizations and laws that are linear, with readily identifiable causes and effects. The positivist approach so dominates quality of life research across all areas that its assumptions are frequently not even recognized by those working in the quality of life field.

In contrast, the realist uses observations to support theoretical concepts that explain underlying mechanisms existing within a society. The most obvious example of the realistic approach in sociology is Marxist analysis, which examines the effects of the means of economic production on individual consciousness and considers social reality as reflecting the ongoing struggle between social classes. In psychology, a realist example is the grand structural model of psychoanalysis and associated interpretations of social and individual phenomena within the psychoanalytical framework.

As an illustration, in the quality of life area, positivists would observe that powerlessness is related to quality of life. From this observation, an empirical generalization would be generated predicting that quality of life will be enhanced when greater control is available. A theory might be developed that would expand this specific observation into a proposition for understanding aspects of the quality of life of a variety of marginalized individuals, such as the poor, those with disabilities, or those with illness.

The realist, however, would set his or her sights on trying to understand the societal or personal mechanisms responsible for the development of, perpetuation of, and perhaps even justification for the marginalization $\rightarrow$ powerlessness $\rightarrow$ poor quality of life relationship. These analyses might be particularly appropriate for understanding the especially strong variation in financial income (and also quality of life) between the richest and poorest in North America or the differing approaches in providing transportation access between Scandinavia and North America for those with disabilities, for example. Any discussion of the quality of life of extremely marginalized populations, such as persons with acquired immunodeficiency syndrome, would need to have a strong realist sense of the mechanisms (societal and personal) by which stigma operates within a society. Wolfensberger's (1972) analysis of the concept of deviancy throughout history is a particularly interesting analysis of a realist perspective. Simmons (1982) analyzed the treatment of persons with developmental disabilities in Canada and England from a similar perspective. Woodill (1992, 1994) has analyzed the role that medical and social science practice has played in marginalizing persons with disabilities.

Idealists study phenomena as primarily social constructions heavily influenced by specific historical times and places. The focus of inquiry is on meanings, and these meanings can be found in government documents, individual perspectives, and observations of individual behaviors (Wilson, 1983). Wolfensberger's (1972) analysis of deviancy also has a strong idealist tinge, and recent work producing life history narratives of persons with disabilities (Martinez, 1990; Ward, 1990) shows aspects of an idealist perspective. Generally, idealist work emphasizes that those things that positivists and realists assume to be "out there in the real world" are actually social constructions based on individual and societal interpretations. Relatively little published research has investigated the potential value of idealism for studying quality of life.

The positivist-idealist-realist debate rarely occurs in quality of life inquiry. As noted, recent work in the disabilities area (see Simmons, 1982; Woodill, 1994) shows a strong realist perspective as well as a critical approach. Unlike the critical approach (discussion to follow), the realist as well as the positivist and idealist viewpoints are not necessarily emancipating but usually focus on understanding and analysis.

DEBATE 3: NATURALISTIC
VERSUS POSITIVIST METHODOLOGIES

Existing at a somewhat more concrete level, an increasingly prominent debate concerns the naturalistic (sharing some similarity with idealism) versus positivist paradigms (as just described). As outlined by Lincoln and Guba (1985), the debate concerns five general axioms: the nature of reality, the relationship of knower to the known, the possibility of generalization, the possibility of causal linkages, and the role of values. The naturalistic and positivist paradigms have different assumptions concerning these axioms and each has implications for conducting research. I like to consider this debate as existing at the level of methodology rather than methods; the differing assumptions of these paradigms are especially relevant to the conduct of quality of life measurements.

*Contrasting the Positivist
and Naturalist Approaches*

More specifically, consider the implications of adopting the positivist approach to reality. According to Lincoln and Guba (1985), the positivist stance (and most quality of life conceptualizations appear to conform to this approach) would see quality of life as existing within the world and capable of being defined, operationalized, and measured. The quality of life researcher would set himself or herself apart from the research subject and need not enter into any interaction beyond that of data collection. The research would provide time- and context-free generalizations (nomothetic statements) concerning quality of life and its determinants. The predictors of quality of life would be identified as temporally precedent causes producing predictable effects. Finally, quality of life research would be value free, with the researcher collecting "facts" and hesitantly providing interpretations and value judgments based on collection of these data.

The naturalistic approach would see reality as multiple, constructed, and holistic. To discover these realities, the researcher and subject would need to be interactive, and the data obtained would result from this close interaction. Only time- and context-bound working hypotheses (idiographic statements) would be possible because the existence of common realities across time would be questioned. Because all entities are seen as in a state of mutual simultaneous shaping, demarcation of causes and effects is impossible. The view that inquiry is value free is dismissed as naive; values are made explicit throughout the research endeavor.

Most quality of life research—psychological or sociological, individual or system oriented—has a strong positivist emphasis. This emphasis is seen across all areas of quality of life inquiry. Recent work in the disabilities and aging areas has seen some application of the naturalistic paradigm with emphasis on narratives and personal stories. The recent Schalock (1990a) and Goode (1994a) volumes on quality of life of persons with disabilities provide examples of this emphasis, and Woodill (1992) provides a critical analysis of the naturalistic and positivist paradigms and their implications for work in the disabilities areas.

The distinguishing characteristics of the naturalistic paradigm are the integration of the social construction assumptions of idealism, a distrust of the natural science inquiry-related assumptions of the positivistic viewpoint, and a rejection of the hypothesis-testing research procedures associated with traditional research. The distrust of universal laws and theories said to be common across time and place also leads to an emphasis on emergent research design. The emphasis on emergent design sees its realization in qualitative research methods.

DEBATE 4: QUANTITATIVE VERSUS QUALITATIVE METHODS

The quantitative versus qualitative debate takes place closer to the actual methods used to conduct research than the previous debates. The linkages between this debate and the preceding debates are obvious, with strong associations existing among the idealist, naturalistic, and qualitative positions and between the positivist and quantitative approaches. At this level, the determining issues are ones of hypothesis testing, statistical generalizability, and the potential usefulness of the inquiry for evaluating government and agency policies and programs.

Quantitative Approaches

It is generally accepted that the positivist paradigm of quantitatively oriented inquiry is useful for describing operationally defined aspects of individuals and their environments (Kerlinger, 1986). These methods include questionnaires, surveys, and experiments with the distinguishing characteristic being the use of operationally defined concepts with associated numerical measurements. They offer much to commend them, particularly the requirement of acceptable evidence of reliability and associations with commonly agreed-on measures of interest, their ease of use, the facility with which data can be manipulated, and the power of well-accepted psychometric scripts.

Five assumptions lead to use of these instruments (Argyris, Putnam, & Smith, 1987). These assumptions are (a) agreement that reality exists "out there" and can be measured by observers using a common yardstick, (b) measures developed and applied have equal meaning and appropriateness for most subjects, (c) the responses elicited are accurate and truthful, (d) the commonalities among subjects are more important than their differences, and (e) the focus of inquiry has been well delineated before carrying out the actual research.

Qualitative Approaches

The qualitative approach questions all of these assumptions. Qualitative approaches usually eschew the use of numbers and, rather than relying on reliability and validity coefficients to provide credence to findings, rely on "thick description" (Lincoln & Guba, 1985). Thick description is essentially the demonstration of consistent patterns of occurrences arising through multiple sources of data. These approaches allow for the identification and documentation of unique life circumstances of individuals. Open-ended approaches allow for the uniqueness of cases to emerge. Importantly, open-ended approaches allow for the communication of life's successes and failures, an especially important aspect of inquiry when the study of marginalized populations is undertaken. The methods included within the qualitative basket include participant observation, depth interviewing, document analysis, focus groups, and personal narratives or life histories.

The qualitative approach has weaknesses as well. These occur primarily in communicating generalizable findings from a sample to a population and testing specific hypotheses developed from policy, theoretical, or practical concerns. As well, the lack of emphasis on traditional notions of reliability and validity is a shortcoming, especially in relation to the need for governments and agencies to provide hard evidence of effectiveness of policies and programs.

Not surprisingly, almost all published quality of life research is quantitative rather than qualitative. This is a situation not unique to quality of life research but reflects the slow emergence and acceptance of the value of qualitative methods. An important contribution to this debate was made by Bryman (1988), who argued for a distinction between philosophical and technical components of the debate. Specifically, Bryman argued that although much is written about the differing assumptions concerning the nature of reality between these camps, many social scientists are more concerned with the question, Which method will best answer the specific question that I have? Qualitative methods are especially useful for delineating new, complex areas of inquiry, whereas quantitative methods are most appropriate for hypothesis testing and generalizing to populations from samples. The implication for quality of life research of qualitative approaches, especially research among marginalized populations, is to let individuals tell their own stories rather than imposing a structure driven by theory or professional concerns and possibly devoid of the human perspective.

DEBATE 5: VALUES-BASED VERSUS
VALUES-FREE APPROACHES

Another debate is whether measures should be value laden (e.g., personal control, integration, and independence are fundamental quality of life indicators) or value neutral (e.g., personal control, integration, and independence can be operationally defined, but value judgments about their importance must be determined empirically). It is becoming increasingly apparent that no inquiry can be value free. Every theorist or researcher makes decisions on what is worth studying and measuring. Although this may be the case, some conceptualizations are particularly explicit not only concerning the values influencing measurement approach but also in discussing the social forces influencing many of their findings. This is especially the case in critical research that has a strong emancipating element. The asking of certain questions by researchers reflects the extent to which explicit values are translated into measurement activities.

Many quality of life theorists, however, maintain the posture of going about creating models and collecting data to contribute to the accumulated store of knowledge, ignoring the effect of their work on individuals. For these basic researchers, the main focus is on the creation of theoretically solid models based on empirically sound (either quantitative or qualitative) measurement approaches. This is especially true in health-related quality of life research (Tilson & Spilker, 1990). Even in the gerontology literature, where the importance of personal control and autonomy is an increasing concern, there is a reliance on empirical findings of advantage for such occurrences rather than an explicit statement of values (Birren et al., 1991).

In contrast, within the disabilities area, the exposition of quality of life values is particularly important. In recent volumes on quality of life and disability (Goode, 1994b; Schalock, 1990c) virtually every chapter contains strong explicit statements of principles and values. For example, Schalock (1990b) outlines a number of quality of life principles, such as the following: Quality of life for persons with disabilities is composed of those same factors and relationships that are important to persons without disabilities. Quality of life is experienced when a person's basic needs are met and when he or she has the same opportunity as anyone else to pursue and achieve goals in the major life settings of home, community, and work. And quality of life is based on a set of values that emphasize consumer and family strengths.

Similar expositions of values and principles are present in the quality of life model developed by the University of Toronto's Centre for Health Promotion (Renwick & Brown, this volume; Raphael, Renwick, & Brown, 1993; Woodill, Renwick, Brown, & Raphael, 1994). These principles include the belief that quality of life issues are similar for persons with and without disabilities and include aspects of personal being, social and community belonging, and personal development and growth. There is also an emphasis on personal control of life circumstances and presence of opportunities. This specific model of quality of life grew out of initial work within the developmental disabilities area but has been expanded into a general model.

In contrast, quality of life work in the aging area represents the more typical nonexplicit presentation of values and principles. Lawton, for example, defined quality of life as "the multidimensional evaluation, by both intrapersonal and social-normative criteria, of the person-environment system of an individual in time past, current, and anticipated" (Lawton, 1991, p. 6). The content domains of "the good life," behavioral competence, perceived quality of life, objective environment, and psychological well-being, represent a relatively values-free approach to assessing quality of life. Empirical findings are expected to determine what makes for the good life.

DEBATE 6: SOCIAL POLICY VERSUS BASIC RESEARCH ORIENTATIONS

Another debate is whether quality of life measurements should be related to social policy (either health-related or otherwise) and change goals. The social indicator movement, as a quality of life strategy, developed out of a strong social policy and social reform emphasis (Raphael et al., 1994b). During the 1960s and 1970s, social indicators were developed to evaluate public programs, establish a system of social accounts, and help establish social goals and social policy (Land, 1975). Social reporting was also seen as an important end in itself as it would help predict future social events and aspects of social life. Unfortunately, because the social indicators approach is closely tied to activist political styles, the onset of the 1980s with its increasing economic crises and fiscal conservatism has been related to a decline in social indicator activities (Miles, 1985).

Not surprisingly, the extent to which other quality of life work has a strong social policy emphasis is a function of a variety of factors frequently independent of the technical quality of the research enterprise. Usually a strong relationship between researcher and government makes the social policy application of findings more likely. In Goode's (1994a) recent volume, collaborations between researchers and government in the disabilities areas in a number of countries are documented. In the Canadian province of Ontario, the quality of life among persons with developmental disabilities project (Woodill et al., 1994) has benefited from funding and collaboration with the Ontario Ministry of Community and Social Services.

A similar social policy application can be expected to result from ongoing work (Raphael, Robinson, Renwick, & Cho, 1994) with the local health planning agency in Metropolitan Toronto, the District Health Council, on community-level quality of life indicators. These indicators may be used to assess community health concerns. The receptiveness to this thrust most likely results from the current period of health care restructuring in Ontario. Most other quality of life work, especially such individually based ones as health-related quality of life, although containing within them the seeds of social policy implications, rarely addresses social policy or social reform issues. Quality of life research among the elderly may also have strong social policy and social reform implications but these are rarely explicitly noted.

DEBATE 7: SYSTEM VERSUS INDIVIDUAL DATA COLLECTIONS

Another issue is whether quality of life data should be collected from individuals (e.g., microlevel data, either objective or subjective, possibly aggregated up to population units) or describe the functioning of systems (e.g., macro-level data, such as income distribution, availability of senior residences, and quality of public transportation). Outside of data collected through social indicators, system-level data are rarely collected by most quality of life researchers. In the social indicators literature, some system-level indicators include employment figures, percentage of children living in poverty, government expenditures on welfare, or gross national product (Miles, 1985).

Many studies that work within a quality of life framework and employ true system-level indicators are found in the journal *Social Indicators Research: An International and Interdisciplinary Journal for Quality of Life Measurement.* These studies employ a wide range of indicators and greatly contribute to our thinking about quality of life issues. Lindstrom (1994), for example, has outlined a wide range of system-level indicators of quality of life that affect the quality of life of Nordic children. These concern issues of income distribution, type of housing, education and employment levels, and availability of leave for family-related matters.

Within the more traditional quality of life areas, system-level indicators could include availability of housing for seniors, meeting of transportation needs for people with disabilities, availability of community living for persons with developmental disabilities, or any of a range of others. Although all of these indicators may exist and may be available, these are not normally subsumed under the rubric of quality of life research. Moreover, these data are normally not presented together with quality of life research within the health-related, psychological, disabilities, gerontology, or other areas.

There is also a role for using individually generated data, aggregated up to the system level, to illuminate quality of life issues. A particularly interesting example of individual-level aggregated up to system-level approach is provided by the *Swedish Level of Living Surveys* (see Erikson, 1993).

In this approach, nine areas are outlined (I provide just two examples of indicators for each area in parentheses): (a) health and access to health care (ability to walk 100 meters, contacts with nurses and doctors), (b) employment and working conditions (unemployment experiences, possibilities of leaving work during work hours), (c) economic resources (income and wealth, ability to cover unforeseen expenses of up to $1,000 within a week), (d) education and skills (years of education, level of education reached), (e) family and social integration (marital status, contacts with friends and neighbors), (f) housing (number of persons per room, amenities), (g) security of life and property (exposure to violence and theft), (h) recreation and culture (leisure time pursuits, vacation trips), and (i) political resources (voting in elections, ability to file complaints).

With the increasing awareness of the important roles that societal and group structures and institutions play in determining quality of life, creation and application of system-level indicators seem essential. Narrow focus on individual-level data collection to the exclusion of system-level indicators ignores an important ingredient in the quality of life recipe.

DEBATE 8: OBJECTIVE VERSUS SUBJECTIVE MEASUREMENTS

There is also debate on whether focus should be on objective measures, such as health status defined by a professional in terms of mobility or quality of housing, or on subjective indicators, such as self-reported health status, self-rated mobility, or satisfaction with housing.

The Case for Objective Indicators

Focusing on objective measures has a number of strengths. First, use of objective measures allows for the application of an extensive body of research from various disciplines. From the health sciences area, measures of health status, including medical and functional status, are well developed and provide important information. Similar contributions are available from the nursing, psychology, occupational therapy, and gerontology areas. Second, use of objective measures allows for the incorporation of community standards into quality of life assessments. Issues such as cleanliness, attractiveness, safety, friendliness, and acceptance of diversity are important considerations that can be objectively defined and measured. Third, objective measures allow for the determination of normative statements concerning the functioning of groups and societies. Indeed, this rationale underlies the social indicators approach to quality of life: "A social indicator, as the term is used here, may be defined to be a statistic of direct normative interest that facilitates concise, comprehensive and balanced judgments about the conditions of major aspects of a society" (U.S. Department of Health, Education, and Welfare, 1969, p. 97). Fourth, objective measures can be directly related to the development and implementation of social policies and programs. This is so because it is probably easier to detect, within a shorter time perspective, the effect of policies and programs on objective rather than subjective indicators of quality.

The Case for Subjective Indicators

The recent emphasis in much quality of life research has been on subjective reports. This has occurred even within the health-related quality of life area: "Quality of life represents the functional effect of an illness and its consequent therapy on a patient, as perceived by the patient" (Schipper, Clinch, & Powell, 1990, p. 16). There are a number of reasons for the attractiveness of subjective measures. First, there has been an awareness that frequently patient, client, or consumer reports of satisfaction and well-being do not correlate well with objective indicators. This is most striking in the case of well-being research in which subjective reports of health, housing, and social contacts are better predictors of happiness and overall satisfaction than objective indicators (Kozma, Stones, & McNeil, 1991).

Second, use of subjective measures allows the recipient of services or a research participant to play a greater role in the data collection exercise. The effect of the consumer movement in both the disabilities and aging areas has supported this shift away from the objective measurement approach. Third, there is increasing concern that the currently available objective measures, in a variety of disciplines, may have been missing the mark by focusing on what may be important for researchers and professionals steeped within their own discipline but not important for consumers or research subjects. This criticism is especially relevant regarding concepts of health and well-being (Labonté, 1993).

A last reason for increasing use of subjective measures has been the effect of researchers working within the naturalistic or qualitative traditions. The need to allow for the emergence of unforeseen effects, the uniqueness of individual cases, and the complexity of social reality has also made the use of subjective measures mandatory in many quality of life measurements. Unfortunately, there are also strong concerns about reliance on subjective measures of quality of life. The finding that subjective and objective measures are frequently poorly related raises an especially troubling issue, especially concerning marginalized populations, such as the poor, persons with disabilities, or people dependent on services. The importance of this issue is seen when it is considered how capable humans are of lowering their aspirations and levels of dissatisfaction in the absence of any hope of realizing specific goals or attainments (Campbell, Converse, & Rodgers, 1976).

This issue of "false awareness" is most apparent in the disabilities area in which social structures have been so deficient as to make false awareness among persons with disabilities a rather ubiquitous issue (see Raphael et al., 1993; Zigler & Balla, 1977). It appears to be common within the aging literature as well, especially in relation to care of seniors who may be frail (Birren et al., 1991). For Naess (1987), this suggests the necessity of identifying the core of human needs and assessing these needs through objective measures as well as gathering data concerning satisfaction. For quality of life measurement, it highlights the importance of combining objective normative judgments of quality together with subjective ratings collected from individuals (Raphael et al., 1994b).

DEBATE 9: SELF-REPORTS
VERSUS REPORTS BY OTHERS

Similar considerations arise in the collection of self-reports versus reports by others. Whether these measures are objective (e.g., a diary of a person's daily activities) or subjective (e.g., a person's satisfaction with these daily activities), data can be provided by individuals, their case workers, other professionals, spouses, parents, friends, or others. Besides the issues of false consciousness raised earlier, additional considerations include the capacity of the individual to respond to the demands of the inquiry, differences between perceptions of others and those of the individual, divergence between the values of the individual and the other person, and dependence of the individual on the other person for either care or support.

The capacity of the individual to respond to the demands of an inquiry is especially important when individuals may have difficulty understanding questions or language. In the most extreme cases, individuals may lack verbal communication ability or have severe cognitive impairments or disabilities (see Oullette-Kuntz & McCreary, Chapter 19, this volume). In many other cases, the individual may be unable to comprehend some of the issues being raised by the assessment, such as access to community resources, satisfaction with their care, or ability to control anger. Second, there is frequently divergence of perceptions between an individual and another person familiar with the person. This may occur for any of a number of reasons, such as lack of familiarity with the daily routine of the individual, attempts by the individual to please the caregiver, or differing baselines between the individual and the caregiver. Rather than identify all of the reasons why this might be the case, it might be best to assume that divergence in perceptions concerning quality of life issues is likely to be the norm rather than the exception.

The third consideration, divergence in values between the individual and other person, is especially important when dealing with individuals with disabilities or impairments and service providers. But it is also relevant when dealing with parents and their children, consumers and their doctors or nurses, or even an individual and spouse or friends. A good example of divergence in perceptions, possibly resulting from differences in values, was a broadcast on the public Canadian Broadcasting Corporation a few years ago, in which a manager of a sheltered workshop for persons with developmental disabilities in Winnipeg provided his perceptions of the satisfaction of the workers who attended his workshop. Although the manager stated that his workers were very happy there, the workers themselves indicated a high degree of unhappiness and dissatisfaction with their daily activities.

Last, recipients of services are especially loathe to indicate dissatisfaction for fear of loss of these services. An unwillingness to express dissatisfaction appears to be especially common among vulnerable populations or groups. This problem arose, for example, in one study of quality of life among seniors who are receiving services from community agencies or public health departments (Brown, Renwick, & Raphael, 1995). Many researchers deal with these complexities by including both self-reports and reports of others in quality of life measurements. These efforts appear essential.

DEBATE 10: TRADITIONAL VERSUS PARTICIPATORY APPROACHES

Traditionally, research is theory driven, designed by professionals, and carried out through scientific, methodologically sound methods. There has been harsh criticism of the traditional approach because of doubtful validity of positivist assumptions concerning the nature of reality, reliance on easily measurable aspects of reality rather than more complex phenomena (e.g., looking for lost car keys under street lamps because of the illumination that is present), and, most important, the view that much medical and social science research not only has not helped persons but has maintained the marginal status of persons who may be poor, with disabilities, or in need of services (Rioux & Bach, 1994; Woodill, 1992).

A strong argument for participatory research, especially when it involves persons with disabilities, was made by Woodill (1992) in a monograph prepared for a consumer organization of persons with disabilities. The monograph examined the role that medical and social science research has played in maintaining the marginal status of persons with disabilities and handicaps. Oliver (1990) argued that traditional research in disability has (a) tended to reduce the problems that disabled or handicapped people have to their own inadequacies or functional limitations, (b) failed to improve the quality of life of disabled or handicapped populations, and (c) been so divorced from the everyday experience of disabled people that many disabled or handicapped people rightly feel victimized by researchers.

Woodill (1992) further developed the argument that in a society in which categorization is common and frequently related to inequality, the disability category is used to isolate populations from the mainstream and has associated consequences. An emphasis on action or participatory research—that is, movement away from the common scientist-subject distinction—could equalize the power relationships in social science research. In addition, action and participatory research approaches are recommended as more likely to empower individuals and be used to improve individuals' lives.

DEBATE 11: CRITICAL APPROACHES

The final issue is best summarized by the question, What is the story behind the story? The critical approach is seen by some as emancipating and appears to add an action component to the realist analysis of societal structures and power (Bredo & Feinberg, 1982). Critical approaches urge the researcher to consider that "knowledge generated is a part of a process of mutual growth or evolution on the part of both parties. The researcher is inevitably an agent of change or a reinforcer of the status quo" (Bredo & Feinberg, p. 6). Guba (1990) saw the goals of the critical perspective as involving the transformation of the world through the raising of consciousness of those most affected (usually adversely) by the structures of society. Critical approaches have been especially fruitful in the education and medical sociology areas and most recently in the disabilities area. In the quality of life area, these analyses are rarely seen, with the exception of Raphael et al.'s (1993) and Woodill et al.'s (1994) work in the disabilities area. This is puzzling as quality of life as a research area, especially in relation to marginalized groups, appears an especially fertile area for such analyses.

Implications for Quality of Life
Measurement and Interventions

Eleven debates related to measuring quality of life have been outlined. These debates ranged from fundamental notions concerning the nature of reality to the nuts and bolts of measuring quality of life. The positions that one takes on these debates have profound ramifications for the development of quality of life measurements and use of these assessments for health promotion and rehabilitation efforts. I illustrate some of these implications by focusing on three general dimensions related to quality of life measurement: individual versus system-level measurement, control of the measurement enterprise, and the increasing recognition of the value of qualitative methods.

INDIVIDUAL-LEVEL VERSUS
SYSTEM-LEVEL MEASUREMENT

A reliance on individual-level measurement of quality of life and neglect of societal factors may lead to attention being directed solely to individual adjustment. Robertson (1990) suggested that such an approach toward understanding the lives of elderly people, for example, may lead to seeing aging as individual pathology to be treated and cured by doctors and other health professionals, thereby ignoring societal issues such as poverty, isolation, and the loss of role and status. A similar analysis can be undertaken concerning the problems of adolescence, which, when analyzed solely at the individual level, may ignore important societal determinants of quality of life (Raphael, this volume). The study of societal-level determinants on health status is gaining increasing importance (Evans, Barer, & Marmor, 1994) and health promotion efforts generally are increasingly focusing on the community and structural levels (Pederson, O'Neill, & Rootman, 1994). The debates concerning sociological versus psychological perspectives, individual versus system-level data collection, and subjective versus objective measurement are especially relevant to this issue.

CONTROL OF THE QUALITY
OF LIFE MEASUREMENT ENTERPRISE

Another particularly important dimension to consider, especially in relation to the quality of life of persons with disabilities or other marginalized groups, is the issue of power and control of the quality of life research agenda. The recognition of the role of control and power outlined by those with a critical perspective is especially important, as are the debates concerning qualitative versus quantitative methods, use of participatory approaches, and taking a values-based versus values-free approach toward the quality of life research enterprise. The recent volume *Disability Is Not Measles: New Research Paradigms in Disability* (Rioux & Bach, 1994) explicitly deals with many of these issues of power and control and the effect of these on persons' lives. The Woodill (1992) monograph is especially useful as well.

THE CONTRIBUTION
OF QUALITATIVE METHODS

Because quality of life measurement is so embedded within the notion of what it is to be a human being, it is surprising that so little of the work is carried out within the qualitative paradigm. This deficiency becomes especially important when the quality of life of vulnerable persons, such as older adults, persons with disabilities or illness, or those who are poor, is measured, because their lives may be especially affected by these assessments. Means must be employed to allow people to tell their own stories in ways that are meaningful to them. Any quality of life measurement, especially those that have the potential to directly affect individuals' lives, should have a qualitative component to supplement quantitative measurements that may be taking place.

Conclusion

Any presentations of quality of life measurements or reviews of quality of life measurements should be examined through the 11 debates presented here. Those conducting quality of life measurements should use them to help make explicit their assumptions and ways of construing quality of life. Such an explication will identify the limitations of a particular model or measurement approach to quality of life as well as identify areas of further inquiry. It seems especially important for those carrying out measurements of quality of life of marginalized or vulnerable populations to consider these issues.

For those reading or considering results of quality of life measurements, these 11 debates allow for a critical appraisal of the approach. Although it cannot be expected that every quality of life measurement exercise will include all aspects of these debates, it is important to be able to identify the assumptions underlying a particular approach. These analyses are essential in the quality of life area, especially when measurements are likely to affect individuals' lives directly.

PART
IV

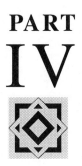

APPLICATIONS OF QUALITY OF LIFE IN HEALTH PROMOTION AND REHABILITATION

PART

IV

A: CURRENT SOCIAL ISSUES

13

Quality of Life Experienced by a Sample of Adults With HIV

Rebecca Renwick
Judith Friedland

The dominant themes in the literature on HIV and AIDS focus on the treatment and a cure for this disease. Of course, this is not surprising given the nature of HIV and the eventual terminal outcome for individuals with this diagnosis. Meanwhile, the number of people worldwide contracting HIV continues to grow rapidly (All & Fried, 1994) and the length of survival time following diagnosis is increasing (Mann, Tarantola, & Netter, 1994). In general, treatment advances in Europe and North America have resulted in a life expectancy of about 10 years (Mann et al., 1994) so that HIV infection is now considered a chronic illness (All & Fried, 1994). These developments are accompanied by a growing concern about the quality of life experienced by

AUTHORS' NOTE: This research was funded by the National Health Research and Development Program of the Government of Canada through a grant (6606-4337-AIDS) to Judith Friedland, Rebecca Renwick, and MaryAnn McColl. The authors thank Tracy Halpen (project manager), Debbie Rudman, and Azmina Habib for their assistance in preparing this chapter.

171

persons living with HIV (Friedland, Renwick, & McColl, in press). Quality of life issues are important in and of themselves but they have also been associated with improved immune system functioning for HIV-positive individuals (Goodkin et al., 1992) and a longer survival time for individuals with several disorders, including HIV (e.g., Namir, Wolcott, Fawzy, & Alumbaugh, 1990; Rabkin, Remien, Katoff, & Williams, 1993). Therefore, it is essential that research be directed toward understanding the quality of life experienced by individuals with HIV rather than making assumptions about its nature and patterns. Major factors that are likely to influence quality of life, such as coping strategies and social support, constitute an important area of research that can enrich this understanding. Knowledge about the relationships among quality of life, coping, and social support has the potential to guide health promotion and rehabilitation interventions that focus on maintaining and enhancing quality of life for individuals with HIV (e.g., see Chesney, 1993). However, to date, the literature on quality of life for persons who are HIV-positive is relatively sparse and not very systematic. Furthermore, much of it is related to its incorporation as an outcome measure in clinical trials for medical interventions (e.g., see Collier, 1994; Kaplan et al., 1989).

This chapter briefly reviews the relevant literature. It then focuses on some of the findings of a cross-sectional study conducted between 1991 and 1993. The purpose of the study was to assess the relationships among quality of life, coping, and social support in men and women who had been diagnosed as HIV-positive (see Friedland et al., in press). The results presented here focus on (a) quality of life as experienced by the study participants and (b) an examination of their quality of life as a function of their available social support and coping strategies as well as important demographic and health-related factors. Implications for research, policy, and service provision are also discussed.

Terminology associated with HIV has changed and continues to do so. Unless stated otherwise, the terms *HIV* and *HIV-positive,* as used here, are descriptive of persons who have been diagnosed with HIV (whether or not they have experienced symptoms) or AIDS.

Quality of Life Issues

Individuals living with HIV must deal with an uncertain future. They do not know whether, when, or to what degree they will experience particular symptoms or the extent of their functional level in the future (Ostrow et al., 1989; Weitz, 1989). Nor do they know whether a cure will be available before they encounter these issues (Ostrow et al., 1989). They are also faced with the very real possibility of their own death at a relatively early age (All & Fried, 1994).

Furthermore, multiple losses and the need for ongoing adjustments are common for individuals living with HIV (Rabkin et al., 1993). Due to the consequences of their infection, they could lose their lifestyle and way of life (e.g., employment, housing, and insurance) (Corthell & Oliverio, 1989). For those individuals who have not disclosed their HIV status, there is the risk that others will discover their stigmatizing diagnosis (Kraft & Rise, 1995). They are aware of the general public's "hostility against persons with AIDS" and that they are perceived as "social deviants" (All & Fried, 1994, p. 9). They may also worry that disclosure of their diagnosis will result in the loss of others significant to them (e.g., partner, family, friends) (Ostrow et al., 1989). Thus, it is not surprising that several studies indicate a relatively high degree of psychological distress in individuals with HIV (see Fleishman & Fogel, 1994).

Studies concerning quality of life are few, however, and the findings are mixed. For example, Cleary et al. (1993) found that overall health status and mental health status were positively associated with and significantly predicted life satisfaction. On the other hand, Chuang, Devins, Hunsley, and Gill (1989) found that, although individuals who are HIV-positive report relatively high levels of psychological distress, they do not have low levels of psychological well-being. Further, their results indicate that overall life happiness was similar for individuals in the various stages of the illness. Rabkin et al. (1993) found that the degree of physical impairment was not associated with life satisfaction.

Quality of life is seldom explicitly defined or thoroughly conceptualized in the literature. It is usually discussed in terms of its operational definition or the measures used to tap the construct (Renwick, Brown, & Raphael, 1994). Furthermore, measures of quality of life vary from study to study. Some focus on health and functional issues, whereas others tap well-being or happiness (Chuang et al., 1989; Cleary et al., 1993). Measures for general populations are typically employed, however, and HIV-specific measures are rare (but see Fanning & Emmott, 1994).

Social Support

People typically experience stress on a daily basis but for people with serious illness or disability, this stress is exacerbated (DiMatteo & Hays, 1981). Persons living with HIV encounter a multiplicity of stressors (Rabkin et al., 1993), as noted earlier. Social support, however, can buffer the negative effects that stressors have on health (Cobb, 1976; Cohen & Wills, 1985), even the stressors associated with serious and chronic illness (DiMatteo & Hays, 1981; Sherbourne, Meredith, Rogers, & Ware, 1992; Turner & Noh, 1988).

Obtaining adequate social support to mediate the effects of stress may be problematic for individuals living with HIV because their disease often affects members of their social networks (Lennon, Martin, & Dean, 1990) and their potential sources of support. Wolcott (1986) notes that they frequently live at a distance from their nuclear families and are not emotionally close with them. For gay men, HIV may have already resulted in the death or serious illness of partners and friends who could have offered support (Lennon et al., 1990). Others who can offer caregiving find that the uncertain and protracted course of HIV makes it difficult to meet the extensive needs for support (Folkman, Chesney, & Christopher-Richards, 1994).

Different patterns (i.e., types and degrees) of support may be associated with different aspects of quality of life. For instance, health and functional components of quality of life may be more positively influenced by different kinds and levels of support than perceived satisfaction with life components. Several major types of social support have been identified in the literature— namely, informational, instrumental (practical), and emotional (Friedland et al., in press).

Social support interventions have been used to decrease the stress and improve the outcomes for persons with chronic disabilities and illnesses. The results of these have not always been successful, however (Cwikel & Israel, 1987). This may be due, in part, to gaps in our knowledge concerning the complexity of both social support and quality of life and the ways in which they are related to health.

Coping

Coping is another resource that, like social support, may positively influence health and quality of life. A variety of coping strategies have been examined in the literature, including those used by individuals who are HIV-positive (e.g., Folkman, Chesney, Pollack, & Coates, 1993). Typically, different coping strategies are associated with different outcomes for persons with HIV. For instance, Fleishman and Fogel (1994) found that avoidance coping (i.e., denial of or self-distraction from negative feelings) was linked with elevated levels of psychological distress. They also reported that positive coping behaviors were associated with lower levels of distress. Other research (Folkman et al., 1993) indicates that involvement coping (i.e., planful problem solving, information seeking, and positive reappraisal of stress) is associated with lower levels of depression, but detachment strategies (i.e., not expressing feelings, distancing, and cognitive escape-avoidance) are related to higher levels of stress and depression.

Given the foregoing findings, coping may be a valuable factor to incorporate in interventions aimed at maintaining and enhancing quality of life of individuals with HIV, especially in combination with social support interventions (Chesney, 1993). To do this effectively, more knowledge is needed concerning which strategies are likely to positively influence which aspects of quality of life and the relative contributions of coping and social support to experienced quality of life. These issues were examined in a study of coping, social support, and quality of life in persons with HIV that is discussed in this chapter.

Research Questions

The results presented here addressed several research questions, as follows:

What is the nature of quality of life experienced by individuals who are HIV-positive?

What is the relationship between their health status and their quality of life?

To what extent is their experienced quality of life a function of social support and coping strategies as well as important demographic and health-related factors?

Method

PARTICIPANTS

Participants were recruited from five clinics and drop-in centers for persons with HIV in Metropolitan Toronto, the most populous urban area in Canada. Most of the sample (63%) was recruited from HIV clinics and 37% from community drop-in centers. Participants were 107 males and 13 females who had an average age of 36.89 ($SD = 8.07$; range: 22 to 63) years. A diagnosis of AIDS was reported by 29% and the rest were HIV-positive with half of this latter group being asymptomatic. The typical time since an HIV diagnosis was 3.50 ($SD = 1.77$) years and 1.90 ($SD = 2.28$) years since an AIDS diagnosis.

Most were single (74%), reported their sexual orientation as gay (75%), and lived alone (61%). The majority (62%) had postsecondary education, yet

67% were unemployed despite a relatively good health status. More than half (54%) of the participants had an annual income of $20,000 Canadian (approximately $14,300 American) or less.

At the time of data collection, participants reported mild HIV-symptom severity, scoring a mean of 2.03 ($SD = 0.51$; range: 1 to 4) on the Symptom Checklist (Fanning & Emmott, 1994), out of a possible score of 4. Only 28% had ever been hospitalized for an HIV-related illness. Participants experienced the range of HIV symptoms, with fatigue, depression, and difficulty sleeping being rated as most severe. Stress reported in the past year was most commonly associated with changes in relationships with people other than partners as well as changes in health, finances, and social activities.

PROCEDURE

Questionnaire packages were made available by personnel at the clinics and organizations taking part. They informed potential participants about the study. They used a nonaggressive recruiting method developed through consultation with consumers (see Friedland et al., in press). A consent form was included in the package that gave potential participants the opportunity to have an interviewer administer the questionnaires. Only one participant requested an interview.

A total of 120 complete data sets were provided by the participants. When compared with the data from the study participants, data on the general characteristics of HIV-positive consumers of services in each of the five settings indicated similarities in age, gender, and sexual orientation. The participants' educational level was somewhat higher than the average for the consumer group at each setting. This may be due to the fact that those with more education were more able to complete and return the whole questionnaire. Study participants from the drop-in centers had somewhat higher rates of unemployment than the drop-in center group as a whole. This suggests that participants who were unemployed may have had more opportunity to access the questionnaires and more time to complete them. These factors and the overall sample size need to be considered when generalizing the findings of the study.

INSTRUMENTATION

The major measures employed to gather the data discussed here are described in the sections that follows. Other quantitative and qualitative measures were also used in the study (see Friedland et al., in press).

Quality of Life

The quality of life construct encompasses people's material resources as well as "overall subjective feelings of well-being that are also closely related to morale, happiness and satisfaction" (McDowell & Newell, 1987, p. 206). Health, however, is also considered to be one of the most important contributing factors to overall life quality (Ware, 1993) and it may be uniquely affected by specific illness processes, such as those associated with HIV (Fanning & Emmott, 1994).

Because of the lack of clarity concerning the definition of this construct and the resulting difficulty in operationalizing it (see Renwick et al., 1994; Wolfensberger, 1994), as well as its multidimensional nature, different instruments were used to tap it. Specifically, measures (to be described) of its behavioral, health-related, and subjective dimensions were employed. This broad-based, comprehensive approach to measurement is consistent with the one advocated by Cleary et al. (1993) for obtaining a better understanding of the effect of illness factors on persons who are HIV-positive.

The Quality of Life Questionnaire (QOLQ). The QOLQ (Evans & Cope, 1989) measures behavioral aspects of quality of life on the assumption that "certain actions or behaviors of an individual in response to particular environmental domains can be considered to represent a good quality of life" (Evans & Cope, 1989, p. 1). It is a psychometrically sound (Evans, Burns, Robinson, & Garrett, 1985; Evans, Hearn, Levy, & Shatford, 1988), multidimensional, 192-item self-report questionnaire consisting of 16 scales, including a social desirability scale. Its generalizability and usefulness as an evaluative measure have been demonstrated with several populations (Evans et al., 1988). In the study reported here, an abbreviated version (i.e., 64 items; four items from each scale) was used (see Evans & Cope, 1989). Wording of the questionnaire was modified slightly to ensure meaningfulness to individuals with HIV. Higher QOLQ scores indicate a better quality of life.

The Fanning Quality of Life Scale (FQOLS). The FQOLS (Fanning & Emmott, 1994) taps health-related quality of life in persons with HIV. It was developed on the basis of information about quality of life issues reported by HIV-positive individuals in the context of clinical interviews. This has contributed to its face and content validity. The FQOLS consists of 37 self-report items concerning different aspects of life that have been affected by HIV. Ratings are made on a 7-point Likert-type scale ranging from 1 (*completely negative*) to 7 (*completely positive*). When used as a diagnosis-specific measure of quality of life, total scores have significantly discriminated among persons at different stages of illness and symptom severity (Fanning et al., 1993). Higher scores indicate a better quality of life.

The Life Appraisal and Life Satisfaction Questionnaires (LAQ and LSQ). The LAQ and LSQ (Campbell, Converse, & Rodgers, 1976) were used together to yield an index of well-being (IWB) or composite score of perceived life satisfaction (see Campbell et al., 1976). This IWB assessed the subjective aspect of quality of life. The LAQ consists of 10 semantic differential items, whereas the LSQ has 10 Likert-type-scale items. Both have acceptable psychometric properties (Campbell et al., 1976). Higher IWB scores indicate greater life satisfaction.

Social Support

Social support is defined as the feeling of being cared for and loved, valued and esteemed, and able to count on others should the need arise (Cobb, 1976; Turner, Frankel, & Levin, 1983). It was measured by two instruments, but only the data from the Interpersonal Support Evaluation List (ISEL) (Cohen, Mermelstein, Kamarck, & Hoberman, 1985) are reported here. The ISEL is a psychometrically sound instrument consisting of 40 true-false questions about the perceived availability of others to provide specific kinds of support if needed (e.g., "When I feel lonely, there are several people I could call and talk to") (Cohen et al., 1985). Its four subscales pertain to four types of support: tangible, appraisal, belonging, and self-esteem. In the current study, the latter two scales were combined to form an emotional support scale in keeping with the three types of support commonly referred to in the literature. Higher scores on the ISEL indicate greater social support.

Coping

The Ways of Coping Questionnaire (WOCQ) is a 66-item questionnaire that assesses the "thoughts and actions individuals use to cope with the stressful encounters of everyday living" (Folkman & Lazarus, 1988, p. 1). It is based on the cognitive-phenomenological theory of stress and coping (Lazarus & Folkman, 1984) and it has good psychometric properties (Folkman & Lazarus, 1988). Higher scores on any WOCQ subscale indicate greater uses of the coping strategy it taps.

Other Measures

Other measures concerning demographics and health status, including recent life changes (indicative of number of stressors experienced), were used. These included closed- and open-ended items as well as the HIV-specific symptom checklist (which taps symptom severity) developed by Fanning and Emmott (1994) and an adapted version of the Recent Life Changes Questionnaire (adapted from Rahe, 1975).

Results

DESCRIPTIVE ANALYSES

Quality of Life

Except as noted, the total scores for the three measures of quality of life presented here are expressed as percentages for ease of interpretation. The mean total score on the behavioral measure (QOLQ) (Evans & Cope, 1989) (excluding the social desirability scale) was 51.81 (SD = 14.98; range: 13.00 to 90.00). This is slightly lower than the norm for samples from the general population, which was 59. Participants' scores for 15 of the subscales (in descending order of magnitude) appear in Table 13.1. On all but four of these scales, participants scored lower than the normative group (Evans & Cope, 1989). They had only slightly higher than normative scores on job satisfiers, creative-aesthetic behavior, altruistic behavior, and relations with others (besides their partners). There were particularly large differences compared with the normative sample on the scales concerned with material well-being, physical well-being, and vacation behavior.

The mean score on the health-related measure (FQOLS) (Fanning & Emmott, 1994) was 55.43 (SD = 15.43; range: 27.40 to 94.00). The items were rated on a 7-point scale ranging from 1 (*completely negative*) to 7 (*completely positive*), but at present, no norms are available for the FQOLS. A differential effect of HIV was reported on the areas of life assessed. Of the 37 areas of life included in the FQOLS, those reported to be most positively and most negatively affected by HIV are presented in Table 13.2.

Participants' mean perceived satisfaction with life, as indicated by the IWB (Campbell et al., 1976), was 56.73 (SD = 13.26; range: 28.90 to 81.30). This score is considerably lower than the norm of 80.07 derived from samples of the general population reported by Campbell et al. (1976). Some of this difference may be accounted for, however, by dissimilarities in income and employment status between the normative and the current samples (for details, see Campbell et al., 1976, pp. 53-57).

Scores for the three measures differed as expected, because they tap different aspects of quality of life. It is interesting to note, however, that the total scores for all three measures exceeded 50% and, thus, were slightly positive.

TABLE 13.1 Behavioral Measure of Quality of Life (QOLQ): Means and Standard Deviations

Scales (Descending Order)	M	SD	n
Job satisfiers	65.68	32.83	59
Relations with others (extramarital)	64.53	25.46	117
Occupational relations	62.71	26.63	59
Altruistic behavior	61.78	34.68	116
Creative-aesthetic behavior	60.85	28.89	116
Relations with significant others	60.79	38.86	64
Marital (partner) relations	55.21	31.62	64
Job characteristics	54.89	34.77	63
Political behavior	54.86	31.06	115
Extended family relations	47.56	36.68	116
Vacation behavior	46.42	36.45	114
Personal growth	45.86	29.27	117
Material well-being	41.88	36.78	118
Sports activity	35.90	25.84	107
Physical well-being	31.47	28.13	116

NOTE: Means and standard deviations are expressed as percentages.

Health Status and Quality of Life

There were few significant correlations among measures of health status and total scores for the three quality of life measures. These significant correlations, however, were only weak to moderate. There were no significant correlations between any of the three quality of life measures and number of hospitalizations. Time since receiving a diagnosis of AIDS was positively and significantly associated with two of the quality of life measures: the FQOLS (Fanning & Emmott, 1994) ($r = .32$; $df = 38$; $p < .05$) and the IWB (Campbell et al., 1976) ($r = .41$; $df = 36$; $p < .01$). Time since receiving an HIV-positive diagnosis was not significantly associated with any of the overall quality of life scores. Participants' symptom severity scores on the symptom checklist (Fanning & Emmott, 1994) were negatively and significantly associated with two of the quality of life measures: the QOLQ ($r = -.31$; $df = 112$; $p < .005$) and the IWB ($r = -.23$; $df = 112$; $p < .02$). The number of stressors they experienced, as indicated by their Recent Life Changes Questionnaire (Rahe, 1975) scores, was not significantly correlated with any of the three quality of life measures.

Analyses of variance (ANOVAs) were conducted comparing participants in three diagnostic groups (HIV asymptomatic, HIV symptomatic, and

TABLE 13.2 Health-Related Measure of Quality of Life (FQOLS): Aspects of Life Most Positively and Negatively Affected by HIV

Aspect of Life	M	SD	n
Most positively affected			
Commitment to present lover	4.93	2.00	57
Openness as a gay individual	4.88	1.66	90
Satisfaction with time spent alone	4.81	1.52	116
Sense of affirmation with gay community	4.64	1.61	88
Spiritual beliefs	4.61	1.61	100
Interest in life	4.57	1.96	115
Most negatively affected			
Future school-career-work-job opportunities	2.60	1.71	104
Creation of new intimate friendships	3.09	1.94	100
Physical strength and stamina	3.31	1.65	115
Sense of optimism for the future	3.37	1.85	115
Psychological-emotional health and well-being	3.41	1.80	116
Sexual desire	3.42	1.84	112
Physical health and well-being	3.47	1.68	116
Control over own life	3.48	1.82	116

NOTE: Participants' ratings were on a 7-point scale ranging from 1 (*completely negative*) to 7 (*completely positive*).

AIDS) for each of the three quality of life measures. None of these results was significant.

REGRESSION ANALYSES

Three models incorporating the major study variables were developed and tested in the context of multiple regression analyses. For each model, one aspect of quality of life—behavioral (QOLQ), health-related (FQOLS), or perceived satisfaction (IWB)—was the outcome or dependent variable. Each dependent variable was examined as a function of demographics, health status, and number of stressors as well as social support and coping. Each model included 10 determinants or independent variables: three demographic variables (income, age, and employment), three social support variables (tangible, emotional, and appraisal support), three coping variables (problem-oriented, emotion-oriented, and perception-oriented coping), and a health status variable (symptom severity).

Each model was tested using hierarchical block regression. In all three analyses, three blocks of variables were entered into the model in the following order: demographics, social support and coping, and health status. Because of their demonstrated relationship with quality of life (Campbell et al., 1976), the demographic variables were entered as the first block. Given their salience in the current study, the social support and coping variables were entered as the second block. Because health status could be a confounding factor and is also considered to be important to quality of life (Spitzer et al., 1981; Ware, 1993), this constituted the third block entered into the model.

Only data from the male participants ($n = 107$) were used in the regression analyses due to the small number of women in the study and preliminary analyses indicated gender differences in coping and social support. Because of the relatively small sample remaining after pairwise deletion of missing data, parsimony and careful development of the models were important considerations. Therefore, the independent variables were included in the analyses on theoretical grounds, but empirical salience was also confirmed through correlational analyses (i.e., correlations of each independent variable with each dependent variable). Evaluation of parameter estimates was based on the criterion of $p < .05$.

Determinants of Behavioral
Quality of Life (Model 1)

The results of the analysis with the behavioral aspect of quality of life (QOLQ) as the dependent variable appear in Table 13.3. By themselves, the demographic variables constitute a significant model, but it explains only 11.1% of the variance. Furthermore, only the income variable is statistically significant. The model is significantly improved by the entry of the social support and coping variables. Three determinants are significant here: emotional social support, problem-oriented coping, and emotion-oriented coping. The first two of these determinants are positively related to quality of life and the third is negatively related. This model accounts for 48.3% of the variance in the behavioral aspect of quality of life, and the addition of the third block (health status) does not enhance the overall fit of the model.

Determinants of Health-Related
Quality of Life (Model 2)

The results for the analysis with the health-related measure of quality of life (FQOLS) as the dependent variable are presented in Table 13.3. Only

3.7% of the variance is explained by demographic factors. The beta coefficient for income is significant but the F ratio for the overall model is not. A significantly better fit is achieved with the addition of the social support and coping variables. This model and three additional determinants are significant: tangible and emotional social support and perception-oriented coping. The first determinant is negatively related to quality of life but the second and third are positively related. This model accounts for 29.2% of the variance in health-related quality of life, and the addition of the health status variable does not improve the overall fit of the model.

Determinants of Perceived Satisfaction
Aspect of Quality of Life (Model 3)

The results of the regression analysis employing the perceived satisfaction measure of quality of life (IWB) as the dependent variable are shown in Table 13.3. The demographic variables do not yield a significant model and together they account for only 2.5% of the variance. Entry of the social support and coping variables significantly enhances the fit, and the resulting model is significant. The model includes only one variable that is even close to significance (i.e., emotional social support with $p = .07$), however, and accounts for only 10.5% of the variance in quality of life. Addition of the health status variable results in the loss of a significant fit for the overall model. Thus Block 2 constitutes the best model but it does not offer much information concerning determinants of the perceived satisfaction aspect of quality of life.

Discussion

OVERALL QUALITY OF LIFE

Overall scores for the three aspects of quality of life examined were slightly positive. This contradicts a common assumption by the general public that persons living with AIDS experience a very impoverished quality of life. In general, researchers have tended to perceive that their study participants who have illnesses and disabilities experience a lower quality of life than the participants do themselves (Rabkin et al., 1993; Weinberg, 1984). There is some evidence that quality of life may even be increased when individuals become seriously ill. Such findings are noted in the literatures on HIV (Chuang et al., 1989; Gloerson et al., 1993; Rabkin et al., 1993) and palliative care (Cohen & Mount, 1992; Loew & Rapin, 1994). These previous findings, together with the current ones, raise some interesting questions. Do individuals who have serious illnesses, such as HIV, lower their expectations concerning quality of life? Alternatively, do they begin to focus on and find enjoyment in areas of their lives to which they previously gave little attention? Or do they use both strategies? Longitudinal studies that examine these questions could provide clearer information about this phenomenon.

SPECIFIC LIFE AREAS
AND QUALITY OF LIFE

The study participants report somewhat lower overall quality of life than the norm groups did on both the behavioral measure (QOLQ) and the perceived satisfaction measure (IWB). There was a more noticeable gap between normative scores and the latter measure. Taken together with the information on quality participants experienced in specific aspects of their lives (Tables 13.1 and 13.2), these findings indicate that quality of life is an important focus for assessment and intervention with individuals who have HIV. Such interventions might be planned to include attention to particular strategies that could be most helpful to individuals with respect to the areas of life that they experience as least enjoyable. Renwick et al. (1994) provide an example of this kind of approach to assessment and intervention with another population who have disabilities.

Table 13.1 indicates specific areas of life (as measured by the QOLQ) in which the participants are experiencing diminished enjoyment. The areas of particular concern are physical well-being and material well-being because participants' scores are much lower than the normative group's (Evans & Cope, 1989). These findings are consistent with earlier themes in the literature concerning the nature of stressors related to physical well-being and financial issues (e.g., loss of employment and income) (All & Fried, 1994; Corthell & Oliverio, 1989; Ostrow et al., 1989; Weitz, 1989). The other areas for which their QOLQ scores are considerably lower than the norms are vacation behavior and marital (partner) relations. The findings concerning vacation behavior (i.e., not taking a vacation or vacation is not relaxing) may be related to financial difficulties. They are also interesting, however, given that leisure and recreational aspects of life are not addressed in the literature on HIV. This is an area that has potential to contribute to the coping process (e.g., provide time for reflection and more positive reappraisal of one's situation or spend more time with close others who may provide support). Given the tremendous pressures on partner relationships associated with HIV (Ostrow et al., 1989), perhaps the lower quality in this area of life is not too surprising.

Table 13.2 indicates that participants found several areas of life to be positively affected by HIV. Collectively, these areas are related to increased commitment to partner, affirmation of gay aspects of identity, and personal growth. Such specific, positive aspects of quality of life have not been discussed in the literature on HIV and are worth examining in future studies of quality of life. Table 13.2 also indicates those areas of life most negatively affected by HIV that, taken together, are concerned with career and future, physical and psychological health, sexuality, and sense of control. Most of these themes have already been discussed in the literature, but, of particular note, is the issue of personal control, which needs more attention with regard to this population (see Folkman et al., 1993; Picherack, 1988), especially as it relates to the process of and strategies for coping and the enhancement of quality of life.

HEALTH STATUS AND QUALITY OF LIFE

In this study, health status was examined using several measures (e.g., diagnostic category, time since diagnosis, and number of stressors experienced). Few of these measures are significantly related to quality of life, however. When there is a significant relationship, the magnitude of the correlations is small to moderate. Furthermore, the health status measure (i.e., symptom severity) used in Block 3 of each regression analysis was not significantly related to any of the three dimensions of quality of life (see Table 13.3).

Using health status measures to tap the construct of quality of life or to make inferences about quality of life are common approaches in the health literature (Bowling, 1991). The kinds of measures employed in the current study did constitute a relatively narrow approach to health status (see Bergner, 1989). Nevertheless, collectively, the current findings concerning health status and quality of life do not support the assumption that health status instruments alone are useful indicators of or good tools for direct assessment of quality of life. These results, taken together with other discussions concerning health status and quality of life (Bergner, 1989; Bowling, 1991), indicate the need for further research on the relationship between the two constructs based on clear conceptualizations of both.

DEMOGRAPHIC FACTORS AND QUALITY OF LIFE

In 1993 (the last year of the study), the Canadian government considered $15,452 for a single person and $30,655 for a family of four persons living in large cities to be poverty-level incomes (National Council of Welfare,

TABLE 13.3 Regression Analyses for Three Measures of Quality of Life

Blocks	Behavioral (QOLQ)			Health (FQOLS)			Satisfaction (IWB)		
	Beta	F	ΔF	Beta	F	ΔF	Beta	F	ΔF
Block 1									
Income	.18*	4.60**		−.26*	2.12		−.09	0.71	
Age	.06			.10			.08		
Employment	−.04			.18			.08		
Block 2									
Tangible support	.14	9.92**	10.93**	−.36**	4.95**	5.99**	−.18	2.12*	2.78*
Emotional support	.30*			.42**			.31		
Appraisal support	.12			.12			.22		
Problem-oriented coping	.39**			−.12			.05		
Emotion-oriented coping	−.21*			−.12			−.04		
Perception-oriented coping	−.13			.50**			.10		
Block 3									
Symptom severity	.00	8.81**	0.00	.07	4.46**	0.42	−.09	1.94	0.47

NOTE: Degrees of freedom associated with F values for each analysis: Block 1 = 3.83; Block 2 = 9.77; Block 3 = 10.76.
*p > .05; **p > .01.

1994). Thus the annual income level ($20,000 or less) for the majority of the participants seems rather low, especially given their high educational levels and reasonably good health.

Income was the most influential demographic factor in the outcome of the regression analyses. It is no surprise that it is positively related to the behavioral aspect of quality of life (Model 1) because many of the items measured by the QOLQ refer or are connected to material goods. At first glance, the inverse relationship of income to health-related quality of life (Model 2) is more difficult to understand. The 37-item FQOLS, however, includes only three questions that could be tied to having a good income. Furthermore, factor analysis of the FQOLS by Fanning et al. (1993) has identified two factors: a sense of self-worth and wholeness and personal desirability in intimate relationships. The difference in the valence of the relationship between income and quality of life for regression models 1 and 2 underscores the implications of differences in instruments that measure quality of life.

Although employment did not appear in the best-fit models for any of the regression analyses, it is important to note that the unemployment rate for this sample is very high (67%), particularly considering their educational backgrounds and health. According to Statistics Canada (1992), the unemployment rate in Toronto at the time of this study was 11.8%.

Clearly, advocacy efforts should be directed toward ensuring that individuals with HIV can continue to work for as long as they are able to do so, free from harassment and with appropriate accommodations in the workplace. Policy makers need to take into account these work-related quality of life issues for persons who are HIV-positive.

SOCIAL SUPPORT, COPING, AND QUALITY OF LIFE

The results of the three regression analyses (Table 13.3) suggest that particular aspects of social support and coping may contribute to enhancing quality of life in this population. Collectively, these findings indicate that different aspects of quality of life are most strongly influenced by different types and combinations of social support and coping strategies. Emotional social support is an important contributor to behavioral (QOLQ) and health-related (FQOLS) aspects of quality of life, however, and this relationship approached significance ($p = .07$) for the perceived satisfaction (IWB) dimension as well.

Problem-oriented coping (e.g., planning and taking action, seeking solutions) and the absence of emotion-oriented coping (e.g., denial and distancing self from problems) also operate together with emotional social support to positively influence the behavioral dimension of quality of life. This finding regarding the absence of emotion-oriented coping is consistent with other HIV research that identified it as a maladaptive strategy (Rabkin et al., 1993).

Health-related quality of life is positively affected by perception-oriented coping (e.g., positive reappraisal of one's situation) and emotional support in combination with the absence of tangible (practical) support. This finding concerning the inverse relationship of tangible social support and health-related quality of life is consistent with earlier research. Specifically, a study by McColl and Rosenthal (1994) suggests that when greater tangible support is required, individuals perceive themselves as more ill and their quality of life as poorer. It may be that although tangible social support is important and necessary, it should be assessed more carefully in studies where participants have chronic illnesses or disabilities.

The major implication of the foregoing findings is twofold. First, as Chesney (1993) suggests, there is great potential value in incorporating coping and social support in interventions centered around the maintenance and enhancement of quality of life for persons living with HIV. Second, coping and social support need to be tailored to the specific aspects of life identified as most needing maintenance or enhancement. Such interventions would need to be based on the results of assessment of the individual's available social supports, patterns of coping strategies, and perceptions about enjoyment and quality in the various areas of life. Research evaluating the efficacy of such interventions would be a valuable source of information for service providers.

Picherack (1988) argues that strengthening social support and coping strategies of persons with HIV constitutes an important aspect of health promotion for this population. Such an approach emphasizes personal strategies and supportive social environments that contribute to quality of life by fostering personal empowerment and increasing feelings of control. This is particularly important because participants in this study report control over their own lives as one of the areas most negatively affected by HIV (Table 13.2). The relationship between perceived control and quality of life needs to be examined in future research, however. Furthermore, the recent literature on HIV seems to have ignored the great potential of a health promotion approach and strategies focused on enhancing the quality of life of individuals living with HIV.

Conclusion

This chapter presented the results of a study of quality of life for 120 adults with HIV. The relationships of coping, social support, demographic, and health status factors with quality of life were examined. Implications for assessment and intervention focused on quality of life, with attention to coping strategies and social supports, were discussed. For example, one major implication of the study for assessment and intervention was that different combinations of coping strategies and social supports are potentially valuable for improving different aspects of quality of life. The importance of social support and coping and their contributions to quality of life for persons with HIV were also discussed in the context of health promotion. Implications of findings concerning employment, income, and quality of life, which are of particular interest to policy developers, were highlighted.

Future directions for research on quality of life were suggested. For instance, further study of the complex relationship between health status and quality of life, based on clear conceptualizations of both constructs, is recommended. Research is also needed to further illuminate the relationship between perceived control and quality of life. In the current study, participants identified some areas of life that were favorably affected by their HIV diagnosis. Such positive aspects of quality of life for persons with HIV have not received adequate attention in the literature and need to be better understood, particularly through the use of qualitative methods. The efficacy of combining coping and social support strategies, tailored to individual needs and targeted to enhancing particular aspects of quality of life experienced by persons with HIV, also needs to be tested in the context of future research.

14

Quality of Life of People With Disabilities Who Have Experienced Sexual Abuse

Mark Nagler

As illustrated in some of the previous chapters, there are many parameters that can be productively used to indicate, if not measure, quality of life. For people who have been victimized by various patterns of deviance, including sexual abuse, rehabilitation and subsequent adjustment are often difficult and, in some cases impossible to achieve. This chapter will examine quality of life issues that affect the victimology of those who have experienced sexual exploitation. The analysis will be on people with disabilities who have experienced sexual abuse because their victimization has been effectively camouflaged, but mirrors, in many respects, the factors associated with the sexual abuse of people who are usually defined as "normal."

Sexual abuse can induce marginality because victims of sexual abuse find it difficult to integrate into society and to enjoy experiences that people who have not been victimized take for granted. People who have been subjected to sexual exploitation may experience lifelong patterns that can be characterized in Durkheimian (1951) terms as *anomie.* The ramifications of this anomie are illustrated in a variety of ways. There may be an inability to form and maintain trusting relationships, especially with members of the opposite sex, or even with members of the same sex if homosexual abuse is involved. Some victims of abuse encounter difficulties in obtaining education and employment because they trust neither their educators nor their employers. Some victims find it difficult to commit to ongoing employment because they believe they cannot trust anyone. Therefore, it seems unimportant to honor obligations. Some victims feel that it is difficult to commit emotionally to long-term relationships. If a relationship does develop, they are inclined to sever their involvement.

Many individuals with disabilities, like their able-bodied counterparts, are traumatized by their sexual abuse. It is difficult for them to identify their abusers because they expose themselves to ridicule and loss of self-esteem. This is illustrated by two factors. Some segments of society demonstrate tendencies to blame victims, even victims of sexual abuse. Second, when victims have the courage to bring their abusers before the courts, the courts appear to pass minimum sentences.

As the discipline of victimology illustrates, some victims of sexual abuse are able to put the experience behind them and live normal lives. Many others, however, find it very difficult to adjust. In terms of physical and emotional health and social well-being, these individuals continue to experience psychological pain, compromised self-esteem, and stigma—all of which are consequences of victimization. Many of the victims of sexual abuse, including the sample of people with disabilities who form the population of an ongoing study by this author, continue to experience flashbacks years and even decades after their sexual assault.

Quality of life among the sexually abused is an oxymoron. Society expresses abhorrence to the suggestion of the widespread practice of sexual abuse as a pattern of deviance. Power theory states that those with the least power are most vulnerable to all aspects of abuse, including sexual abuse. The theme of this analysis is to illustrate the extent of sexual abuse, to describe the victims and their perpetrators, and to illustrate the patterns of adjustment illustrated by the victims.

Most of the data in this analysis came from an ongoing study on the abuse of people with disabilities. First, data examining 39 individuals with various disabilities who had experienced various forms of sexual abuse were used. The participants represent 11 different ethnic groups, four racial groups and range in age from 18 to 73 years old. Five of the participants had not received high school graduation, whereas six of the individuals are enrolled or have graduated from postsecondary educational institutions. Only one was male.

It is extremely unlikely that the lack of males represents the legitimate population because their victimization tends to be closeted for reasons pertaining to the traditional male image.

Second, 12 interviews were supplemented with data from psychologists, psychiatrists, social workers, and the clergy. The participants directed the investigator to consult the individuals from whom they had sought professional counseling, and in all cases, the data gathered were authenticated by the participants. The remaining 27 participants claimed that the author was the only one with whom they had discussed their sexual abuse.

The people interviewed in this study had disabilities that included hearing deficit disorder, sight impairment, muscular dystrophy, cerebral palsy, multiple sclerosis, attention deficit disorder, AIDS, paraplegia, and quadriplegia.

Frequency of Sexual Violence
Against Persons With Disabilities

Sexual violence is very widespread, especially against those with disabilities. According to the Minister of Health and Welfare on Child Sexual Abuse in Canada (1990),

> Family violence in this context refers to physical, psychological or sexual maltreatment, abuse and neglect of women (but also men with disabilities) by a relative or caregiver. It is a violation of trust and an abuse of power in a relationship where women (people) should have the right to absolute safety. (p. 20)

Many investigations have revealed that sexual violence against those with disabilities was once considered a taboo topic because most people genuinely believed that such excessive deviance was so reprehensible that indeed it would seldom, if ever, be practiced. In Canadian society, two women in three are victims of unwanted sexual acts (Badgley, 1984). Data on any type of sexual violence always underestimate the extent of the problem because the majority of victims are reluctant to reveal their victimization.

Contemporary data reveal that one woman in six is physically or sexually abused by her husband, ex-husband, or live-in partner. What is particularly revealing is that 14.7% of women in the general population have disabilities and women with disabilities are much more prone to all types of abuse, including sexual abuse, because in addition to being members of the female gender, they are doubly victimized by being perceived as disabled. The sexual violence becomes further insulated by the fact that most of the abuse is inflicted by individuals known to the victim. Of the victims of spousal assault, 95% are women, and at least 89% of the abusers are men. More men with disabilities are abused than nondisabled men. The incidence of abuse is 20% or higher among people who are deaf or have developmental disabilities (Senn, 1988).

Who Are the Abusers?

The vulnerability of people with disabilities tends to be camouflaged because most of the perpetrators of sexual abuse against people with and without disabilities tend to be members of the family (Cole, 1986; Rinear, 1985). Females with disabilities are exceptionally reliant on their family members and very often on their caregivers for various aspects of care (Boyle, Rioux, Ticoll, & Feiske, 1988). Being in a dependent relationship increases the vulnerability of individuals because they are reluctant to expose their abusers due to the possibility of incarceration of the abuser as well as the economic, social, and psychological ramifications of family breakdown. Family dissolution exposes people with disabilities to the possibility of relinquishing substantial if not the entire means of economic, social, and psychological support on which all members of the family rely. In addition, people with disabilities depend on a number of others for the necessities of life. Family members, boyfriends, other relatives, acquaintances, neighbors, attendants, medical and paramedical personnel, homemakers, interpreters, counselors, and hospital and institutional workers have been identified as violating their positions of trust. In their positions of power, they influence the economic, social, physical, sexual identities, and self-esteem of the individuals with whom they are in "professional" contact. The more dependent individuals are, the greater the risk they experience in being exposed to all forms of abuse. Because they depend on a host of individuals for many of their needs, it becomes too costly for them to expose their perpetrators to the consequences of being identified as abusers. Perpetrators know that their victims are literally chained to this dependency syndrome and are therefore prone to continue their violation of trust in the belief that they will rarely be identified (Caparulo, 1987).

Vulnerability

Individuals, particularly women and children, living in institutional environments are most vulnerable (Bourgeois, 1975; Burgess & Hartman, 1986). Caregivers within an institutional environment are usually freed from the possibility of exposure by the social, psychological, and physical insulation and isolation of being within an institutional domain. Residents may be further victimized by institutional rules and union agreements that inhibit, if not prohibit, the exposure of abusive employees who are in positions of power and responsibility (Ammerman, Van Hasselt, Hersen, McGonigle, & Lubetsky, 1989; Blatt, 1980; Comfort, 1978; Sundram, 1984). It is estimated that women with disabilities are 1.5 to 10 times as likely to be abused as women without disabilities, depending on whether they live in the community or in institutions (Harris, 1990; Sobsey, 1988).

Those with disabilities are not as well protected as the mainstream population. People with disabilities are often defined as asexual and, in many cases, are much less likely to receive any sex education. There are many people with disabilities who are being abused and have no realization that what is taking place is abuse, and there are others who are absolutely powerless to do anything about it (Bellamy, Clark, Hamre-Nietupski, & Williams, 1977; Pettis & Hughes, 1985). The compromised status of people with disabilities becomes more insidious when one realizes that many segments of the so-called normal community, which include the police, judiciary, family, and friends, frequently consider people with disabilities to be incompetent witnesses. Thus, when many victims report the fact that they have been abused, they are seldom believed because they are seen to lack legitimacy. Those with disabilities are vulnerable at all stages of their lives and their vulnerability tends to increase with age. Only 20% of the cases involving abuse of individuals with disabilities are ever reported to the police or any other authority (Sobsey, 1988).

The Consequences of Victimization

Lenore Walker uses the term *learned helplessness* to describe why women are at best reluctant to leave an abusive situation. The term, as originally defined by Seligman (1975), illustrated that nondisabled women are very reluctant to leave abusive situations because of the social, economic, and psychological consequences of losing a spouse or familial support or both. Victims, including individuals with disabilities, are prone to remain in abusive situations for a variety of factors. Blaming the victim is a generally perceived phenomenon that maintains that the victim invited the abuse, intentionally or unintentionally. Members of the judiciary have commented that female victims, including females with disabilities, were partially responsible for their abuse because they dressed in an inappropriate manner or visited bars or male residential premises at inappropriate times. One must reflect on the legitimacy of blaming the victim in view of the fact that many members of the judiciary perceive diminished responsibility on the part of the perpetrator and illustrate tendencies to pass minimum sentences. The length and severity of the penalties illustrate the lack of credibility and the image that women, particularly women with disabilities, are accorded when they attempt to obtain justice from the courts. Many victims of sexual violence often believe that it is inappropriate and often impossible for them to obtain legal redress and hence are deterred from seeking the intervention and protection of the courts (Bauer, 1983; Lerner & Simmons, 1966).

Some victims of sexual violence feel that they are in a position of learned helplessness (Gunn, 1989). Being the most powerless, they believe that it becomes inappropriate or dangerous to seek justice. The process of seeking justice involves "coming out of the closet"—self-identification as a victim—and exposure to the wrath of family or others. This attack on the self-esteem of the victims acts as a further deterrent to their protection.

One major characteristic that serves to insulate perpetrators of sexual violence is the fact that they often represent positions of power and prestige. These abusers take advantage of their positions of power when they exploit the most vulnerable—those with disabilities—by rationalizing that they are doing the victim a favor because no one else would be sexually interested in her or him. Husbands, male acquaintances, and other individuals are often prone to be the abuser because they believe that the victim will seldom divulge the event because of the stigmatizing implications. Power, shame, and stigma insulate abusers from the social, legal, and moral responsibilities.

Forms of Abuse

There are many forms of abuse experienced by victims. These include verbal abuse, physical abuse, unwanted physical contact, rape, incest, and, in some instances, sterilization. Individuals with cerebral palsy, Down syndrome, and a variety of other conditions were often sterilized as a matter of routine (Adam & Gudalefsky, 1986; Chakraborti, 1987). These policies reflected the science of eugenics not to mention the fact that people with disabilities were often denied legitimate opportunity for sexual expression.

Alleviating the Sexual Abuse of Victims and Its Implications

The social science of victimology is only in its infant stages. The rights and opportunities of redress for those who have been victims of sexual violence are often compromised.

Beginning in the 1970s, the philosophy evolved that nondisabled victims of sexual violence and those with disabilities had to be believed when they had the courage to identify their abusers. This idea was encouraged by the development and influence of women's liberation groups, women's rights advocates, and the medical and paramedical establishments. This philosophy instilled a widespread belief that victims of abuse should always convey the truth. The legal, social work, psychology, and psychiatry professions are now establishing factors that ought to be considered when analyzing the credibility of victims. A current concern is the false memory syndrome. Many authorities have established that in some cases, victims may believe abuse has taken place when it in fact has not. According to experts on the false memory syndrome, therapists and others may implant ideas in vulnerable people, consequently engendering the belief that they have been victims (Ames & Boyle, 1980). It has been established that many victims of incest and other forms of sexual violence understandably repress these experiences. Some recall these experiences decades after the abuse. Abusers now have another form of defense in their arsenal of protection. It is sometimes impossible to establish whether or not an individual has been a victim, and the false memory syndrome can be used to attack the victim's credibility (Adler, 1986).

The women's liberation movement has been instrumental in motivating large segments of the female population, including persons with disabilities, to advocate for their rights and protection. The women's movement has been accused of ignoring the rights of women of color and women with disabilities. It appears that most women's rights groups are in the process of genuinely attempting to include the demands of the population consisting of females with disabilities. In the United States and Canada, a movement has been established that can be defined as a network for women with disabilities. These groups state that they are still considered to be marginal in the mainstream women's movement but believe it is mandatory for them to establish their separate presence in order to advocate for the rights of women with disabilities.

The recognition of family violence and sexual violence has become prominent in the past four decades. The evolution of the gender movement, expanding civil rights legislation, and the adoption of the Americans with Disabilities Act (1990) in the United States creates a social psychological mandate for the protection of all groups. On an individual basis, however, it becomes increasingly difficult for people to seek redress for their victimization. In the past, native people across North America were institutionalized in residential schools where all patterns of sexual perversion were widely practiced by employees of church-related institutions. It was not until the late 1980s that their victimization was acknowledged and investigated by the mass media, the judiciary, and other governmental realms. Similarly, orphans and juvenile inmates were often victimized during their period of institutionalization, confinement, or imprisonment.

Individuals who were victims of sexual abuse in institutional environments believed that they could not trust anyone—teachers, family, clerics, doctors, and, in fact, any other caregiver or individual in a position of authority. Because of this lack of trust, many victims encountered difficulty in obtaining education and employment. The majority of individuals who experienced institutional abuse tend to be unemployed. Many of these persons are unlikely to receive education, counseling, and support that would qualify them for positions in a technologically advanced society. Victims of sexual abuse often possess poor interpersonal skills and subsequently experience many forms of family pathology. However, the resources necessary to formulate strategies and organizations to mainstream these victims are seldom in place. Some victims of institutional abuse are now receiving financial compensation but this seldom benefits those who have been victims of sexual abuse.

The foregoing discussion has illustrated the fact that sexual victimization is widespread. One can begin to address quality of life issues in analyzing the reactions of people to the violence that they have encountered.

Sexual abuse in all its forms has only recently entered the public arena. On the one hand, the public and the judiciary profess to be shocked and outraged by the practice of sexual abuse, especially by those in positions of trust. On the other hand, the judiciary gives expressions of outrage that are subsequently manifested in very light sentences. In fact, seldom are maximum sentences imposed on the transgressors, and in most instances minimum sentences and probation tend to be the standard patterns of sentencing. This practice conveys to victims of sexual abuse that they are not protected by society (Harris, 1990).

Quality of Life and
Victims of Sexual Abuse

Quality of life is defined, for the purpose of this text, as a matter of degree rather than as an absolute. Quality of life, to be understood in personal terms, must be evaluated and illustrated in terms of how the individuals who have experienced this victimization subsequently adjust. Some victims are able, through processes of restitution and counseling, to alleviate the consequences of their victimization, but others demonstrate varying degrees of stress and shattering of personal esteem and identity (Goffman, 1963). They become, in Goffman's term, *stigmatized*. In publicly identifying their victimization through efforts of seeking counseling and redress, many of these victims are assaulted by their perpetrators for having the audacity to charge so-called well-meaning caregivers with sexual abuse. Many are unable to shed the consequences of their victimization. Some, in addition to their disability, are stigmatized as possessing psychiatric problems signifying their ineptitude. In a Marxian sense, people who have experienced sexual violence demonstrate varying degrees of alienation. They find themselves to be occupants of marginal status positions. For many of these individuals, living becomes characterized by anomie because, for the duration of their lives, they encounter difficulties in normal functioning (i.e., they have learned never to trust anyone).

Applications to Sexual Abuse

As stated, quality of life is not an absolute and therefore it is possible, by gauging patterns of adaptation of those who have experienced abuse, to recognize their patterns of adjustment. Many individuals are able to overcome the experience and live normal or near-normal lives. There are others who are unable to overcome the social, physical, and psychological consequences of their abuse. It must be acknowledged that many of the difficulties that were accrued to the individuals with disabilities were not only consequences of the abuse but also consequences of their physical disability. Conceptually, it is difficult to illustrate the precise consequences of sexual abuse. Ongoing research locating individuals with similar backgrounds, status, and disabilities may shed light on the uniformity of adaptation illustrated by those who have experienced the described patterns of abuse. Preliminary analysis of the data illustrates several patterns of adjustment by individuals who have experienced disability and various patterns of sexual violence.

Patterns of Adjustment

The first group, consisting of those abused by family members, claim to have never disclosed their abuse to anyone else. Failure to disclose was due to the stigma of being abused; fear of family dissolution; fear of exposing the perpetrator because of the economic, social, and psychological consequences; the stigma of being a victim; the shame and sense of alienation of not being protected by their families (e.g., siblings, mothers, and other family members); and the resulting lack of self-esteem. These individuals had never belonged to support groups. Four individuals belonged to organizations for the blind, paraplegics, those with cerebral palsy, and those with multiple sclerosis. They belonged to these organizations only to seek information regarding their specific disability and in no instance did they discuss the abuse to which they were subjected. These persons claimed that as long as nobody knew, their life would be as acceptable as possible. These victims of sexual abuse would not identify their abusers because of the fear of personal costs. Despite evolving societal philosophy, they feared any stigma resulting from identification to expose victimization and deal with the perpetrators. The possible ramifications of exposure were perceived as further victimization and a threat of their quality of life. Four of the individuals who had experienced sexual abuse maintained that they would never identify their family members who were the perpetrators because, in all likelihood, there would be social, economic, and psychological costs as a result of being separated from their families.

A second distinct group are individuals with disabilities who have been victimized by individuals outside their families. These victims typically report their abuse to their parents. Parents are becoming advocates for their children and are encouraging them to seek compensation for their victimization. They advocate prosecuting and penalizing the offenders. Two of the interviewees who belonged to this group feared that outside relatives would take matters into their own hands in a violent way. Other parents refused to discuss the assault and pressured their children never to discuss the issues because it "will only cause trouble." Victimized children tend to be very reliant on their parents but experience anomie when their parents demonstrate reluctance to effectively manage the ramifications of abuse. The individuals in this group had been subject to abuse within the previous 4 years and were very much aware that the abuse was a significant problem not only for nondisabled people but for people with disabilities as well. They all desired legal intervention but were sometimes reluctant to pursue legal options because of the expense and because court penalties were deemed trivial. The people with disabilities in this category assumed that their experiences with regard to sexual abuse have been undermined in the eyes of the authorities by the fact that they happen to have a disability. For these individuals, pursuing action was seen as a costly pursuit because not only would they suffer the effects of public exposure but their credibility would have been questioned.

A third group of individuals, be they able-bodied or individuals with disabilities, attempt to deal with their abuse many years after the event. They identify their victimization with the encouragement of support groups and

the evolvement of societal philosophy, which maintains that it is advanta-
geous for individuals to cope with their abuse even decades after the event.
Many discover that they can benefit from professionals, family members,
and others. Six individuals who were interviewed in this category, however,
maintained that disclosures initiated unnecessary family discord. Their
credibility is often held in question as a consequence of factors associated
with the false memory syndrome. This is a source of much disappointment
because there are a multitude of anxieties associated with disclosure and the
complainant often discovers that his or her credibility and self-esteem are
trampled on by the abusers and by those who represent the abusers before
the courts.

A group of the abused population has evolved over the past two decades
that is very similar to the militants in black power organizations or the
militants in feminist groups who are bent on achieving self-esteem, self-respect,
power, and redress. These people are not stigmatized by their abused or
disabled status. As a consequence of their empowerment, they are now
striving to educate the public that sexual abuse of people with disabilities is
widespread and should be dealt with in a forthright manner. Not only are they
endeavoring to attain justice for themselves but they are encouraging others
to take charge of their lives, to accuse their abusers, and to attempt by
whatever means deemed necessary to obtain justice. Like their able-bodied
compatriots, a growing number of abused people across North America now
believe themselves to be members of a legitimate minority within a democratic society. The focus of all minorities within this democratic framework
is to achieve protection, integration, and acceptance. For these citizens,
obtaining justice is considered to be a right to which all people are entitled.

A fifth group can be described as people with disabilities who are totally
victimized by their interpretation of disabled status. These people have been
socialized to "know their place." According to one individual, "I must accept
anything and everything or they will put me out on the street." These persons
represent the classic illustration of learned helplessness because they believe
there is no viable strategy of obtaining justice, respect, safety, and fairness.
(The author received seven unsigned letters from individuals representing
this pattern detailing long patterns of sexual assault by family members and
institutional staff.)

Another category that appears to be similar to a previous group are those
who were abused in the past and recalled it years after the event. Their
victimization was so severe that they totally repressed their negative experiences for periods of time ranging from 7 to 55 years. As a consequence of a
multitude of triggering events (including marriage, dating, sexual activities,
the reading of a book, the viewing of a program or movie, meeting the abuser,

or a combination of these), the subject recalled his or her abuse. This group included four females and one male. In analyzing their difficulties, they maintained that their problems in all phases of living were probably related to the fact that they had experienced severe sexual abuse characterized by physical and psychological torture. One victim, in seeking justice, subsequently brought charges against his perpetrator and was accused in court of being a victim of the false memory syndrome. The supposed perpetrator maintained that not only was the victim alienated and isolated as a consequence of being disabled but the victim brought forth the action because he genuinely believed that the abuse had taken place despite the fact that it had not. The accused expressed sympathy for the victim. The case was dropped. Cases of this nature pressure all those who have experienced these patterns of violence to refrain from actions designed to obtain reparation.

Another group represents individuals who are able to live normal or near-normal lives despite the abuse they have experienced. "You have to put it behind you. You have no choice," was the response of a 38-year-old woman, married with three children and affected by cerebral palsy. She conveyed the fact that she was the victim of incest for over 14 years. After she left home and graduated from a university, she was fortunate to have been surrounded by supportive friends and a particular religious group. They provided acceptance and the social support that allowed her to change her self-concept. In fact, this woman became a resolute and outspoken individual. She maintains that her most difficult episodes stem from the fact that at various times, for no apparent reason, she continues to experience flashbacks of the abuse to which she was subjected. She stated,

> I cannot explain why, but in class, in church, at weddings and even once when I was bathing my own child, I had the flashback. It always affects me, but now I know I have a wonderful life. I cannot afford to dwell on the past.

On reviewing the data, one dramatic factor was revealed. All of the participants, for reasons they could not identify, experienced flashbacks. These flashbacks occurred at all times. One articulate woman, 24 years after her abuse, maintained that at her wedding, at the birth of all of her children, at funerals, at New Year's Eve parties, in the middle of the night, and indeed at all times, she experienced the flashbacks. They would come at moments of depression and at moments of joy.

Many victims find that it is difficult to come to terms with their past abuse. They know they should not feel responsible, but the majority of them express some feelings of culpability. Many victims express the belief that no one can really be relied on. The woman just described, having been married for 20 years, still feels anxiety when her husband comes home late, believing that he may be having an affair. She admitted to the researcher that there were no grounds for this belief because her husband has never done anything to indicate unfaithfulness. The problem stemmed from her childhood experiences. She learned never to trust anybody and this feeling still persists. This individual obviously indicates the capacity to live a successful life but still experiences the psychological trauma of being a victim. As she stated, when you have been victimized and you reflect on its consequences, it is like constantly experiencing the death of a loved one. The other participants in this study also revealed ongoing dissonance. Their capacity to develop relationships, undertake responsibility, and accept others was damaged by their being victims of abuse.

These case studies were illustrated to demonstrate the effect of sexual abuse on victims. Victims traditionally seek empathy, support, and justice. Inevitably in their search, they become angry, disenchanted, and disappointed because their legitimate identities are called into question and occasionally ridiculed.

Many of the victims claimed it was difficult to establish rapport with counselors, be they social workers, psychologists, sexual abuse specialists, family physicians, or psychotherapists. They indicated that they believed these professionals were competent but were unable to relate to them the extreme personal crisis they experienced as victims of sexual assault. Seven individuals became disillusioned with the counseling process and subsequently dealt with their problems without professional assistance. Most of the others continued with the counseling. Nine individuals indicated that they might have adjusted in a shorter period of time if they had had access to counselors who were more cognizant of the consequences of their abuse. Many of these victims claimed they would have liked to have seen different counselors but that would have caused them more anxieties because many counselors are inclined to assume stewardship of their clients.

A new thrust in counseling has been in the area of complementarity. Complementarity requires that counselors and clients have to be matched not only by the traditional factors of professionalism but also by interpersonal factors that establish a positive and trusting relationship between therapist and client.

Conclusion

In promoting health and quality-equality of life, professionals seek to maximize adjustment. Some individuals who have experienced sexual abuse, whether or not they have disabilities, are able to get on with their lives and do not allow the experience to dramatically affect their well-being. Others who have experienced similar trauma encounter ongoing difficulties that have continuing and long-range effects on their lives. Thus, many victims are reluctant to pursue justice and experience ongoing personal problems. In many cases, the best professional interventions are not entirely productive, but some do receive support and encouragement from professionals and others with whom they interact.

Sexual violence is any form of sexually related traumatic event. Sociologically, it has been illustrated that the value of sympathetic parents, peer groups, and support groups of all kinds is immeasurable in motivating victims to adjust. Despite the intervention of professionals and well-meaning others, it is often difficult for victims to respond in a positive manner. Negative responses include the emergence and growth of psychiatric disorders; substance abuse; a distrust of others, particularly those in positions of authority and power; a distrust of the opposite sex; aggressive tendencies toward others; and last, suicide.

Many victims, particularly those who have experienced this form of violence at a young age within an institutional environment, demonstrate ongoing difficulties with regard to the acquisition of education, employment, and the ability to establish permanent relationships. Thus, their adjustment patterns can be best described in terms of Merton's (1967) depiction of anomie, which conveys isolation, alienation, and meaninglessness.

There is a widespread belief that society abhors sexual violence in any form. Sometimes there is the inclination to believe that this abhorrence is more a myth than a reality. If one surveys the penalties imposed by the judiciary on perpetrators of sexual violence against people without disabilities as well as the disabled survivors of sexual abuse, one discovers the rarity of the imposition of maximum sentences. Hence, victims are becoming reluctant to pursue their perpetrators in the courts of law.

In the fall of 1994, Richard Sobsey published an eloquent work titled *Violence and Abuse in the Lives of People With Disabilities: The End of Silent Acceptance?* The question mark indicates a number of concerns outlined in the preceding analysis. As one survivor maintained, "Having been sexually abused is like having terminal cancer. It always affects you and it will affect you until the end." All of the respondents maintained that they often reflect on the abuse, and, hence, the abuse colors their adaptation to society.

15

The Quality of Life
of Marginal Citizens

Homelessness

Ivan Brown

It has often been said in recent years that a society can be judged by the way it treats its marginal citizens. Current Western values, at least, support the notion that all citizens of societies, regardless of their ability to contribute to their societies, have the right to have access to the resources that provide the basic necessities of life. But values held by societies vary in their degree of strength and are not always equally held across societies. To the extent, then, that this particular value is actually held strongly within Western societies and to the extent that it is equally held across those societies, treatment of marginal citizens is one important measuring stick we can use to evaluate societies as a whole.

Most modern societies make explicit in their formal laws, their literatures, and in the ways they organize their social institutions what subgroups they consider to comprise their marginal citizens. In general, these are people who have tried but failed to attain the dominant way of life practiced by most people, people who make no attempt to attain this way of life despite apparent ability to do so, or people who do not (apparently) have the ability to attain this way of life. Marginal people are those who do not contribute to the dominant way of life of a society, or they are those who do contribute but the cost of such contribution exceeds the contributions they make. People with a wide variety of disabilities, people with both acute and chronic health problems that arise from lifestyle factors (e.g., alcoholism, drug use, sexual activity, and poverty), and people who live in ways that differ from the vast majority are usually described as marginal citizens.

The question of whether or not modern societies should even be thinking in terms of marginal citizens has been raised. For example, Rioux (this volume) has argued that because all societies have some citizens who do not or cannot meet general standards on their own, it should be a given that societies' roles include providing the necessary supports and access to resources that enable such people to lead the types of lives that are best for them within their general cultures and that such lives should be readily accepted as part of what a society is all about. This is a view that appears to be gaining acceptance both in theory and research (e.g., Goode, 1994a) and in practice (e.g., Brown, 1994; Schalock, 1994b). Despite these recent changes in our thinking, though, the fact remains that we do still think in terms of marginal citizens within our societies, and it seems unlikely that this will change without some rather lengthy transition period. Thus the concept of marginal citizens, although perhaps not desirable in the long term, is still viable in the short term.

The fields of rehabilitation and health promotion focus on broader issues than just marginal people, but both include within the issues they address the physical, psychological, and social well-being of marginal people. The general goal of rehabilitation is to work to support quality within the lives of all people (Johnson & Jaffe, 1989), and that of health promotion is to enable people to take charge of and improve their lives, especially as it relates to their physical, emotional, and social well-being (Epp, 1986; World Health Organization, 1986). Jointly, these two fields appear to represent a good venue within which to examine and promote quality within the lives of marginal people.

Marginal people are not a homogeneous group, and as such, it has often been considered difficult to address marginality in general except in broad conceptual terms or at the macro-level of analysis (Jones, Levine, & Rosenberg, 1991). For this reason, marginal peoples are often placed into subcategories for ease in studying and analyzing specific issues and problems. This practice has the advantage of containing the issues in question to a manageable size but often results in separate analyses of the various subgroups. This is somewhat unfortunate, for the analyses of subgroups of marginal peoples are seldom connected, even though it seems evident that many of the problems that underlie how we treat marginal citizens are common across subgroups. Thus in this chapter, I will focus on homelessness with a view to identifying some conceptual and practical problems the fields of rehabilitation and health promotion encounter when they attempt to improve quality within the lives of people who are homeless, but such problems pertain very much to other groups of marginal people as well.

What Is Homelessness?

An important conceptual distinction that needs to be made in the vast literature on homelessness is between *home*lessness and *house*lessness (Momeni, 1990). To be houseless is simply not to have a place of dwelling, whereas to be homeless entails not being in a place that is considered to be "home." A person who is temporarily or permanently houseless may feel homeless or may not feel homeless at all; both of these conditions have been described very clearly by a great many authors among so-called street people (e.g., O'Reilly-Fleming, 1993). Conversely, a person could be homeless even though he has a house in which to dwell, such as living in a city or country where there is almost no social or cultural integration (see Table 15.1).

Homelessness is a broader concept than houselessness but it is somewhat different and may or may not subsume it. Despite this, the term *homeless* is commonly used in the literature to describe either homelessness or house-lessness or both. More than that, the term is often used to describe people who do not have permanent homes (e.g., Sahlin, 1992), people who use temporary shelters (e.g., Timmer, 1988), or simply people who are inade-quately housed (e.g., Kearns, Smith, & Abbott, 1991). These usages appear to represent various degrees of houselessness and perhaps homelessness. The lack of a clear distinction in conceptualizing and using terms has resulted in some confusion within the overall literature because the implications for policy development, resource allocation, and service delivery are clearly different for various degrees of houselessness than they are for homelessness. Such distinctions are valuable when addressing policy and pragmatic issues that relate to individual people or groups of individuals, and because almost all of the literature on homelessness does address these issues, it seems important to provide clear conceptualizations and to promote their use.

There is a broader view of homelessness, however. It is rooted in the ancient notions of tribal identity, cultural tradition, and integration within the environment in which one lives that are inherent to the human condition (Morris, 1967) and considers how these are played out in the context of the ever-changing present (Morris, 1971). Baudelaire's comment that "moder-

TABLE 15.1 Conceptual Distinction Between Houselessness and Homelessness

	Homed	*Homeless*
Housed	Having a dwelling place that is considered home	Having a dwelling place that is not considered home
Houseless	Not having a dwelling place but being in a place that is considered home	Not having a dwelling place and being in a place that is not considered home

nity is the transient, the fleeting, the contingent; it is one half of art, the other being the eternal and the immovable" (quoted in Ignatieff, 1984, p. 135) illustrates that considerations of this kind are neither recent nor new to human thinking. Still, they are always new in the sense that the modernity, because it is fleeting by nature, keeps changing.

In our current modernity, a large, powerful, but impersonal public structure has assumed that it can see to most human needs. Seemingly contrary to its intentions, however, it has created a number of troublesome paradoxes (Ignatieff, 1984). Ignatieff claimed, for example, that this public structure promotes freedom of individual choice, but to equalize people's opportunities to put their choices into effect, agents of the state (experts) need to advocate on behalf of individuals' choices, thereby alienating people from their own choices. Similarly, sharing of state resources among all citizens is promoted, but because social solidarity is not supported by such sharing, competition is actually encouraged. These and other forces work within our current modernity to alienate people, moving them away from a sense of identity, integration, tradition, and social belonging and resulting in a psychological homelessness for individuals and in a cultural or moral homelessness in a broader sense (Ignatieff, 1984).

Such homelessness is often camouflaged by constant innovation and motion. It may even be invisible, in many cases, because we claim to value both innovation and motion. But moving frenetically from one innovative experience to another leaves little time or energy to integrate one's own human needs. Indeed, one of the very functions of such movement is to enable one to enjoy activities without having to integrate one's own human needs. But the resulting enjoyment is hollow because not being connected solidly to tradition, to others, or to the environment, it has little or no intrinsic substance. In turn, it becomes all the more difficult to integrate such experiences with one's own human needs. One has only to move on to new innovative experiences, and thus the cycle is perpetuated.

It is within this context that many people become homeless in our modernity, and it is within this context that homelessness is perpetuated for many people. To be housed without addressing the human needs associated with social interaction, connection with one's cultural past and present, or feelings of belonging within one's environment is to ensure that homelessness will persist. This has been widely recognized in the literature, perhaps not explicitly, but numerous policies and programs have been developed and implemented that address specific factors related to interconnection and homelessness. These include substance use (e.g., Linn, Gelberg, & Leake, 1990), crime (e.g., McCarthy & Hagan, 1991), psychiatric disorders (e.g., Rife, First, Greenlee, Miller, & Feichter, 1991), health problems (e.g., Institute of Medicine, 1988), poverty (e.g., O'Reilly-Fleming, 1993), alienated youth (e.g., Hier, Korboot, & Schweitzer, 1990), and others.

These efforts, however, overwhelmingly support the medical and social problem approaches to homelessness. That is, they view being homeless as the fault and responsibility of the homeless person and homelessness as a social problem that can be redressed and that needs to be dealt with by eradicating the problem in the most expedient way. The view that homelessness may arise because of forces within our sociopolitical structure and that systemic structural and attitudinal changes are the best way to include people who are homeless is only beginning to emerge (see Rioux, this volume). If the latter view has more merit than the former, then there may be little value in studying factors associated with homelessness and designing programs that address these factors because the answers lie within our own attitudes toward homelessness and within the functioning of our economic and sociopolitical systems, not within the people themselves (van Vliet, 1989).

All this suggests that the meaning of homelessness as a concept is embedded within the social context where it is used. Homelessness exists primarily because, and to the extent that, we place social value on all people having a place of residence and on feeling at home where we live. It also exists because, and to the extent that, we are willing to tolerate variation and divergence from the norm of being housed and homed. The nuances of these social values change over time and vary from one culture or subculture to another, and in turn, the meaning of homelessness itself changes. The danger in assuming that other social contexts attach the same meaning to homelessness as we do is apparent enough, but there is also danger in changing its meaning because such changes may not be supported by other people within other social contexts. On the other hand, there is danger in underrating the meaning of homelessness because, in so doing, we may very well overlook or underestimate a social inequity that could be redressed.

Homelessness and Quality of Life

No matter how homelessness has been conceptualized or which approach has been taken toward it, there can be little doubt from the literature that there has been a considerable commitment to deal with homelessness over the past several decades (Burt & Cohen, 1989) and that the overall intent of these efforts has been to enable people to lead better lives, lives that have more quality. Despite these efforts and their intent, the number of people who are considered to be homeless, in North America at least, appears to have risen rather dramatically in recent years (Milburn & D'Ercole, 1991). For this reason, it does not seem likely that attention to homelessness will diminish in the near future. If quality is to be enhanced in the lives of people who are homeless, however, a number of conceptual and practical problems need first to be taken into account. Four such problems are raised in the subsections that follow and are summarized in Table 15.2. They are purposely ordered for they move from basic to more general, and thus they might be thought of as levels at which to think. It is not the contention here that these four are exhaustive but, rather, that focus needs to be placed on at least these and perhaps others.

WHAT ASSUMPTIONS UNDERLIE "QUALITY" OF LIFE?

By its very definition and popular usage, the word *quality* means the degree to which something is excellent. But it is also a description of something that is excellent. When we use the phrase "quality of life," we generally refer to the degree to which life has achieved excellence or the degree to which life can be considered to be a quality (excellent) life.

Quality within one's life is moveable rather than fixed at any one point in time. There is a generally held underlying assumption that, given choice, people will want to move the quality of their lives toward quality (excellence) rather than toward nonquality. There is also an assumption that such movement toward attaining and maintaining a quality life is something that is possible for all people. Both these assumptions are based on the broader assumption that having a quality life is a good thing, something worth striving for. These assumptions are in keeping with the general thrust of the social indicators movement but need to be made explicit in rehabilitation and health promotion programs that endeavor to improve the quality of people's lives because they may or may not be held by individual people whose lives we are attempting to improve. For example, a person who is homeless may

TABLE 15.2 Conceptual Levels and Practical Actions in Improving Quality of
Life for Individuals and Groups of People Who Are Homeless

Conceptual Level	Practical Action
The approach to "quality" in life	Determine the assumptions relating to the phrase "improving quality" by asking, Is quality a good thing worth striving for? Is movement toward better quality wanted? Is movement toward better quality thought to be possible?
Personal meaning of "quality" in life	Determine the meaning attached to the word *quality* as it relates to overall life by asking, What things are highly valued for their ability to contribute to quality or excellence in life?
Personal choice	Determine the degree to which personal choices reflect the personal value system and thus improve quality by asking, Do the personal choices result in behaviors that are in keeping with what is valued? Determine the degree to which personal choices will be permitted to improve quality by asking, Do they cause harm to self or others? Do they enhance quality from the point of view of others in the environment?
Acceptance of marginality	Determine the degree to which potential improvements in quality are accepted as part of the makeup of the general society by asking, To what degree, and how, are marginal people set apart? To what extent do the criteria for determining quality for marginal people overlap with similar criteria for the general population? How clear are the criteria for determining quality, both for marginal people and for the general population? What structural barriers need to be reshaped to promote inclusion?

not want his life to be better and may not consider that having a quality life
is a good thing or something worth striving for. Such assumptions may need
to be re-examined or transformed for some individuals or groups of individuals. A first crucial step when attempting to improve quality within the lives

of people who are homeless is to consider and respect their individual and group assumptions regarding the phrase "improving quality" itself.

PERSONAL MEANING OF "QUALITY" IN LIFE

When we use the phrase "quality of life," the question of what constitutes quality or excellence arises. Quality is ultimately a judgment that derives from current social-cultural and personal values applied to opportunities that are available in people's living environments. Because of this, the meaning of quality differs from culture to culture within human life, from subculture to subculture within cultures, and from person to person within subcultures. What constitutes quality cannot be precisely described because it is constituted by whatever is deemed to be excellent by particular people who hold particular values and who live in particular circumstances. Consequently, the phrase "quality of life" cannot be precisely described because it is whatever is considered to be quality by people applied to the lives that they are living.

What can be said, though, is that there are no doubt cultural, subcultural, and individual influences on the understanding and interpretation of both quality and quality of life. Moreover, both for people in the general culture and for such marginalized people as those who are homeless, the relative importance of these three influences differs from person to person. For some homeless people, individual influences may be particularly strong, whereas for others, cultural and subcultural influences may be more important.

In any consideration of improving quality within the lives of people who are homeless, the meaning of quality or excellence needs to be established in conjunction with the environmental opportunities and the personal and social values that contribute to that meaning. In addition, the relative importance of the cultural, subcultural, and individual influences needs to be determined.

PERSONAL CHOICE

Personal choices, presumably, are made within the context of the set of values that are currently held by individuals. Personal choices do not always make sense in terms of the sets of values held by others but are in keeping with those of the person. If a choice feels right to a person, it probably is right in terms of the set of values he or she holds. Thus those choices represent what, on balance, are in the best interests of the person.

To the extent that this analysis is valid, a rationale can be set out for why personal choice must always be respected. Personal choice that individuals consider to be improving their lives represents improvement within the contexts of their own assumptions toward quality, their own meanings of quality, and their own value structures.

An interesting issue that arises from personal choice with regard to behaviors is the degree to which they are in accordance with personal value systems. All people, but especially those who are homeless, may choose behaviors that are not at all in keeping with their own value systems but do them anyway because of the benefits they entail. Spending a night in a shelter with strangers on a cold night and having to take a shower before a free meal is served are simple examples but there are many others. Here, behavior that is in keeping with the value system (what the individual would do if given real, or unfettered, choice) is forsworn for other behavior that brings with it immediate benefits. People who are homeless probably vary considerably in the degree to which their behaviors reflect their actual value systems, and thus this degree is likely to be best assessed at the individual level.

Another issue concerned with respecting personal choice is the degree to which it can be permitted at all. All nations set limits on behavior and enact laws to describe in detail those that are not permitted, such as theft, assault, kidnaping, and murder. In a less formal way, all cultures devalue other behaviors by frowning on them. For example, taking a bus seat before an elderly person has an opportunity to do so does not contravene any law in most regions but it is usually frowned on as a devalued behavior. Illegal or devalued activities may be very much in keeping with an individual's personal value system and may, in fact, improve the quality of that person's life but they are still not permitted as acceptable.

Within the social and health services fields of most Western nations, it has become customary to think that individually motivated behavior is accept-able if it does not bring harm to the self or others, but that it is unacceptable if it does result in such harm. The idea here, then, is that a personal choice can be considered acceptable, and thus respected, even if it does not work toward what others think of as improvement; however, it cannot be consid-ered acceptable, and thus cannot be respected, if it brings with it harm of any kind, even if it does work toward what the person thinks of as improvement.

The result of this thinking is that many behaviors that arise from personal choice are thought of as not constructive but still allowed and others are simply not allowed, whether they are constructive to the person or not.

This guideline, though not without obvious problems, seems simple enough to follow but it can result in dilemma. Take, for example, a woman who is homeless, is apparently physically healthy, but who chooses to take little nourishment other than doughnuts and coffee. Her behavior is not harming others and it is not readily apparent that it is harmful to her. Should her choice be respected or not? Another example is a man who is homeless and washes very infrequently. Does the odor that results from his not washing constitute harm to self or to others? Does the fact that few people associate closely with him because of his odor constitute harm to self? Answers to these kinds of questions are not easy and probably need to be made at the individual level, after social and personal values have been weighed carefully.

The larger issue, though, is that if personal choices are truly in keeping with people's approaches to quality and truly represent the movement toward quality or nonquality that is in keeping with their own views and values, then such choices should clearly result in better quality in their lives as they see it. On the other hand, it is difficult if not impossible for most of us to think how harmful, illegal, or self-destructive behavior can be quality-enhancing. If we are correct in assuming that these behaviors are in fact not quality enhancing, then the difficulty lies in individuals' assumptions about quality and the meanings they attach to it based on their own social values and the environments in which they live. Personal choices based on assumptions that quality is not worthwhile and not possible result in behaviors that do not contribute to quality. Personal choices based on meanings attached to quality that relate harm to self or others result in behaviors that bring harm to others. For example, if quality means defying social conventions to the extreme—as it does for some people—harm may be brought to the self by not attending to nutrition, shelter, and other things; if quality means finding joy in committing illegal acts—as it does for others—harm may be brought to others by cheating, robbing, or more serious acts. Thus, although personal choice is quality enhancing in the sense that it supports personal views and values, it is not always quality enhancing, from the point of view of other people, to the very person who is exercising it or to other people in the environment.

Who should decide whether or not personal choices are quality enhancing and, if so, the extent to which they may be, are difficult questions. However the questions are answered and however decisions are made about whether or not to permit behavior that results from personal choices, it seems essential that if professionals in rehabilitation and health promotion wish to improve the quality of life of people who are homeless, they first need to consider the degree to which personal choices are in keeping with an individual's own value system and the degree to which personal choices enhance quality within the individual's life. They then need to weigh carefully the extent to which behaviors that result from personal choices can be respected and permitted.

ACCEPTANCE OF MARGINALITY

A fourth key conceptual-practical problem in homelessness is the degree to which marginality in its many forms is accepted within the general society as part of that society's own makeup. The issue here for people who are homeless is, even if they want to make personal choices to improve the quality of their lives (as they see it) and are permitted to do so, whether any changes they make to that quality are considered by the social environment in which they live to form a part of that environment. If they are not, the incentive for making such changes may be substantially lessened.

People who do not or cannot contribute significantly to the dominant ways of life of a society have been treated in a variety of ways in the past, including being set apart and valued as special and even magical (Brown, in press), being devalued through derision and institutionalization, and being included as one sector of the makeup of the culture's population.

Being set apart, whether in a valued or a nonvalued way, suggests that marginal people are not accepted as part of the makeup of a society but, rather, are thought of as outside of it. In institutionalization, one formal way of setting marginal people apart, the intent seemed on the surface to be honorable; that is, people were said to be housed apart for their own well-being. In fact, strong exclusion (setting apart) may well make improving quality within the lives of those set apart easier to achieve because the criteria for doing so can be clearly laid out and followed. The difficulty with housing apart as a method of improving people's lives, though, is that these criteria that are used to determine what constitutes a "good life," and hence the permissibility of the behaviors of those people set apart, are almost always different from the criteria used for the general population. The general social-cultural values that determine what constitutes quality are not fully accessible to those who do not live within it and contribute to it.

Homeless people may be physically situated in our midst but they are very often set apart socially, psychologically, and morally. This setting apart is typically accomplished within the context of the anonymity that exists in most large urban centers where homeless people often congregate. Hence it becomes okay for people who are homeless to use a bus shelter as a lodging, to wear the same clothes for many months, and to pull all their life belongings around in a cart when they are already set apart either formally or informally.

On the other hand, these things are not okay for people who are included as part of the very makeup of a society because they are not okay for those who are doing the judging. In other words, when marginal people are thought of as being included within the makeup of the general society, there is an overlap in the criteria that are used to judge what quality is and what behaviors work toward quality. Here, quality for marginal people is still different but not so different.

Inclusion, then, tolerates difference, but it goes beyond that. It tolerates difference within some general criteria that are used for all people within the society and, because these are general, they are based naturally on the common needs of human beings in most cultures. Thus, where marginal people are included in the makeup of a society, there is concern that the basic necessities of life are available and accessible and that the physical, psychological, and social well-being of marginal people is being addressed. There is also concern that these things are occurring according to the same standards for all people. Thus where homeless people are included, there is a general understanding and acceptance that they have the same physical, psychological, social, and basic life needs that we all do and that these needs are met in ways that are not dissimilar to those used by all others in the society.

Within Western nations, to varying degrees, there has been movement in recent years toward acceptance of the philosophy of inclusion. But many social structures that were put in place to improve quality within the lives of people who were set apart are still in operation and currently act as barriers to improving quality for those who are included. For this reason, if we are to adopt and follow the philosophy of inclusion, we need to reshape the social structures that function as barriers to it in a timely manner. By doing so, we should make improving quality much more accessible to marginal people than it is at present.

Summary and Conclusion

It seems apparent that the problem of homelessness can be dealt with at the surface level by providing shelters, food, and a variety of programs but that these treat the symptoms rather than the roots of homelessness (van Vliet, 1989). The four conceptual-practical problems have been described in an attempt to try to understand some of the very basics of quality as it pertains to marginal people. There may well be other problems that have not been explored here that are of equal significance.

The overall goals of rehabilitation and health promotion speak to improving quality within various areas of the lives of all people, including those who are homeless. But if quality is to be improved within the lives of people who are homeless, these disciplines need to have a firm understanding of whether improving quality is seen as a good thing, what is meant by quality for individuals who are homeless, to what degree their personal choices can lead to quality, and to what degree their behavior is included as part of the overall makeup of the society in which they live.

PART

IV

B: ABILITIES AND DISABILITIES

16

Communication Disorders

Just Minor Inconveniences?

Bernard M. O'Keefe

You all know people like Tom. He had a stroke about 4 months ago, but everyone pretty much agrees that Tom is doing pretty well. He's walking now without his cane. The headaches are gone. Sure, he has trouble finding some of the words he wants to use, and when he does speak, it's hard to tell what he's saying. Some of the words are slurred, and he can't seem to "get his mouth around" a few of them, but what's the big deal? Tom is retired; he has his family. So his life is pretty good, wouldn't you say? Well, maybe not.

Individuals like Tom who have severe (and even not-so-severe) communicative disabilities experience real limitations in their vocational, social, and cultural environments. The combination of difficulties in being understood plus the frequent unwillingness of communicative partners to fully interact can have a ruinous effect on the quality and consistency of in-the-world contacts, personal relationships, and the support received from others.

For many disabled people, communication problems are at the heart of their disablement and central to their personal struggle to learn to overcome their disabilities. This is true whether they are young or old, whether they are male or female, and whether they are disabled from birth or become disabled later in life. They are often left isolated, powerless, and dependent. They are deprived of important ways of expressing their individuality (Hawkridge, Vincent, & Hale, 1985, p. 3).

Invisible Barriers

Severe communicative disabilities hold a special frustration for those persons who experience them. All too often, people simply have no idea to what an extent the degree of enjoyment of many of life's meaningful activities can be restricted when people attend to the manner of speaking more than the message it carries. After all, speech and language are not merely practical tools. They are integral parts of our personal identities. They allow us to exhibit intelligence, modify our surroundings, and affirm our very existence in this world (Létourneau, 1993).

Communicative disabilities, like other disabilities, interfere with an individual's ability to interact with his or her environment, a critical determinant of the quality of life (cf. Wright, 1983). Consider the following scenario. It's a hot night and you'd like to order an ice cream cone at the local Baskin-Robbins store. There's a bit of a line, and everyone is anxious to get their double-scoop raspberry ripple or cherry cheesecake. You're just dying for a mint chocolate. But you know that when you order, your breathing will stop. Then your face will turn red, your head will move forward as your brow furrows and your eyes squint. Your lips will feel welded shut but you know that eventually you'll be able to produce a strangled "m—m-m____." And then you'll start all over again for the next part of the word. Will you get in that line and, come what may, order that cone?

That unsettling depiction makes it immediately apparent that communicative difficulties can most certainly restrict the degree to which one enjoys the important possibilities of life—that is, to participate successfully in those aspects of life that are important and possible. The reality is that all of the immediate environments in a person's life can be deleteriously affected by difficulties in communicating. This is important because the prospects for a good quality of life are intensified when the physical, social, and community aspects of a person's immediate environment encourage the creation and enjoyment of life's possibilities (see the Renwick & Brown chapter, this volume).

PHYSICAL SURROUNDINGS

Speech and language allow each of us a certain measure of control over the so-called concrete aspects of our home, school, and work environments.

It is important to most of us that these places be attractive, clean, safe, private (at least to a degree), and personalized. But what of the person in a nursing home with severe aphasia? Or the child with cerebral palsy who is nonspeaking? It can be difficult or even impossible for them to influence those around them to provide surroundings that meet their needs and desires.

COMMUNITY STANDARDS

Many people have experienced the need to have a little talk with a neighbor about some bothersome noise or for a chat with a canvasser about the value of the local neighborhood watch. But how does the person with advanced amyotrophic lateral sclerosis (ALS) (Lou Gehrig's disease) or spastic dysphonia (a condition that causes the voice to tremble and break uncontrollably) work effectively yet tactfully to ensure that the neighborhood is clean, attractive, safe, friendly, and accepting?

SERVICES AND RESOURCES

You may not think twice about calling the town office about a broken street light or the local hockey arena about junior programs. But what if you had severely hypernasal speech as a result of a cleft palate or were embarrassed because you weren't able to produce an *r* or *s* sound? You might just pass up those calls. People with severe communicative disabilities often do and consequently may suffer a diminution in the quality of their lives. They settle for less in the way of the community services and resources that are relevant and available to them. Health care, social services, educational opportunities, vocational training, leisure activities, recreational services—any or all of these may be affected because of difficulty in communicating.

SOCIOCULTURAL ENVIRONMENT

Perhaps the sociocultural area is the environment most negatively affected by communication disabilities. Many (even most) people are uncomfortable when interacting with individuals who have trouble expressing themselves verbally (Beukelman & Mirenda, 1992). It becomes more difficult to attain a desirable measure of enjoyment in life when consistently high-quality interactions are not available from those persons who are most important to us, people such as family members, roommates, neighbors, coworkers, and classmates. Likewise, the ability and opportunity for comfortable conversation with members of a religious organization, clerks, people of the same cultural or ethnic group, casual acquaintances, and even perfect strangers are important ingredients in a fully lived life.

Types of Communication Disorders

In general, communication disorders might be thought of as falling into the categories of speech, language, voice, and fluency.

> *Speech disorders* include articulation disorders, dysarthria (the slurring often present in the speech of people with neurological disorders), and apraxia of speech (problems in putting together and in sequence all of the correct components of a word).
>
> *Language disorders* include delay in the development of language in general, specific language disabilities, and aphasia.
>
> *Voice problems* include dysphonias related to laryngeal pathologies or anomalies and resonance problems related to difficulties such as palatal control.
>
> *Fluency disorders* include stuttering and cluttering (which, although somewhat similar to stuttering, has different origins and effects).

Some persons are so severely communicatively disabled that they are not able to speak at all or are not able to communicate in at least some situations that are important to them. These persons use *augmentative* and *alternative communication techniques* to communicate, including the use of time-saving codes, special symbols, communication boards, and high-technology devices.

Causes of Communication Disorders

Some communication disorders develop along with speech and language. These *developmental disorders* include delayed articulation and delayed language development. Other disorders have an *organic* origin, such as a cleft palate or other maxillo-facial conditions. Congenital or acquired *neurological* problems, such as cerebral palsy or ALS, often result in communicative disabilities. Some difficulties in speech and language are *idiopathic*; that is, their causes cannot be pinpointed—many childhood articulation problems or specific language problems are examples. Stuttering has traditionally been thought of as being the result of environmental influences, but recent evidence indicates that stuttering, like other fluency disorders, may be of neurological origin or at least have a neurological component.

Communication disorders are common disabilities (perhaps this is one reason why people with normal speech tend to underestimate their effects on the individual). There are at least 2,000,000 Americans aged 21 or younger with serious speech or language problems (Gibbons, 1982). The total prevalence of speech and language disorders across all ages includes millions more (Van Riper & Emerick, 1984).

How Quality of Life Is Affected
by Communication Disorders

How much of an impediment can a communication disorder be to attaining a desirable quality of life? Here is how Metellus, Lefebvre-des-Noettes-Gisquet, and Vendeuvre (1993) described the effects of aphasia on the individual:

> Persons with aphasia are often overcome by feelings of degradation, regardless of their age at the onset of the illness. Whether viewed as a physiological, linguistic, or psychological problem or as a difficulty in social situations that may necessitate psychiatric intervention, to this day the motor deficits caused by aphasia are still considered a challenge to physical medicine and its related disciplines that appeared in the past few decades to treat the diverse repercussions of severe strokes. (p. 62)

Hawkridge, Vincent, and Hale (1985) have written that

> blind, deaf and speech-impaired people are all seriously handicapped, but of the three, speech-impaired people are at a special and different disadvantage. This is because blind and deaf people have a dysfunction in receptive (passive) modes, whereas speech loss involves a dysfunction in expressive (active) modes. (p. 33)

There is no question that the seemingly endless requirements for interpersonal communication that all persons experience place those with communication disorders under more stress than others. Such a constant strain can cause the development of undesirable forms of behaviors that go beyond the limitations caused by the speech and language problem itself. An environment that is perceived as threatening or an environment that fails to meet the individual's needs can be exceptionally anxiety producing (Rustin & Kuhr, 1989).

Communication disorders that have developed along with the person, such as misarticulations, delayed language, stuttering, or dysarthria due to cerebral palsy, carry with them a number of barriers to the attainment of a desirable life. For example, half or more of all children with speech, language, and communication disorders also have significant socioemotional difficulties (Cantwell & Baker, 1991; Prizant et al., 1990). These difficulties may include limited social interaction, mood disturbances, inappropriate affective expression, difficulties in relationships with caregivers or peers, irritability, and behavioral problems (Prizant & Meyer, 1993).

It is possible, however, that communication disorders that are acquired, such as aphasia or dysarthria due to a neurological disease, may be even more threatening to a personally satisfactory life. Aphasia may be the most serious disability related to brain injury in general because it so often results in personal, social, and economic troubles. Furthermore, treatment can be difficult and its results unpredictable. Relapses are not unusual, especially in elderly persons. Its unexpected and frequently instantaneous appearance can be devastating to both the individual and family. As Létourneau (1993) noted, "aphasia hammers in the reality of aging in a single sudden blow. Patients seemingly age overnight. And they thought this only happens to other people! It is almost like dying" (p. 68). The patient and family naturally (and probably correctly) feel that an injustice has occurred. They are left with feelings of impotence, disbelief frustration, anger, and many, many unanswered questions.

What effect on your quality of life would you experience if it took you an average of 12 seconds to activate a single key on a communication aid using a head-mounted light pointer because your ALS made it impossible for you to speak or use your hands? But even so-called minor speech problems extract their pound of flesh. What if you were a young male with puberphonia (a female-like, high-pitched voice)? Remember when you were in high school how fitting in was the most important aspect of your life? What would it have been like if, whenever you spoke, you made glottal stop sounds (an explosive sound produced by the sudden release of air pressure) because of the limitations of your cleft palate repair? And would life be tougher for you if your *r* sounded like a *w* and you always had half an ear open for the Elmer Fudd jokes behind your back?

Penalties Associated With Communication Disorders

Many people with severe communication disabilities have been hurt deeply and repeatedly—all because they did not (actually, could not) conform to the speech standards of our society. They are not at fault for their disabilities, but they are treated as if they were (Van Riper & Emerick, 1984). People with disabilities are often perceived as dependent, isolated, depressed, emotionally unstable, and socially inadequate (Furnham & Pendred, 1983). What do persons with communication disorders face from the communication partners they encounter? Unfortunately all too often, it is impatience, embarrassed withdrawal, or, worst of all, distant politeness. Small children often encounter taunting and imitative behavior from their peers.

Van Riper and Emerick (1984) recorded the reaction of a new university student:

> It was quite a shock when I came to college from the small home town where everyone knew me. My articulation is so garbled that I had to take off my freshman beanie and show people my name tag when I introduced myself. The worst part is the stares I got in stores. Speech is so public, so self-revealing, and I'm sure people think I'm either drunk or retarded. (p. 7)

Difficulties in communication may affect an individual in ways that we might not ordinarily consider. For example, communication is vital to the success of a sexual relationship. Sexual problems can stem from an inability to communicate worries and needs. It is difficult to achieve a satisfactory intimacy when a person has difficulty expressing sexual needs appropriately (Létourneau, 1993).

There are some other very practical penalties associated with communication disabilities. For example, consider the secure feeling we get from the knowledge that by dialing 911, help is only a phone call away. But what about the person whose stuttering, aphasia, or severe dysarthria makes the immediate use of the telephone impossible? They don't feel so secure, and in fact, they are not.

For many people with disabilities, enormous amounts of energy may be used up merely to cope with daily life. Struggling each day with nondisabled peers can be exhausting and stressful. The feeling of never fitting in can sap self-confidence and the sense of personal worth.

Personality Changes

Communication problems can cause drastic changes in a person following onset of an acquired severe communication disorder. Such personality changes arise not only from etiologic factors such as brain damage but also from a person's reaction to newly acquired limitations. Changes can include anxiety, denial, regression, egocentrism, damage to self-esteem, isolation, emotional lability, lack of inhibition, aggression, shame and guilt, and dependence and passivity (Létourneau, 1993). Sadly, the person who has suffered a loss of communication skills may be tempted to just give in and entrust themselves to others. There may follow a heightened need for affection and search for secondary gains. The effect of these changes can be so severe that it becomes the predominant element in a person's daily life.

Sometimes the person the family knew is barely recognizable. In essence, they may have to learn to live with someone new!

Limitations on Life's Possibilities and Opportunities

Even if a person who stutters wants to pursue a career in sales, potential employers may refuse the opportunity based on speech skills alone. An aphasic person may not be allowed to return to her old job as a secretary because her boss cannot see past her word-finding problems. The person whose speech is marked by nasality may not be taken seriously in his desire to try out for the school play. The person who uses a computer to speak may be discouraged from her desire for placement in a regular classroom.

Communication Disabilities Do Not Equal Poor Quality of Life

Though we have been examining the negative effects of communication disabilities on the pursuit of a good quality of life, there may be reason to challenge the assumption that persons with severe disabilities, such as aphasia or stuttering, are necessarily less happy, cheerful, and popular than the able-bodied (Cameron, Titus, Kostin, & Kostin, 1973). Weinberg and Williams (1978) reported that persons with disabilities do not necessarily view their disabilities as a great tragedy that has befallen them. Only 49% wished to be no longer disabled; 11% of 88 persons sampled viewed disability as a terrible thing, and only 7% saw it as the worst thing that has happened to them; most viewed disability as simply a fact of life. Most people hold the traditional view that foremost in importance are physical appearance and ability but for many persons with disabilities, other values have superseded these. Individual personality factors and attitudes, however, play major roles in how persons with disabilities perceive their own physical circumstances (Weinberg & Williams, 1978).

The Interaction of the Person With a Communication Disorder and the Environment

Difficulties with communication have some serious implications for those characteristics of quality of life that are related to the human condition: being, belonging, and becoming (see the Renwick & Brown chapter, this volume).

BEING

Being is the most personal aspect of who one is. How does restricted speech and language affect the *physical aspects* of being, such as physical health, nutrition, exercise, hygiene, grooming, clothing, and overall physical appearance? All of these features of self should be under the control of the individual, but if the individual cannot exercise such control because he or she cannot influence others via speech, then the nature of these aspects may be imposed on the individual or merely ignored.

Likewise, the *psychological aspects* of being, including the person's psychological well-being, may be adversely affected. As with other persons with disabilities, individuals with communication disorders may have negative evaluations concerning self and a negative view of personal sexuality. It isn't difficult to understand how a person with a severe stuttering problem can have a poor sense of locus of control.

Some of the *spiritual aspects* of being may also suffer as a result of difficulties in communicating. One can see how a person born with a severe physical disability that makes speech impossible might react bitterly to a perceived capriciousness of fate and develop a distorted set of personal values and personal standards or even suffer crises in spiritual beliefs.

BELONGING

Perhaps no prerequisite of a quality life is placed more at risk by communicative disability than that of belonging. It can be very difficult for the child who uses a communication board, the young man with puberphonia, or the career woman who communicates via esophageal speech (due to removal of a cancerous larynx) to fit comfortably with the social, physical, and resource-related aspects of their various environments.

In some cases, a communication disability may result in an individual being required to live away from home and neighborhood (it may also follow that personal space and privacy are compromised). It may exclude a person from the local school or from a job.

Conversational interaction is a key component in establishing an individual's bonds with his or her social environments. Without the ability to effectively and efficiently influence others through intelligible speech and a constructive use of language, it can be difficult to attain a true sense of acceptance and belonging. People with severe difficulties in speech, especially those with neurologically based disabilities and fluency disorders, often sense an incompleteness in their relationships with intimate others, family members, friends, coworkers, neighbors, and other members of their cultural and ethnic groups.

We live in an era in which we depend increasingly on the various resources typically available to members of the community to meet some of our needs. All of us can tell horror stories of how we had to wend our way through great reels of red tape before we were able to reach someone who even might be of help to us in arranging for a merited service. Imagine, then, the frustration that must be experienced by the person with distorted speech or confused language when that person attempts to locate information about sources of adequate income, employment, educational and recreational programs, medical and social services, and community activities.

BECOMING

No society can guarantee its members pleasurable and fulfilling lives. It is enough that the society provides its members the opportunity for the "pursuit of happiness." Certainly, people with severe communication disabilities have the same hopes and aspirations for a full and useful life as everyone else. But are they really provided such opportunity? There is little question that individuals with severe communicative problems encounter at least some limitations in experiencing many of the practical activities requisite to a full life, experiences such as purposeful work, going to school, helping others, and seeking out services. Similarly, there may be real restrictions on leisure activities. These activities may not be of practical value but they can encourage relaxation and help reduce stress. Certainly, difficulties in communicating can change usually pleasurable social activities, such as games and visits, into highly stressful situations.

The idea of going on a vacation, with its attendant requirements for communicating with numerous strangers, may be anything but appealing. Imagine for a moment that your speech is distorted to the point that it is sometimes unintelligible because oral cancer has resulted in a partial glossectomy (surgical removal of the tongue). You simply want to fly to Disney World, check into the hotel, and enjoy the theme parks. How many difficult, wearying speaking situations might this entail? Dozens, actually, from the time you call the travel agent until the time you hail a cab at the airport on the way home. Unless you are a person of resolve and courage, you may not be willing to expose yourself to so many arduous and exhausting situations. Perhaps you have a travelling companion and that person can look after most communicative interactions, but after a while, what kind of toll will this take on your self-esteem?

For the person who cannot communicate orally, there is always that hesitation before entering into activities, many of which help a person to grow. Yet, what is life if we don't explore new things, learn new skills, expand our knowledge, and work actively to solve our problems?

Quality of Life and the
Speech-Language Pathologist

Although behavioral changes in speech and language are the immediate targets of the speech-language pathologist (SLP), it is improvement of the chances for the person with a communication disorder to achieve a better life that is the true goal of treatment. It is immediately apparent that the degree to which the person enjoys the important possibilities of life is strongly influenced by that person's ability to influence others through the creative and persuasive use of speech and language. In the presence of communication disabilities, opportunities are reduced and constraints are increased. The individual who stutters severely will not be provided the opportunity to compete for a broadcasting job. The person with a language disorder will not be considered as club secretary. Lamentably, these same people may not be invited to join the local service group or even be asked to join the crowd for an after-work beer. Even when they do attain the diploma, get the job, join the club, or go along for the beer, the level of satisfaction or pleasure experienced may be far lower on the continuum than it would be if they didn't live in an atmosphere tainted by anxiety and frustration.

It is a given that a disability, by itself, does not necessarily lead to an increased or decreased quality of life. The SLP, then, needs to do more than just help an individual express himself or herself more clearly. The clinician must also aid the individual to cope more successfully even when speech remains slurred or dysfluent or when just the right words cannot be readily retrieved. The clinician must also remember that every individual is in continual interaction with the environment. Therefore, the SLP must provide treatment designed to teach the individual not merely to speak better with others but to interact better with them. The child with a severe language disability will be helped to a degree by learning to produce the *ks* blend (as in *excuse*). The child will be helped much more, however, by learning when to use the word *excuse* (as in "excuse me") as a part of a program to teach the social use of language.

Enhancing Quality of Life of the
Person With Communication Disability

What can individuals with communicative disorders do to seek a more personally desirable and fulfilling quality of life? First and foremost, these individuals (and the clinicians who work with them) must understand and accept that the handicapping effects of communication disabilities can be reduced by focused, goal-oriented, highly practical approaches to remediation. People with disabilities must live with the realities that attitudinal barriers exist and must be dealt with on an ongoing basis. Unfortunately, society overvalues human factors, such as rationale, intellect, and physique, and undervalues qualities such as compassion and spirituality.

If disability cannot be changed, then the affected individual must adapt to it. The unnecessary handicap imposed by an unwillingness to recognize what is and to go on from there need not be accepted, however. The handicap related to disabilities is often generated by either the human-made parts of the physical environment or social customs, values, attitudes, and expectations. Therefore, physical objects and people must be reckoned with (Vash, 1981).

Therapy must focus not solely on compensatory programs but also on adjustment to disability, social participation, and community integration (Kerr, 1977). Changing communication behaviors must, of course, be a major goal of treatment. Certainly, the opportunities to achieve personal growth, social growth, and abilities at cooperative action are enhanced as communication skills increase (Brooks & Heath, 1993).

Speech-Language Therapy and
"Being, Belonging, Becoming"

It is a wonderful thing for an SLP to help a young man to lower his inappropriately high voice, to aid the person who stutters to control phonation, or to assist the lady with aphasia to learn new strategies for summoning words held deep within her memory. It is equally important, however, for the clinician to suggest ideas about how individuals who are coping with communication disabilities can improve the ways in which they fit with the social, physical, and resource-related aspects of their various environments.

BEING

Individuals with a communication disorder must be encouraged to stay physically strong and active, be well rested, and look after themselves emotionally. The man who stutters who is healthy and rested and who approaches speech with an affirmative attitude is likely to control breathing for phonation more efficiently, and his mental alertness will help him to apply principles acquired in therapy more successfully in the "real" world. At a time when many religious and other spiritual beliefs are often met with suspicion, the clinician should also remember how powerful such beliefs can be as motivators, antidepressants, and, most important, comforters.

BELONGING

Therapy should be designed to meet the specific, practical, everyday needs of the individual with a communication disorder. As a young clinician, I worked with a man with articulation and resonance problems. Patrick was a nuclear physicist who worked for a major public utility. Therapy was going along reasonably well, but keeping Patrick's interest level high and, especially, getting him to work outside of clinic time, was like pulling teeth. I just couldn't keep him enthused. On the suggestion of a wise clinical director, I asked Patrick to bring me some basic reading material on nuclear-generated electricity. I learned what I could (embarrassingly little, really) and worked with Patrick to design therapy that centered around what he did, the people he worked with, and those situations that he identified as of particular importance to him. The results were remarkable, and the importance of keying therapy to the individual's physical, social, and community needs remained with me thereafter.

BECOMING

It must always be remembered that people communicate for a number of reasons with none being more important than fitting in with the rest of the world. Patrick's performance in therapy improved because we began to deal with the practical things that were important to him—in his case, work and leisure activities. Though it didn't strike me at the time, Patrick's abilities to confidently manage the communicative situations that he encountered each day provided a foundation for growth as well. It allowed him to explore new interests, meet new people, and develop new ideas—all those things that people do to make themselves into better persons.

Beginning Speech and Language Therapy

It is easy, in the clinician's eagerness to get to the symptoms of the communication disorder, to forget that the person with the symptoms (and that person's family) may not be as ready as the clinician to get at them. The man who has just learned that his dysarthria is related to a progressive neurological condition, such as Parkinson's disease, or the mother who has just learned that the unblemished child she thought she had is falling behind in developing language, may rationalize the symptoms while they absorb the shock of discovery. Associated avoidance, depression, or other strong reactions must be accepted. The SLP cannot rush the active cooperation of either the individual with a communication disorder or significant others. But the clinician can take comfort in realizing that grief eventually subsides as people adapt to losses and find new ways of meeting their needs, and fortunately, most depression fades with time.

Once a person with an acquired severe communication disorder concedes its presence, it is natural for him or her to want things to be like they used to be and to concentrate fully on "getting back to normal." The clinician often tends to unconsciously cooperate with this overriding but often inappropriate goal of treatment. Instead, the SLP should work toward accommodation rather than acceptance.

Components of the Therapy Program

Therapy should be designed with practical outcomes in mind. In planning therapy, clinicians must always be careful to consider the uniqueness of each individual. Age of onset, length of time the individual has had the disability, age, cognitive level and literacy, and the person's need to communicate are only a few of the many personal factors that must be taken into consideration. It may be necessary to deal with males and females differently because they often have very different views of what is important to them. Consider esophageal speech. The sound produced might be considered as harsh and turbulent by some listeners. But males who have lost their larynx don't seem to be as concerned about this as women. As a consequence, men are more successful in learning esophageal speech than women (Gardner, 1966). Apparently, woman find the sound of the new voice embarrassing. As a consequence, they are self-conscious about using it (Stam, Koopmans, & Mathieson, 1991). Perhaps they also fear a loss of their feminine identities (Shanks, 1979).

When planning and carrying out a therapy program, the SLP, the individual with a communication disorder, and the family should constantly monitor their activities to ensure that activities are aimed at providing the highest level of practical communication skills possible to meet the individual's desires in life. If the aim of therapy is not merely to raise measurable levels of speech and language but, rather, to help prepare individuals to use speech and language to exert a measure of control in important and desirable aspects of life, then the outcome of treatment is far more likely to really matter. Usually, these aspects of life are those prosaic activities that make up the bulk of everyday life for all of us. They include attempts at increasing our levels of physical well-being; improving our relations with other people; getting involved in social, community, and civic activities; expanding our personal development and fulfillment; and enjoying recreational activities (Flanagan, 1982).

Of what use is technically accurate speech if a person is a self-centered conversationalist? What is the value of fluency if a person doesn't know how to use speech effectively for courting and intimacy? How helpful is a mellifluous voice if its owner doesn't know how to communicate when interviewing for a job? There is a cardinal rule for SLPs and probably for other helping professionals as well: Every activity should have a practical, functional objective.

Communication Partners: Friends and Foes

The desire to communicate with others is an integral part of being human. We all want to express our feelings, our opinions, our wants, and our needs. But it is difficult to find satisfaction in personal interactions when the speaker experiences constant anxiety over the reactions of communicative partners (cf. Zola, 1981).

Meaningful integration with our fellow humans is an important component of a meaningful and enjoyable life. When people pay less attention to what is said than to how one says it, however, the degree of enjoyment of many of life's meaningful activities is restricted. Imagine the little boy with a cleft palate who asks some of the neighborhood kids if he can play with them but is greeted with taunts about his funny mouth and talking through his nose. And the woman with ALS who uses a voice output communication aid whose efforts to speak via her machine are often greeted with the kind of body language and facial expressions that scream, "I'm uncomfortable; let me out of here." Or the dysfluent man whose simple response to a request for directions includes stoppages in breathing, repetitions, interjections, and facial contortions that are received by the listener with distrustful looks or no looking at all. How about the man with aphasia who struggles valiantly to request a second cup of coffee only to have the waitress respond to his wife, "Does he want anything else, Dear?"

SOME SUGGESTIONS FOR
COMMUNICATION PARTNERS

We have painted a rather chilling picture of ourselves—the people who interact with persons with communication disorders. But a knowledgeable and compassionate communication partner can also represent a potentially invaluable asset. The family member or friend who understands how to react to disordered communication, who knows how to help improve communicative skills, and who can help teach how to neutralize a potentially distant or even hostile communication partner is undoubtedly the best tool that the SLP has in the big bag of tricks.

In planning and carrying out therapy, the suggestions of significant others, friends, coworkers, and fellow students should be sought out and considered carefully. Nobody knows the individual better than family and friends. The physical therapist, occupational therapist, teacher, counselor, and other professionals who work with the individual with a communication disorder also have valuable knowledge about his or her capabilities and needs that should be solicited and incorporated into speech and language therapy.

Research Issues

Research in communication disorders, like the research in many disability disciplines, has tended to focus on the cause and remediation of disorders. Until recently, little had been written about the effects of communication disability on quality of life. We need to know more about the ways in which communication partners interact communicatively with individuals with speech and language disabilities and how they perceive them overall. It is also essential to document differences in the ways those with communication disorders interact with their environment in comparison to the general population.

The development of instruments designed to specifically measure the effects of communication disorders on quality of life and outcome effects of speech and language therapy on the quality of life would be of special value.

Implications for Policy Development
and Service Provision

Those who determine health policy have frequently overlooked the needs for well-equipped, fully staffed, fully funded speech and language programs. It may be that some tend to consider speech and language problems as mere annoyances. They must learn to recognize that communication disorders, even those perceived as mild, can have seriously deleterious effects on the way in which individuals can strive to gain the best life possible.

Advocates for individuals with communication disabilities need to lobby for antidiscrimination laws that ensure that persons with communication disorders are not unfairly excluded from educational and vocational opportunities. Professional organizations and governments need to bring to the attention of the general population not only the potentially handicapping effects of communication disorders but also (and more important) the abilities of those with communication disorders to perform socially and vocationally at levels commensurate with the general population.

It is the responsibility of all of society to ensure that inequities in resources and services provided to those with communication impairment are reduced to ensure that they may function in an environment free of artificial barriers. Persons with communication disorders must be provided access to a full range of educational choices and services, relevant community and peer groups, and community services.

Those who determine the curricula for training programs in speech-language pathology must also reconsider the content of their training programs. They have tended to underestimate the need for training students to work with the whole person, not simply the speech and language symptoms they carry with them. Clinicians need to ensure that the people with whom they work view themselves not as victims but as empowered individuals who can take charge of their lives.

Summary

The serious effects on the quality of life of individuals with communication disorders have gone largely unrecognized by those of us who do not have problems with speech or language. Consequently, many invisible barriers have been erected that make it difficult for individuals with communicative disabilities to pursue and realize a personally satisfying quality of life. Nonetheless, the presence of speech and language disorders, the penalties related to them, and the need to make personal adjustments that they mandate do not necessarily prevent the attainment of a personally satisfying quality of life.

The most profound use of our human communication skills is meaningful and satisfying interaction with other humans. But successful communication and all the benefits that accrue from it require more than reasonably intelligible speech and generally grammatical language. To successfully interact with other humans, we must know and apply pragmatic skills; that is, we must possess and use language in socially appropriate and effective ways. The SLP must, of course, cooperate with individuals with communication disorders, their significant others, and other professionals in designing programs of therapy that help individuals with communication disorders to reach the highest technical levels of speech and language possible. It is equally essential, however, that individuals with speech and language problems be prepared to use those skills in ways that allow them to exercise a measure of control over their own lives.

By now, the reader has repeatedly read that *quality of life* is an elusive concept. It can mean so many things to so many people. But of one thing we can all be sure: A life that is good for an individual will always include other people. And it is through speech and language that we can best know them and they know us.

17

Quality of Life for Deaf and Hard-of-Hearing People

David G. Mason

Why De-Identify the Deaf in the Name of a Mythical Image?

In this chapter, the term *DHHs* (deaf and hard of hearing) refers to culturally deaf persons, hard-of-hearing persons, late-deafened persons, and oral deaf persons. These persons share many common personal and social world views and values. Hearing persons are those who hear and talk and take their spontaneous access to the world of the human sound for granted. Most of them rarely have any contact with DHHs. Many of those who do rarely have an insight into how they affect DHHs' quality of life. Few of them are aware of the differences and similarities between the four DHH categories. They are likely to perceive DHHs as "hearing-impaired persons," which implies that their deafness is a medical concern, or as "differently abled persons," which implies that they are no different from other persons with any types of disabilities. Most of the DHHs this author knows prefer to identify themselves as culturally deaf, oral deaf, hard-of-hearing, or late-deafened persons. This difference has implications for the quality of DHHs' lives. Hearing persons' perspective of DHHs can be said to be somewhat similar to how a typical city dweller perceives and conceptualizes a forest on the basis of his or her limited exposure to a single tree. He or she may never realize that the forest is much more than trees and is full of life.

One objective of this chapter is to stress that it is essential to respect DHHs' need to identify with one or more of the DHH categories. Another is to stress that it is important to distinguish between how DHHs perceive themselves and how hearing persons perceive them. The following thought should be deemed appropriate: Unless the way hearing people perceive DHHs is consistent with how DHHs perceive themselves, the hearing perspectives are likely to have a profound, often adverse, effect on the DHHs' quality of life. Various medical, social, and educational objectives formulated to "address the deafness" generally de-emphasize DHHs' own perspectives and empha-size hearing people's perspectives of what DHHs should be or have.

History shows that many such objectives have adverse effects on DHHs' quality of life (Lane, 1989). Training a culturally deaf child to learn to hear and talk like a hard-of-hearing person and training a hard-of-hearing person to talk like a late-deafened adult exemplify such objectives being pursued in schools. These objectives put an enormous pressure on the culturally deaf and hard-of-hearing children and their families at home. From within the field of psychology, we have seen psychologists who attribute DHHs' mental and social problems to their being deaf, rather than to their struggle in a sociocul-turally or educationally inaccessible or irrelevant environment. In addition, it is crucial to note that many professionals who assess or work with DHH children in such environments do not have the ability to carry out spontane-ous communication, particularly with DHHs who prefer to sign or write.

The term *audists* (Humphries, 1977) refers to certain professionals and laypersons whose mission is to fight against or ignore DHHs' need to stabilize their self-concept and to identify with other DHHs. Typical audists are interested in how they can help DHH children learn what they might have rather than what they already have. As an example, their mission is to teach DHH children to talk; they do not recognize American Sign Language (ASL) and deaf culture. They are not interested in DHHs' ability to become bilin-gual with ASL and English.

Audists typically work with DHH children and their hearing parents but avoid the same DHH persons when they are older and experience difficulties as "oral failures." They rarely, if ever, have DHH adults as friends, consult-ants, or colleagues and avoid contact with DHHs, including culturally deaf persons who have M.A. or even Ph.D. degrees (Soderfeldt, 1991). Their so-called high moral ground and altruistic mission appeal to young parents who have DHH children as well as to the media, foundations, industries, government, and the general public.

Another category of professional and lay persons deals with or relies on indirect knowledge about DHH people. Indirect knowledge implies learning about DHHs through someone else's direct or indirect perspectives. Such perspectives abound in professional journals and books, university class-rooms, professional workshops, and conferences, as well as media and government sources. As a general rule, much of the indirect knowledge about deafness in printed English is read and discussed by these people of whom very few have any meaningful contact with DHHs, let alone having them as their colleagues or friends. They vastly outnumber DHH persons in profes-sions that deal with the way DHHs live; such professions include teachers of the deaf preparation programs (Mason, 1994b). These people as a group have so much power that they often have profound, often adverse, effects on DHHs' quality of life.

Context for the Discussion: The Author's Perspective

As a person who perceives himself as culturally deaf, my perception of the hard of hearing, oral deaf, and late-deafened may be consistent or inconsistent with how other DHHs perceive themselves and their relation-ship with other people. Because I know more than 5,000 DHH persons across North America, however, I assume that my perspectives are more consistent than inconsistent. I have no intention to speak on behalf of all other DHHs through this chapter. I expect that some DHHs will not agree with certain things written in this chapter but know that some others will appreciate it.

The DHH Categorizations

Each of the four categories of DHH—culturally deaf, hard of hearing, late-deafened, and oral deaf—is distinctive, and each has identifiable attributes and values. Such distinctions constitute the basis for the existence of the separate local, regional, and national organizations of the culturally deaf, hard of hearing, late-deafened, or oral deaf (discussed later in this chapter). Individually, many DHHs choose to identify with one or more of the catego-ries; some do not. It is not unusual for a DHH who identifies with one of the four during his or her childhood to identify with a different one during adulthood. Many DHH adolescents experience an identity crisis. They may feel that they are special and unlike the other DHHs or that they are more hearing than deaf. It is not unusual, however, for them to go through this phase and eventually have and value friendships with other DHHs. This is likely to happen when they realize that their relationships with their hearing friends become more superficial and "nice," rather than deeper and more meaningful as they grow older.

Four Sample DHHs

From a series of interviews, conferences, presentations, and articles, the following shared experiences have been noted among DHH persons. The names of the following persons are pseudonyms, and the genders of proper names and pronouns are immaterial.

TOM, A CULTURALLY DEAF PERSON

Tom was born deaf. His parents heeded professional advice that he should learn to talk orally and refrain from signing. He was encouraged to talk at school but was not making progress with his oral communication. As he grew older, he did not make much progress with his written English either. He felt he was treated like a slow learner at the oral school. He made friends with peers who had culturally deaf parents. He was impressed with their ability to sign very well and discuss various topics. Tom quickly acquired sign language and eventually became more confident with himself.

At one point, a high school classmate announced that he was going to take the Gallaudet University entrance examinations. Tom thought he should try the examinations, too; others thought he could not pass them. He took the examinations and passed them. Today, he has a master's degree and is a leader in both the deaf and hearing communities. He admitted with some regret that he and his parents still cannot communicate through either ASL or oral English.

MARY, A HARD-OF-HEARING PERSON

Mary had a wonderful mother who was a former teacher. She made sure that Mary had every opportunity to learn and use oral communication at home and at school. Mary spent much of her childhood and adolescence with hearing people with rare exposure to other DHH persons. As she became older, she felt she was different from her hearing peers and that her world was less accessible than theirs. She did not understand why it seemed that way until she realized that she was hard of hearing. As a young adult, she was determined to acquire sign language and learn about deaf culture, and eventually became acquainted with culturally deaf persons.

As a mature student, she felt that hearing and deaf people did not respect her as a hard-of-hearing person. Hearing people wanted her to be hearing, and her deaf peers encouraged her to come to terms with her identity as a deaf person. She could talk on a one-to-one basis with either hearing or deaf people but found it difficult to take part in group discussions with them. In addition, she also resented hearing people who trivialized her experience as a hard-of-hearing person and used her as a role model to encourage other DHHs to talk as she does. Today, she volunteers in a variety of hard-of-hearing organizations to educate both hard-of-hearing people and the general public. Mary was not happy with certain shortcomings inherent in the frequency modulation (FM) system. It restricted her to listening only to the speaker who carried the microphone and denied her access to the rest of her classmates, whereas the others could hear her talking. Mary became much more relaxed and appreciative, and she was finally able to enjoy class lectures when ASL interpreters were present.

JOHNNY, AN ORAL DEAF PERSON

Johnny was born deaf, and his parents decided that he should go to an oral school for the deaf. He made excellent progress as an oral student, and educational professionals often selected him as a model student. They would, for example, ask him to frequently demonstrate his oral abilities in front of audiences.

As a young child, he saw several deaf signers from a nearby school for the deaf and knew he was different because he was oral and did not sign. As a teenager, he left the oral school for the deaf to attend a small-town high school with his hearing siblings. With his excellent athletic abilities, he was able to participate on high school teams. In a tournament, he happened to find out that culturally deaf athletes from a school for the deaf were also competing. Tom approached them and introduced himself. Incidentally, it was the turning point of his life. He started acquiring ASL and becoming involved in various deaf community activities. When he was a university student, a professor informed him about a school for the deaf not far from the campus. He decided to go to meet people there. Eventually, this led to his participation in one of the World Games for the deaf. During the games, he noticed that hundreds of deaf athletes from all over the world signed, and he could not sign. Within a few years, he acquired ASL and, as an adult, he became a regular sign language instructor. He became very active in the deaf community, much more than in the hearing community, even though he could

use speech in one-to-one dialogue. As an adult, he prefers to use an inter-
preter when he is with a large group of hearing people.

LESLIE, A LATE-DEAFENED PERSON

Leslie grew up a hearing person and became deaf when she was approximately 10 years old. She attended a school for the deaf in a major city before
completing a regular high school program in a small town. She took a job at
a school for the deaf where oral communication was the main educational
objective. Leslie's considerable experience with oral language complemented
the school's objective. As a young adult, she was active in both the hearing
community with her siblings and the deaf community with her deaf friends.

She signed with her deaf friends but tended to stop signing and start
speaking when hearing persons were present. She often apologized for
inadvertently leaving her deaf friends out of the conversation. Although she
signed, she felt that she was superior to DHHs who prefer to sign, basically
because she could speak and the others could not. As a professional employee
at a school, she resented others for trying to show that ASL is a true language
even though she signs.

General Categories

CULTURALLY DEAF PERSONS

Culturally deaf persons are not, or are no longer, concerned about their
being deaf or their inability to hear and speak like hearing people. Audists
call them "oral failures" (Jacobs, 1974, p. 34), even after opportunities to
train them to talk orally. These oral failures typically acquire and use ASL
and become much more involved with the world through printed English, as
well as with their ever-increasing network of contacts through ASL. They
accept, but are not concerned about, their limited oral abilities as they become
older. They appreciate TV captioning, TTY for phone use, and printed materials. Unfortunately, educational professionals rarely recognize or incorporate
such remarkable bilingual abilities as part of school activities. The reason so
many such professionals fail to recognize deaf bilingualism may be traced
to educators' preference for teaching the deaf English skills. Books such as
the one by Gary Bunch (1987) emphasize English-only approaches.

Young culturally deaf children spontaneously acquire and use ASL even
though it is rarely supported at school. At home, most parents do not sign
and feel it is their responsibility to help in teaching their children to learn to

talk and to avoid signing (Ling & Ling, 1978). Incidentally, I know several leading professional oral advocates who, ironically, can and do sign.

Many of my culturally deaf acquaintances are fighting the stigma of being an oral failure or having poor English skills. This negative stigma can be traced to their prior schooling experiences (Mason, 1990). In retrospect, their former teachers or principals should have informed them that they already had a highly sophisticated language with ASL. They could have commended them for being ASL-dominant or balanced bilingual (Kannapell, 1985). Because until recent years most teachers did not realize that ASL was a true language, it is not difficult to understand the oversight or ignorance. Their job was to emphasize English.

It seems that educators do not see the significance of culturally deaf children becoming ASL-English bilingual, often starting as early as their first year at school or before. Typically, DHH children cooperate with their teachers and parents and try to learn oral skills and refrain from signing in classrooms. Many of them sign out of the educators' eyeshot or outside the classrooms. Although their speech may be intelligible to their family members, hearing teachers, speech therapists, and close hearing friends, they rarely use it in casual conversation. They simplify their ASL with hearing people who have limited signing abilities. They would supplement their English-like utterances with gesturing in an attempt to make it easier for hearing people to understand them. Unfortunately, this gives a wrong impression that DHHs' language is underdeveloped or impoverished.

Culturally deaf persons often prefer to communicate through writing, ASL interpreters, or a combination of the two. But when they are with other culturally deaf people, they discuss anything—concrete and abstract—in ASL, depending on their interest in topics. It is not difficult to discuss high-level theories in ASL. Many of them discuss in ASL what they read in English.

Culturally deaf persons are leaders, organizers, followers, and supporters in the deaf community, in addition to having responsibilities as parents at home and employees at work. The quality of their voluntary work in deaf organizations compares well with that of dedicated members of any "hearing" organization. The general public is usually unaware of this remarkable phenomenon.

ORAL DEAF PERSONS

Oral deaf persons and culturally deaf persons have numerous similarities even though their mode of communication is different. Oral deaf persons typically use one language, such as English, whereas culturally deaf people typically use two—ASL and English. Regardless of how deaf these persons are, educational professionals insist that they use their residual hearing and work on their oral communication skills at home and school. They encourage them to use detachable hearing aids, recommend cochlear implants, integrate them into hearing-dominated schools, or a combination of these. Professionals generally discourage DHH children and their parents from seeking contact with deaf adults.

Ideally, the "oral successful" deaf person would become fully included in the hearing world. Even with their excellent oral communication abilities, however, many of them feel comfortable making friends with other oral deaf persons or culturally deaf persons, rather than with hearing people (Leigh & Stinson, 1991). Oral deaf associations exist in Canada and the United States because of this basic need.

I have noticed that oral deaf and culturally deaf persons share many common attributes, experiences, observations, and values. This leads to the following questions: Why do professionals, audists in particular, work diligently to keep oral and culturally deaf persons segregated? What do the same professionals do when oral and culturally deaf persons meet and become lifelong friends and enjoy signing? I know of numerous "ex-oral" deaf adults who have become advocates, activists, or even militants in fighting for the recognition of ASL and deaf culture. They do not fight to preserve audists' objectives. Many of them even seek to identify themselves as culturally deaf. Many of them are angry with their prior schooling experiences. I also recognize that there are oral deaf adults who are satisfied with oral communication and prefer not to sign. These scenarios clearly exemplify a serious conflict between how DHHs perceive themselves and how professionals, mainly hearing professionals, perceive them.

HARD-OF-HEARING PERSONS

Hard-of-hearing persons are the largest single physical disability group (Lutes, cited in Warwick, 1994). The onset of their hearing loss varies from person to person. Some have been hard of hearing since early childhood and others become hard of hearing progressively.

Lutes (as cited in Warwick, 1994) stressed that the hard-of-hearing group does not have a distinct identity. Some can hear and speak reasonably well and others cannot; some others pass as hearing persons. Although Ford (1993) defined the hard of hearing as persons who use speech as their primary means of communication, some of them use ASL and prefer to identify themselves as culturally deaf. Also, some profoundly deaf persons prefer to identify themselves as hard of hearing (Warwick, 1994). Many hard-of-hearing persons do not know where they fit between the culturally deaf and hearing communities until they have met with other hard-of-hearing persons through hard-of-hearing associations. Bruce (1994) wrote, "Upon entry into adulthood, hard-of-hearing adolescents face the tasks ahead—intimacy, generativity, and integrity. Unless they are able to resolve previous crises, particularly identity confusion, they may instead face isolation, stagnation, and despair" (p. 16).

Oral hard-of-hearing persons may feel they do not need to acquire and use ASL or LSQ (Langue des Signes Québecoise, or Québec Sign Language) in certain situations but would find it helpful in others. My hard-of-hearing acquaintances have often said that they prefer one-to-one oral communication situations but dread classroom seminars. They find it difficult to listen to several hearing classmates competing for their turn to speak or receive attention. Hard-of-hearing persons appreciate listening to one speaker at a time with an FM system, reading transcriptions of their speaking on video or computer monitors, or both.

Hard-of-hearing persons generally value their residual hearing and appreciate detachable assistive hearing devices. Korthright and Ford (1993) observed that some hard of hearing persons feel that they are deaf without a hearing aid and hard-of-hearing with it. They are frustrated with noise and electromagnetic interference (EMI) pollution that interferes with their concentration on spoken presentations or lectures. EMI refers to the unwanted sound-related pollution the FM system picks up, particularly when its source is in unknown parts of a building. When two separate FM systems are turned on within the same proximity, the system can wreak havoc, interrupting the person's listening concentration (Korthright & Ford, 1993).

Those who have been hard of hearing since early childhood are more likely to be active in hard-of-hearing associations than those who became hard of hearing progressively or at one point in their adulthood (Ford, 1993). Like culturally deaf persons, hard-of-hearing persons have local, regional, national, and international organizations of hard-of-hearing persons and may become active as leaders, supporters, and advocates of such organizations and their causes.

LATE-DEAFENED ADULTS

Late-deafened adults are basically hearing persons who have become functionally deaf after their childhood (K. Woodcock, personal communication, 1994). Woodcock classified the late-deafened into the four subgroups: progressive; traumatic; medically related, such as viral illnesses; and surgical, such as removal of hearing-related organs or structures. Those late-deafened persons who feel they do not identify with hard-of-hearing or culturally deaf people are likely to meet others of their kind through such organizations as the Association of Late-Deafened Adults (ALDA). During a recent conference sponsored by ALDA, a late-deafened person said, "It was an enjoyable experience being with people of 'my own kind' and meeting newly deafened people who at last found an organization that understood what they were going through" (Barnhart, 1994, p. 6).

Late-deafened adults may experience disadvantages associated with their hearing loss; however, they have many advantages over some other DHHs. Because they qualify as deaf persons, they become eligible for educational programs for the deaf which has some advantages: For example, they have acquired English through their experience as hearing persons (Padden & Humphries, 1988), hence educational professors call them *postlingually deaf* (Jacobs, 1974). They are likely to have the edge when they and other DHH students are required to do the same postsecondary education assignments involving English and "hearing world" values.

The process of adjustment to their hearing loss varies from person to person (Schmitz, 1993). Those who suddenly become deaf are likely to need to adjust more than those who have been becoming progressively deaf over years. Schmitz interviewed several late-deafened students at the National Technical Institute of the Deaf in New York. Their comments included the following: "I miss hearing," "My mind hears the sound," "I remember songs in my head," "I've simply learned to manage it (deafness), not control it. One needs to accommodate to the turn of events, because if not, one suffers." "There are times when I feel hearing and times when I feel deaf" (p. 15). Another late-deafened student has said, "I am proud to say that I know a second language [ASL]" (p. 16). Some quickly acquire ASL and become active in the deaf community, whereas others struggle to preserve their self-concept as hearing persons and remain in the hearing world. Many of them, particularly those who have to come to terms with their hearing loss and acquire signing, eventually expand their network of contacts to include other DHHs. Those who do, often quickly adjust and become active in the deaf community and enjoy lifelong contact with culturally deaf, oral deaf, hard-of-hearing, and hearing persons, depending on their preferred mode of communication.

Like the culturally deaf and hard-of-hearing people, late-deafened adults have their own issues or problems they must address. They are concerned about certain hearing professionals or laypersons who insist that they should think of themselves as hard of hearing or hearing rather than as deaf. In addition, they resent the apparent lack of insight into what it is like to become deaf after being able to hear for years.

What About Other DHHs?

DHH persons with cochlear implants will be likely to identify with one of the four categories of DHHs when they are older and on their own. This is because the cochlear implant does not give them the quality of hearing average hearing people enjoy. DHHs with one or more physical disabilities also identify with whichever DHH category they feel comfortable with. Some of the author's acquaintances have cochlear implants and others have additional physical disabilities.

What Is a Deaf Community, and Do the DHHs of Different Categories Join Forces?

We do! A deaf community is not restricted within any geographic boundaries or to any particular DHH group. It exists when DHH and hearing people who sign get together for local, regional, provincial, national, or even international activities. Many oral DHHs who become involved eventually acquire ASL. It is not unusual for culturally deaf persons to enjoy a lasting network of contact with DHH signers anywhere in Canada and in other countries. During a teachers' conference in Wisconsin, Don Moore (1992) made a comment on the language status of ASL, saying that it did not have a consistent definition. (Does spoken English have one?) For an unexplained reason, he overlooked the fact that he was at the same conference where I, a Canadian, enjoyed conversation in ASL with a number of hearing and deaf Americans I had never met before. One may wonder if his comment reflects the futile educational objective to impose variations of oral-signed systems that resemble English (Wilbur, 1987) as policy methods for DHHs in schools in North America.

There are times when persons of all the different categories unify for common causes, such as the Deaf Ontario Now (DON) movement in 1989, which was inspired by the Deaf President Now (DPN) movement at Gallaudet University in 1988 (Gannon, 1989). The DPN resulted in the unprecedented replacement of an appointed hearing president with a late-deafened president. Likewise, the DON movement eventually led to another unprecedented event: the first-ever election of a culturally deaf person to a major government and the first-ever appointment of another culturally deaf Canadian as a university professor.

The International Committee of Silent Sports sponsors the World Games of the Deaf and the Winter World Games for the Deaf in different countries around the world every 4 years. The culturally deaf, late-deafened, hard of hearing and the oral deaf work together as organizers or teammates; many become lifelong friends. Hearing persons are also supportive and involved in such events.

Likewise, there are times when the DHHs need to address their common issues among themselves. They have the Canadian Association of the Deaf, Canadian Cultural Society of the Deaf, Canadian Deaf Sports Association, Canadian Hard of Hearing Association, ALDA, and the Oral Deaf Association. Some become involved with the World Federation of the Deaf (WFD) and the International Federation of Hard of Hearing (IFHOH). The culturally deaf, hard of hearing, late-deafened, and oral deaf do not restrict themselves to one particular organization. Some become involved with WFD and IFHOH.

External Perspectives as
Quality of Life Issues

Hearing people generally do not perceive DHHs the way they perceive themselves. Such differences in perspectives are expected; however, there is something amiss about a particular category of hearing people—for example, the audists. They impose their experiences, observations, and values on DHHs and show a lack of interest in DHHs' own. The following discussion includes mere samples.

THE DE-IDENTIFYING OF DHHs

Deaf and *hard of hearing* were the basic terms used in the deaf community until the 1970s. In clinical, academic, and research communities, audists used the terms *hearing impaired* (HI) and *hearing handicapped* (HH). HH and HI in essence imply that deafness is a condition to correct. These terms appear in numerous professional books, articles, conferences, and workshops. Typically, more hearing than DHH people consume such information about deafness. This implies that hearing perspectives on DHHs recycle and perpetuate infinitely.

The inclusion movement proponents fight to stop the labeling of persons on the basis of their physical or mental characteristics, or both, and prefer to categorize them as *differently abled* persons. In some ways, the inclusionists of the 1990s, the audists of recent decades, and Alexander Graham Bell and his cohorts are similar. They fight DHH persons' need to identify with the other DHH persons who share common experiences, observations, and values. They also dislike or fight against the signing community. In addition, the inclusionists are, in essence, segregationists because they are instrumental in determining with whom DHH children should or should not be in contact.

De-Identify to Control?

One may wonder why certain professionals seem to encourage segregation of DHH adults and parents of young DHH children. Ritter-Brinton and Stewart (1992) admonished deaf adults that they should maintain "nonjudgmental attitudes toward parents, show patience, offer constructive feedback, and try to understand the parent's position" (p. 89). This admonition seems strange because DHH adults rarely, probably with the exception of "hearinglike" DHHs, have any contact with young hearing parents who have DHH children. This statement seems to reflect a motive to maintain an invisible barrier between DHH adults and young hearing parents who have DHH children. At least 98% of all professionals and their cohorts who have working relationships with such young families are hearing. Most such parents have no contact with DHH adults. Many of the parents eventually realize that they need to sign to improve their relationship with their adolescent children.

The Intrusive Measures Based on External Perspectives

Lane (1989) wrote examples of how the professionals, or paraprofessionals, attempted to "cure" deafness and muteness with chemical, electrical, and mechanical means. Lane compiled traits under the " 'social,' 'cognitive,' 'behavioral' and 'emotional' headings from 350 pieces of professional materials related to deafness" (1992, p. 36). These traits are similar to those that colonizers attributed to uncivilized savages in earlier centuries. The articles and books from which these traits are compiled are on reading lists for teachers of the deaf preparation programs in North America.

Who Are Certified Teachers of the Deaf?

A 1993 survey of 30 of the existing graduate programs for teachers of deaf preparation (Mason, 1994b) shows that at least 95% of instructors and students are hearing. Many more courses categorized as Aural-Oral Communication Science, Psychology, and related fields are required in these programs than those categorized as Foundations and Orientation to Deaf Education. The following statement reflects a hearing perspective on how culturally deaf persons should acquire language: "A deaf person is one whose functional use of hearing precludes successful processing of linguistic information through audition with or without appropriate amplification such as hearing aids" (Bess & McConnell, 1981).

Carver (1989) pointed out that the literacy rate among the DHHs is low. One may wonder if there is a relationship between the low literacy rate and this hearing perspective. Yerker Andersson, president of the WFD, stressed that "the education of the deaf should not be a concern reserved for scientists, educators and other experts" (Andersson, 1994, p. 2). This implies that the serious discrepancy between the hearing and DHH perspectives is a worldwide phenomenon and a concern that should be addressed.

Changing Paradigm?

In recent years, there has been an increase in the public's awareness of DHHs as people with their own unique characteristics. There appears to be a change in the way the general public perceives DHHs. Stewart-Muirhead (1994) points out that researchers, clinicians, and the public have been challenged to address ethical issues regarding the cochlear implant program for young children. This article has stimulated discussion among the members of the medical community.

Ewoldt (1981) showed that DHH children can read English even if they cannot hear and speak it. This study challenges a myth that DHH children need oral skills to read and recognizes that deaf children do learn to read through ASL-English bilingual approaches. Kretschmer and Kretschmer (1990) pointed out that language acquisition by the deaf child must be treated differently from that of hearing peers. Staley, who had stressed the importance of teaching the deaf to hear and talk, in 1994 wrote, "Not every child will develop good oral language. It is just another option to consider and progress depends on the child and the efforts and contributions of the parents and the follow-up team" (p. 2). O'Connor (1994) explained that communication builds the social spheres within itself, the family, and community. This, in turn, affects the individual's psychological state, coping strategies, and the development of a concept of self.

The number of articles that question movements to promote the integration and inclusion of all DHH children, regardless of their disabilities, has been increasing. Ken Weber (1994) posed this thought-provoking question, "Is the integration movement destroying itself?" (p. 1). There is no need to explain what this question implies. Joyce Lorimer (1994) discusses how the inclusion movement affects the academic standards on which universities are built. The onus is on certain leading inclusion movement proponents to explain why true inclusion does not take place in the same universities where they work.

Probably for the first time ever, the government of Canada published literature that put as much, if not more, emphasis on the sociocultural aspects of DHHs than on deafness as a clinical-pathological concern (Health and Welfare Canada, 1994). Dolnick (1993) discussed cultural perspectives in *The Atlantic.*

Reflection and Conclusion

One can postulate that all humans seek to identify with others whom they believe share their common experiences, observations, world views, and values. As social beings, humans need camaraderie with others (examples include hearing parents of deaf children associating with other parents of deaf children, teachers attending conferences together, and students hanging around with their particular peers rather than others). The culturally deaf, hard of hearing, late-deafened, and oral deaf have the same underlying need that Alexander Graham Bell, as an eugenicist, tried to "correct" (Lane, 1989).

Recommendations

DHH children are trained to grow up to fit in the hearing perspective of what they should be or have. In their free environments, these children revert to themselves and become themselves. Likewise, as they become older, they do things that are not consistent with the hearing perspectives. The recommendation is that professionals should not formulate language-communication and educational objectives for DHH children on the basis of their hearing perspectives. Instead, they should learn from DHH adults and empower them to become active in reforming how best to meet young DHHs' educational needs. As long as hearing professionals impose their values on DHH children, the risk of adverse effects on DHH persons' quality of life remains high.

On the basis of my experience with more than 5,000 DHH persons, I recommend that all DHH children be allowed to acquire and use ASL—or

LSQ in francophone society. They should not have to wait until they are teenagers or adults before they are allowed to sign. This does not necessarily mean that they should not be allowed to acquire oral communication skills. The young DHH children should not be required to compromise by mixing oral skills with ASL skills to help make it easier for hearing professionals. In retrospect, it is easier for hearing people to learn ASL than for culturally deaf children to learn oral skills.

I recommend bilingual-bicultural education (BiBi) for all DHH children (Mason, 1994a), simply because almost all the 5,000 DHH persons I know use ASL and read English and are involved in both deaf and hearing communities. Very few use one or another version of English-like sign systems (Wilbur, 1987). Most of them can utter some speech but cannot carry out spontaneous conversation in speech. The educational model should be based on what is happening in the real world rather than on hearing perspectives on what DHHs should be and have. As an example, culturally deaf adults tend to have more confidence with ASL and printed English than with oral English or a variation of signed English or a combination of the two as described by Wilbur (1987). Because BiBi encourages DHHs to become bilingual (ASL and English) and encourages mutual respect between DHH and hearing people, DHH children's families are likely to find it beneficial for them too.

I know some DHHs who succeed with English-only educational approaches in hearing-dominated environments. As long as they feel satisfied with them, they should continue. Because there are more hearing people around the world who know two or more languages than know just one, however, it is reasonable to suggest that all DHHs and their families should not be denied the opportunity to become bilingual with ASL and English. Futhermore, it is likely that hearing and DHH persons will share more common perspectives as ASL-English bilinguals.

18

People With Developmental Disabilities

Applying Quality of Life to Assessment and Intervention

Roy I. Brown

A wide range of research has now been undertaken in the field of quality of life as it relates to people with developmental disabilities (Brown, Bayer, & MacFarlane, 1989; Goode, 1994b, 1994d). The research that has been carried out (e.g., Brown, Bayer, & Brown, 1992; Halpern, 1994) features issues that have not always been considered in quality of life studies in other fields of development (Romney, Brown, & Fry, 1994). For this reason, the material not only has particular relevance to the field of developmental disabilities but also may have implications for research methodology and practice in allied areas.

The Nature of Quality of Life

Some studies have attempted to define quality of life, yet a large number of researchers have ignored this very necessary process. Felce and Perry

(1993) have examined some of the commonalities and differences relating to the quality of life models within the field of developmental difficulties. The definition of quality of life is influenced by the different approaches and content that have been used (Schalock, 1994a). The models (see Brown et al., 1992; Cummins, 1992; Parmenter, 1988) are at once practical and pragmatic, and this probably accounts to some extent for the consensus between different proposers and underscores the stress on subjective as well as objective measures of quality of life.

Quality of life is, at one level, a personal expression of individual behavior, and the concept itself has to reflect perception, variability, and idiosyncrasy, thus making it difficult to measure comprehensively. This complexity, however, in no way negates the use of the construct, although criticism of it has been made by several authors (see Goode, 1994b). It is argued by proponents of quality of life (Brown, Brown, & Bayer, 1994) and conceded by some critics (Taylor, 1994) that quality of life research sensitizes those involved, providing opportunities to look at the field in a fresh way—a new window through which to understand behavior, argument, and intervention. Issues such as choice predominate, and implicit within this function is the notion of providing environments that lead to empowerment of the individual. Although Wolfensberger (1994) chills at the use of such words, here they reflect the ability of individuals to exert their resources effectively over their environment and thereby change the effect of the environment on the individual.

Assessment

There has been some attempt by various research workers to develop assessment scales (Schalock, 1994a). Goode (1988) has suggested that there may be some dangers in starting a new assessment revolution with intensive evaluation of individuals. New techniques are being devised and, because the models of quality of life for these are often holistic, assessment that arises from them tends to be global. Selection of specific areas after screening may help to avoid the problem raised by Goode.

Brown et al. (1989), Cummins (1992), Renwick, Brown, and Raphael (1994), and Schalock, Keith, Hoffman, and Karan (1989) all refer to a variety of domains. Some authors, such as Cummins, not only deal with the challenge of verbal information but attempt to assess quality of life using partially nonverbal techniques—for example, the calibration of quality of life using pictograph differential discriminations. Other scales, such as those of Brown and Bayer (1992), have arisen out of a need to measure quality of life within groups of people with developmental disabilities to gain a better grasp of the constructs involved and also to provide interventions based on personal choice. Cummins's (1992) material provides quantitative scores. It may be argued that a move in quality of life scales to quantitative measures may lose the nuance and detail of program needs and individual choice. But the amount of data obtained in qualitative format may not be easy to process. Brown and Bayer found that it might be easier to measure relative rather than absolute judgments—that is, whether an individual does better at *A* than *B* or likes *A* more than *B*. In carrying out measures of this type, where items can be ranked, Brown and Bayer (1992) found that over a long period of time in stable programs, high reliability scores were obtained (between .6 and .9 for most items).

Evans (1994) has argued that until we develop some normative results on quality of life in the general population, it may be inappropriate to develop such measures for specific populations. This proposition may have little relevance to disability studies in the sense that the perception of quality of life appears to be an important component of the individual's motivation and his or her concerns for future development without reference to norms.

Quality of life measurement can not only provide reliable and valid data but also identify effective goals within specified domains and suggest intervention strategies. Through this approach, the social and educational environment of the individual can be modified. As a result, behavior, performance, and perception can change for the individual and for those around the individual. In this sense, quality of life measurement is highly innovative and can be directed to program needs rather than simply comparing individuals with others. Rather than regarding quality of life measures as normative, it might be more satisfactory to describe them as idiosyncratic scales, which look for specific interests, needs, concerns, and perceived changes of individuals within specific contexts. Furthermore, data from quality of life scales can be used to enable various members of a family and individuals with developmental disabilities to discuss differences on a group basis and come to a more common viewpoint. This should lead to more effective interventions and social relationships and, in turn, to an improvement in quality of life.

Certain ideas emerge as important. It has been argued that quality of life measures can include both subjective and objective measures. There is a sense, however, in which the subjective components may be treated as objective data. Such data can be obtained by different assessors, and measures can be repeated and tested for reliability and validity. This is no different from a wide range of questionnaires that have been employed over the past 50 years. It is the meaning that we, the observers, attach to the data that makes them subjective or objective. Wolfensberger (1994) argued against quality of life measures because, being subjective, they are not scientific. This is to misunderstand the basis on which most quality of life data are collected and the conclusions that are made from such statements. The individuals make statements about themselves and their environments. This is objective. There is no claim that such views match external events or measures. Indeed, the discrepancies between the former and the latter may be very important, and the personal statement may be primary because it links to self-image and motivation.

To some degree, the recommendations that have been developed in the area are not only embedded in quality of life but associated with other constructs such as social role valorization (Wolfensberger, 1983) and societal views of disability itself (Barton, Ballard, & Folcher, 1991). This is, perhaps, not surprising, for quality of life is itself the outcome of a developmental process, which has increasingly considered social attributes to be a source of major handicap. The definitions provided by the World Health Organization (Brown, 1991) regarding impairment, disability, and handicap fit such a model, though even these tend to confuse the fact that handicapping conditions can themselves lead to disability. It is also important to recognize that quality of life is not simply related to a pleasure principle but forms the basis for cognitive and emotional development.

Quality of Life in
Research and Practice

If quality of life is a concept that results from an ongoing developmental process, it is probably much more complex than we have recognized. The work that follows is designed to illustrate this point. It builds on studies reported by Brown et al. (1989, 1992). The definition of quality of life used in those studies was the discrepancy between a person's achieved and current needs and desires (MacFarlane, Brown, & Bayer, 1989). This refers to the subjective or perceived as well as the objective assessment of an individual's demands. The greater the discrepancy, the poorer the quality of life (MacFarlane et al., 1989). This definition is holistic, as it relates to all domains of an individual's life. It recognizes the interaction between the individual and his or her environment.

The study itself was the culmination of 6 years of research into the quality of life of 240 persons with developmental disabilities, mostly with mild to moderate intellectual disability, between the ages of 18 and 63 years, who attended rehabilitation programs in western Canada. The purpose was to look at performance and subjective reflections of individuals about various aspects of their lives. Intelligence testing (Wechsler Adult Intelligence Scale

[WAIS]), scores on the Adaptive Functioning Index (AFI) (Marlett, 1976), and a quality of life scale designed by Brown and Bayer (1992) completed by study participants and sponsors (frequently parents) constituted the major measures. Apart from intelligence testing, the measurements took place each year for the first 3 years of the study, where individuals continued in their rehabilitation programs. Following this period, some of the individuals received intervention where attempts were made, using quality of life concepts and principles derived from the first part of the study, to improve levels of performance and experience of quality of life. The intervention stage provided individuals with choice over activity, place of intervention, and, wherever possible, selection of professional worker. In other words, the individual controlled the issues of choice, whereas process was in the hands of the professional workers. The same assessment techniques were employed following the interventions, supplemented by measures of the effects of interventions of choice.

The results reported suggest very considerable development in those individuals who had such opportunities and exceeded the development of those who were not in such programs: (a) the intervention group improved in performance intelligence (modified WAIS); (b) the intervention group decreased in ratings of vocational performance on the AFI; (c) the intervention group improved in social education (AFI) scores, particularly in reading, writing, concept attainment, time telling, money handling, and motor movement; (d) on the Quality of Life Questionnaire, the intervention group and their sponsors perceived improvement in skills (18 skills monitored) and home and personal skills (20 skills monitored) and recorded an increase in needed support, although sponsors saw less need of support (16 areas monitored); the sponsors noted improvement in community enrichment, although the consumers recorded a decline in positive feelings about the environment (14 attributes were monitored); and (e) sponsors perceived a decline in leisure activities in the nonintervention group (29 activities monitored).

In addition to the above results, specific interventions for particular individuals showed gains in such activities as vocational management and social performance. It was noted that intervention of choice often resulted in positive transfer to other skills that were not involved in intervention. (For full details of the research model and analysis of results, see Brown et al., 1989, 1992.)

The results gave rise to a wide range of recommendations and also provided some insight into the types of direction that will need to be seriously considered in future quality of life work. Some of the findings initially appeared paradoxical, again illustrating that quality of life is an extremely complex concept and one that does not necessarily follow preconceived notions. For example, improved quality of life does not necessarily improve an individual's level of happiness. In fact, reduced happiness may be recorded. Improved quality of life may result in greater criticism of the environment. Success brings the need for greater success!

It may be expected that this work now applied in other contexts, such as the work of James and Brown (1992), Timmons (in press), and Velde (in press), suggests other applications in relation to specific forms of disability. Yet the principles appear to remain the same. For example, issues of choice in relation to children with Prader-Willi syndrome regarding eating behaviors might at first glance be seen to be a potentially dangerous process, yet quality of life practice can open new opportunities for development of self-image. Quality of life studies in the area of inclusive education (Brown & Timmons, 1994) suggest that inclusive processes are rather more involved than we have presently considered and include a myriad of actions and perceptions that affect learning within a quality of life framework (e.g., who controls bedtime, how pocket money is provided, whom one telephones, where and with whom one eats meals, and choice of school).

Brown and Timmons (1994) found that teenagers with disabilities often stated that they lived highly sheltered and uninvolved lives and wished to participate in a wide range of other events. Interestingly enough, such behavior covered not only educational aspects, such as the types of curriculum they might experience, but whom they wished to involve, during both educational and noneducational parts of the day. They were concerned about isolation in eating meals at school and had a desire to share with others. Within the home, they wanted to be involved with other members of family in simple activities, such as walking the dog. Very often, parents were totally unaware of the requirements of their children in such areas. Able, experienced, and well-meaning parents make assumptions. Timmons (in press) encountered many such examples in the collection of data.

The past three decades in particular have been associated with the development of a series of philosophical positions and mission statements about disabilities (e.g., Wolfensberger, 1983, 1994). These have often been put forward in a form that asserted "vision" as a primary driving force. These developments are important, but without exploration and application of the detailed changes required, negative forces such as "dumping" tend to occur. The results outlined above suggest that quality of life models can provide a wide range of practical recommendations and these have considerable relevance to how rehabilitation professionals are educated within colleges and universities. Last, quality of life models challenge, at a very practical level, the types of management systems that have developed. The basic notions of quality of life as described here contradict the type of hierarchical management systems that many agencies employ and practice in their fields of endeavor.

STAFF IN AGENCIES—THEIR CONCERNS

The study also examined the views of agency personnel. Very often, staff did not know how their agency was functioning nor did they have a clear idea of how they might become promoted or change program activities. Frequently, they saw themselves as worse off than the clientele. Under such circumstances, it is unlikely that progress and changes would take place.

There were a number of issues that arose during the intervention stage. Many agency personnel indicated that they could not, even if they wanted to, support such interventions, largely because of management regulations. It was not sufficient that the activity was the choice of the individual with a disability.

What were these interventions? They were predicated on the wishes of the clients (e.g., cooking specific meals, going out with specific people, obtaining particular work, or living in a particular place). They could indicate where intervention would take place—in their home, local community, or agency. They had some control over the choice of personnel who would work with them. Many of these interventions lasted only a matter of months (several weeks to 2 years). Individual contact with the rehabilitation worker averaged between 1 and 3 hours per week, and this was far more than individual contact within the agency's regular program.

EMPLOYMENT—A SECONDARY AIM?

The data raised a number of other issues. First, individuals in rehabilitation agencies had a wide range of worries and anxieties. These were highly specific and, on the whole, were not about work but about other facets of their life. The image in rehabilitation, which has been generated in Canada, Australia, the United Kingdom, and elsewhere, is that employment is the direct road to rehabilitation. This is not the case if issues of personal choice are taken as a guide. It seems from the data that responding to individual choices, which are frequently other than those regarding employment, results in success that can eventually lead to choices about employment. Thus it may be essential to make use of choice within nonemployment domains to eventually achieve employment or complete inclusion within the community.

PERCEPTION OF LIVING CONDITIONS

It was apparent that individuals became more critical of the conditions under which they were living as they improved in other domains. Yet sponsors, often parents, believed the individuals' circumstances had in fact improved. In other words, interventions involving choice may lead to improved quality of life in objective terms and in the eyes of other observers,

but individuals with disability may become more critical of their environments and therefore indicate greater dissatisfaction and unhappiness.

It seems important not to regard happiness necessarily as a positive
indicator of quality of life. Quality of life appears more related to an ability
to gain power over a situation, to be able to express one's opinion, and then
be able to manipulate the environment to the best of one's ability and
according to one's choice. It also appears to relate to improvement and a
desire to have more effect on the environment. This leads to new challenges
and, often, difficulties. As the individuals become less satisfied with aspects
of their life, they may be seen as more difficult to manage by traditional
trainers in agencies. Such was the view of agency personnel. Indeed, rehabilitation is misguidedly directed to making people quiet when in fact its
strategies should be directed toward people becoming noisy—that is, challenging the system under which they function. As individuals improved their
quality of life, as rated by themselves and sponsors, and as performance
improved, many vocational supervisors rated the consumers as worse (see
earlier discussion). This may have been because the raters saw persons in
intervention less frequently, but it may also suggest that effective community
behavior is not acceptable workshop behavior and the development of
assertive behavior may be viewed critically by personnel. Quality of life
programs do not work for conformity but for individual choice and action.

CHOICES AND PERCEPTION

It has been argued that models based on choice, empowering environments, and control by the individual require a different form of assessment
from traditional normative and criterion-referenced testing. To carry out
interventions of choice, we need to know much about the individuals'
perceptions of situations, including their own performance, and their
choices. Brown and Bayer (1992) have suggested that such choices can form
a basis for intervention goals and strategies. Two of the objections to choice
by agencies have been recognized as the inability of clients to keep to their
choices and the inability for personnel to respect and follow through with
the choices of an individual, regardless of their personal preferences. Results
from the Brown et al. (1988, 1992) studies often showed changes in viewpoint by clients and sponsors over time. Many agencies argue that it is not
possible to use viewpoint and choice when individuals change frequently.
Brown et al. (1992) argued that these changes are the essence of rehabilitation. The quality of life model described by Brown et al. (1992) accommo-
dates and anticipates such changes for they see quality of life as a dynamic
model where change and discrepancy are acceptable. With such a view,

personnel training must be based on the idea that the duty of personnel is to follow through on the choices selected by the individual. Thus the exploration of choice, monitoring its changes, and selecting appropriate means of fulfilling choices result in a client-documented assessment process.

CLIENT AND SPONSOR PERCEPTIONS

High test-retest reliability in quality of life skills may reflect lack of progress and presence of a noneffective intervention. Intervention is choice driven and, therefore, success is likely to produce different effects in different people, reducing test correlation over time. This probability should be followed up in future work. It was also noted that correlations were high between individuals and sponsors recording events at the same time. But this was in terms of item order, not necessarily in terms of quantity. Indeed, one of the changes that occurred, once quality of life interventions took place, was the gradual change in perception of individuals in terms of the magnitude of scores associated with particular events. This brought consumer perceptions closer to those of their sponsors. For example, during traditional intervention, individuals tended to indicate they were happy and did not need much assistance in various activities, whereas sponsors thought assistance was necessary. During intervention, individuals and sponsors came to perceive the needs more similarly. Baer (in press) reported a somewhat analogous finding in the field of head injury where clients saw themselves as ineffective but sponsors saw improvement and effectiveness. With quality of life intervention, where there is a shift to consumer-sponsor agreement, rehabilitation becomes, at least theoretically, easier because as soon as the family agrees on needs and directions and records similar successes and failures, quality of life intervention becomes more practical and more effective.

One of the challenges to personnel in the particular program that Brown et al. (1992) described was to carry out choice intervention when the family was not sure of the needs, desirability, or direction. Because parents and other sponsors have views about the availability and desirability of intervention or the likely success of intervention, Brown et al. noted selection factors that encouraged some people to be involved and others to decline intervention procedures. Indeed, where there was a desire by the sponsor for involvement to take place and to accept the individual's choice, greater progress was obtained. It is therefore important in such work to try, through counseling and demonstration, to bring parties closer together, but the needs of the consumer must be viewed as paramount. The objective correctness of their views is not the issue—the issue is acceptance and resulting dignity of the consumer.

EMOTIONAL NEEDS OF CLIENT

Many of the concerns stated by individuals relate to emotional needs, and this has emerged as a clear issue in quality of life assessment. In the Brown et al. (1992) study, it was noted that in many instances, although parents recognized the need for assertiveness training and emotional support, they often felt unable to provide further emotional support in practice. Whether this was due to the fact that they had become stressed about individuals continuing to live with them over long periods well into adult life, or whether they required quiet and more supportive environments for themselves as they approached retirement, needs to be explored.

In the Brown et al. (1992) study, issues relating to the need for quiet residential environments, the importance of contact with fathers as well as mothers, and the health of relatives were recorded more frequently than issues relating to employment. These are the people's stated interests and form the subject matter of intervention, regardless of issues. Many individuals with disabilities made no or few statements about future events—an aspect of quality of life that might be examined further. Lack of future planning strategies and a paucity of personal possessions relating to the future were very apparent.

Relevance to Professional Training

FRONTLINE PERSONNEL

The development of quality of life models has major significance for the education of professional staff, particularly those, but not only those, at the frontline level. Most new personnel receive their training in university or college programs. But the field is in an early stage of development, and most of the professionals employed in this area come from other areas of expertise; a number are employed by virtue of experience rather than professional training. Most people who train in the rehabilitation field as professional practitioners and developmental educators receive their first experience in traditionally run programs; that is, for the most part, they see individuals in vocational rehabilitation centers, day training programs, sheltered workshops, group homes, and even institutions.

But a quality of life model requires something else. Because choice is relevant and a critical part of an individual's program focus, intervention and support may take place in any environment selected by the individual. Frequently, this will be within the community or his or her own home. In these cases, practitioners have to work on a one-to-one basis where parents or others observe interactions with the individual concerned.

This leads to a wide range of questions and concerns, and personnel must be well equipped to provide explanations as to the methods and use of content. They must be versatile in terms of their knowledge base, be able to think on their feet, and be able to devise individual programs that foster achievement of the individual's own goals. They are also likely to experience individuals who change their goals or interests. Thus the skilled front-line practitioner of the future will elicit, through observation, assessment, discussion, and pilot exploration, the individual's choices of experience, lifestyle, or program, and identify the specific goals and places of intervention.

Personnel will also be scrutinized in terms of whether the client feels they are the right person to facilitate. For younger children who have developmental delays, this will happen within the parental home where parents will act as advocates. Although it may be necessary or desirable that an individual has advocates, however, experience suggests that goals set by parents or others frequently do not lead to progress when they are not the goals of the individual (see Brown et al., 1992).

This also changes the orientation of the practitioner, which is a very strong argument for suggesting that people who receive college or university training gain their primary experience and practice in this choice milieu. Following this, they could be apprenticed through an internship to a field worker who is highly experienced in understanding quality of life programs and who would support and monitor their initial work. New practitioners would then function on their own. Consultants could be employed but would, as their name applies, give advice. It would be left to the client or consumer and his or her worker to implement the advice if it was thought by the consumer to be appropriate.

QUALITY OF LIFE PROGRAMS
AND MANAGEMENT

Other challenges emerge relating to the management of such programs. If personnel at the management level do not endorse and support such programs, it is difficult to ensure that they work in practice. Indeed, following their 6-year study, Brown et al. (1992) were frequently asked whether it was possible to adjust current programs to fit such a model. Their impression was that most current services would not be able to do so easily because of traditional philosophies and methods of operating, which prevent radical change. Where changes have occurred, they are often superficial and do not represent a total revamping of the system. The responses from personnel attending seminars and workshops following the study indicated that the quality of life model could not be implemented for a variety of reasons: because the consumers changed their minds, all personnel or relatives could not agree with the goals of the consumer, or union and management negotiations took up staff time that prevented the flexibility required. Only one of the agencies that Brown et al. (1992) worked with came forward to ask for help in changing their direction of application. This was done with some success and included providing in-service education. Senior personnel from the agency registered in master programs at the university, which provided opportunities to experience and to negotiate developments of the type described at frontline and management levels.

It will be necessary to set up new demonstration projects, and in such instances, the managers, directors, and planners must study alongside frontline staff. It will probably be wise to link this into university and college programs where joint contracts between university and rehabilitation services can foster demonstration models. In most countries, there are now some staff who have this type of experience.

Many will argue that the programs described are now going on in the community, but the type of discussion, counseling, flexibility, sharing with consumers, and dedicated practice in the field at any time of the day are dimensions that, in practice, do not frequently occur. It is, over time, those who have worked in such models who should become the managers of services. It may be effective for such managers to be appointed on a rotating basis, with the front-line system. It is essential that managers are knowledgeable about behavior at a personal level. It is important to realize that although stability of relationships with consumers is very important in quality of life front-line intervention, personnel also require time away from direct client contact. Such situations can be emotionally demanding and individuals can be on call 24 hours a day. Although there are many nuances to work out, all of the above features were included within the demonstration study of Brown et al. (1992) and have been identified in a practical Australian study (Miller & Davey, 1994).

ETHICAL CHALLENGES

A number of ethical challenges arise. Individuals who work with consumers in the field on a one-to-one basis are necessarily involved in close personal relationships. Frequently, individual consumers come to see their field-workers as friends and occasionally this can grow into much stronger personal relationships. It is important that field-workers have opportunities to recognize their own feelings and to have an ethical consultative group that can provide them with advice and support. It is also important that personnel do not leave a situation suddenly and without warning, for when relationships are strong, leaving can create a real sense of personal loss.

Basically, the process outlined does provide the opportunity to develop and deal with emotional support. It is associated with personal choices, which include interventions and environments of choice that enable the development of self-image. Such a process is relevant not just to intellectual or developmental disability. Preliminary work by Baer (in press) and by Velde (in press) indicates the relevance of similar processes with people who have head injuries and those with physical disabilities. Personal experience working with people with severe and profound disabilities suggests that choices and opportunities for personal expression are critical, even though these may be at a very simple level (e.g., choice of positions in a room, a choice of drink at lunch).

COST OF INDIVIDUAL CHOICES

It will be argued that such models are costly, though analysis of a demonstration program suggests that this is not the case (Bayer, Brown, & Brown, 1988). The evidence is that such a model provides more one-to-one relationship time than in present programs. Employment of more highly skilled and experienced personnel is more costly. These skilled personnel, however, though involved on an individual basis, work with a variety of people during the course of a week—each up to several hours. It is not essential that their involvement take place throughout the day, and it is probably the intensity of contact, using a space- and time-distributed model, that makes it of greater relevance. There is no need for purposely designed buildings, and individual field-workers can very frequently operate from their own homes (Lichty & Johnson, 1992). Thus minimal building, heating, and lighting costs and upkeep costs are involved.

The second most heavy cost relates to transportation of workers as they move from place to place. For administrative purposes, a single office at most is required where personnel can meet together to discuss programs and experiences, meet with a service manager from time to time, and receive secretarial help. On such a basis, the cost per client is no more, and frequently, much less expensive than current programs.

POLICY IMPLICATIONS

The model described does not fit with traditional hierarchical structures. It challenges government services to recognize how they can interface with such projects without providing hierarchical structures for reporting. Probably no more than a basic monitoring process is required, although as such models are moved to more and more challenging situations, the duration of intervention and the skills necessary will increase, thus accelerating the costs.

Experience in the past indicates that this is not something that is readily understood within administrative structures. Once demonstrations have been set up, there is a tendency to bureaucratize them and to provide a wide range of rules and regulations that involve a considerable amount of paperwork. It is this that tends to add costs to programs. It is essential that government organizations do not require such intensive administrative work nor should they be required by the services themselves.

It is suggested that governments allow for flexibility in funding demonstration models using individualized funding—strategies that are now going into operation in some countries. Within the Brown et al. (1992) study, interventions took place for several months and were successful, but this did not mean the individuals were then able to function independently. It did mean that clients had a greater number of skills, perceived themselves as improved, and had more concerns about their environment. Though contact with personnel may decrease or increase over time, the ability to monitor ongoing challenges through such contacts must be available.

Relevance to Research

The model that has been described needs to be subjected to further research both to examine the wider implications of applying quality of life models and to clarify the type of processes required in intervention. The type of exploration that is required should accent different research models. First of all, group operations in the traditional sense are not feasible. That is, it is not possible in most instances to have quasi-experimental studies with experimental and control groups where the same treatment is applied to all those in the experimental group. The basis of quality of life is individual choice, so the process of implementation will also differ. It is the model that is undergoing research, not simply a specific intervention. The interventions differ from individual to individual in type, time, place, content, and personnel.

There is, of course, a considerable need to discover what types of knowledge, interaction, and personnel are most effective in such situations and what new aspects should be developed. There is also a need to find the range of issues and choices perceived by individuals and the effects of attending to them. Thus it is expected that variability in intervention and outcome will occur. Research will then be directed to intervention methods rather than intervention per se.

The attitudes and skills of frontline personnel must be examined. The needs and choices of persons need to be assessed in a quality of life context, and the means of such assessment require much further exploration. Experimental studies using individuals as their own control seem highly relevant for the examination of specific effects of intervention. The employment of phenomenological methodology to examine individual perceptions and thoughts about development becomes critical, and such studies, if well carried out, can provide leads for more traditional studies.

The importance of personal exploration of such themes by potential clients cannot be overemphasized. Despite traditional views to the contrary, it appears that personal perceptions are amenable to the standard criteria of scientific methodology. The views of subjects are observable, reliability can be assessed, and the statements can be validated against intervention outcomes. It is apparent that quality of life studies are gradually leading to a better understanding of people's needs and choices and that they are also providing challenges not only for administrators and intervention personnel but also for research workers who are expected to use nontraditional methodologies.

19

Quality of Life Assessment for Persons With Severe Developmental Disabilities

Hélène Ouellette-Kuntz
Bruce McCreary

A number of methods have been described in the literature for concep-tualizing and measuring the quality of life of persons with severe developmental disabilities. In this chapter, we will outline the work we have completed to date to this purpose, namely, the development of the Quality of Life Interview Schedule (QUOLIS). Although QUOLIS can assess the quality of life of all persons with developmental disabilities, it is intended primarily for use in those instances where individuals' intellectual and communication impairments prevent their direct participation in assessment.

No clear definition of quality of life has yet been reached. Many agree, however, that "quality of life has less to do with what and how much we have

AUTHORS' NOTE: The authors thank the Community Services Program at Rideau Regional Centre, Smiths Falls, Ontario; Richard MacLachlan; and the participants, family members, and staff at Ongwanada, Kingston, Ontario. Our work was financially supported in part by the Office of the Dean and Vice Principal, Faculty of Medicine, Queen's University, Kingston, Ontario.

in the way of material goods than with the conditions under which we acquire and use them" (Ackoff, 1976, p. 292). Choice and opportunities for personal decision making also appear to be critical elements—it is important to "fashion one's own fate, to create one's self" (Ackoff, 1976, p. 290).

Although quality of life considerations are prominent in discussions of policy and service provision in the field of developmental disabilities, the best way to conceptualize and measure it remains unclear. This is particularly so for people who have severe intellectual impairments (IQ < 35), major problems in communicating their needs and wishes, or both. Many of these people have had limited life experiences and opportunities to choose where to live, how to spend their time, and with whom to associate. Their lives are often complicated by the effects of other disabilities, such as cerebral palsy, epilepsy, and behavioral disorders, that reflect the presence of severe central nervous system damage. In addition, whatever might have caused this damage may also have affected other organ systems, creating a whole range of congenital anomalies. Terms such as *multiply disabled* and *medically fragile* are used to capture this complexity.

Within the total developmental disability population, approximately 8% are considered to have IQs lower than 35 (American Psychiatric Association, 1987). Although it is recognized that intelligence tests may not accurately measure intelligence in persons with severe disabilities, IQ is used here to give an indication of the population concerned. Individuals classified as severely disabled are unique in their limited expressive and receptive language abilities (Borthwick-Duffy, 1990). About two-thirds are thought to have major problems with speech and language. Because of this, most are unable to complete the type of written questionnaire or individual interview often used to assess quality of life. Many researchers and service providers interested in persons with severe disabilities appear to have concluded that whatever quality of life might be, it can never be assessed accurately without the direct contribution of the individual concerned. In our view, this is short-sighted; it excludes those who cannot provide us with information that we can clearly understand. Although this group represents only a fraction of the total population of those with developmental disabilities, they must not be forgotten in our efforts to improve the quality of life of all persons. We fail them if our conceptual formulations and our measures cannot accommodate their unique characteristics.

Defining Quality of Life

Although it is argued that "the primary dimensions of [q]uality of [l]ife are the same for all people, with or without disabilities" (Rootman, Raphael,

Shewchuk, Renwick, Friefeld, Garber, Talbot, Woodill, & Brown, 1992, p. 7), the necessity of operationalizing quality of life differently for persons with more severe handicaps has also been recognized (Borthwick-Duffy, 1990; Ouellette-Kuntz, 1990). Borthwick-Duffy contended that when individuals are highly dependent on others for the majority of their daily needs, quality of life and quality of care may become inseparable. Goode and Hogg (1994) also stressed the significance of quality medical and educational services in quality of life for persons with profound or multiple developmental disabilities or both.

A document that is of particular relevance to quality of life for persons with disabilities, and one that influenced our work, is the *World Programme of Action Concerning Disabled Persons* (United Nations, 1983). In that document, the United Nations focused on two goals for persons with disabilities: full participation and equality. For persons with profound or multiple developmental disabilities or both, the attainment of these goals must consider both basic needs (such as health, safety, and comfort) and higher-order needs (such as friendship and fulfillment). Furthermore, close attention must be given to the availability and accessibility of a variety of supports for meeting these needs as well as to the extent to which these supports provide enjoyment for the individual.

Approaches to Data Collection

Although it is often argued that individuals are the best judge of their quality of life, some individuals are unable to appraise and communicate aspects of their quality of life reliably. Raphael, Renwick, and Brown (1993) provided an overview of the research concerning difficulties encountered when interviewing individuals with developmental disabilities in general. Selai and Rosser (1993) claimed the following in assessing qualify of life:

> Not only is the [individual] required, through a demanding task of introspection to consider [his or her] physical, psychological and social well-being, but also on some measures to make a higher-order judgment concerning [his or her] attitude to [his or her] [life situation]. (p. 68)

Instances where individuals' ability to assess their own quality of life has been questioned include the case of young children, patients with severe psychotic symptoms, elderly persons with dementia, those suffering from brain damage, and individuals with severe developmental disabilities.

A 1974 study conducted in Massachusetts that stressed the involvement of individuals with developmental disabilities as respondents in a survey concerning deinstitutionalization and community adjustment found that 12.5% of the subjects could not be interviewed (Wyngaarden, 1981). A more recent study in Wales found that only 50% of participants could be interviewed (Lowe & de Paiva, 1988). Furthermore, although 50% were interviewed, the researchers reported that the proportion of participants who provided "appropriate" responses to "yes-no plus comment" questions such as "Are there any rules you don't like? . . . Which ones?" and "Do you like living with everyone in your house or ward? . . . Why?" ranged from 6% to 73%. Participants fared somewhat better when asked opinion-only questions (e.g., "What's it like to live here?" and "What do you like about [day program]?"). The proportion of so-called appropriate responses to this type of question ranged from 24% to 80%. After conducting several studies interviewing individuals with developmental disabilities, Sigelman et al. (1981) concluded that "verbal interviewing techniques appear to be infeasible in the profound retardation range [and] applicable with some severely retarded persons" (p. 127).

What this suggests is that, although objective measures of quality of life usually can be validly and reliably obtained with relative ease, obtaining subjective measures of quality of life is often problematic in instances where the individual cannot be interviewed. Two primary approaches have been described in the literature for capturing the subjective element of quality of life assessment for individuals who are deemed unable to do so reliably for themselves. The first approach is to use caregivers as alternative sources of information. The second is to rely on direct observations of individuals and their expressions of satisfaction or dissatisfaction in various life domains.

THE USE OF CAREGIVERS AS ALTERNATIVE SOURCES OF INFORMATION

Sigelman et al. (1981) have demonstrated through numerous studies on the validity and reliability of interviewing techniques used with individuals with developmental disabilities that "agreement between mentally retarded clients and parents or attendants . . . is low enough to suggest that substantially different information may sometimes be obtained from the two sources" (p. 127). In testing the psychometric properties of the Multifaceted Lifestyle Satisfaction Scale, which assesses the personal satisfaction of adults with limited intelligence, Harner and Heal (1993) concluded that "professional caretakers do not always accurately predict satisfaction reported by individuals in their care" (p. 233). These findings are supported by research in other fields, such as oncology, where physicians are found to be poor judges of their patients' preferences (Slevin, Plant, Lynch, Drinkwater, & Gregory, 1988).

The use of proxy may, however, be an appropriate approach in quality of life assessment when severe receptive or expressive language limitations or cognitive difficulties make interviews with individuals impossible. A reputational surrogate or proxy approach may be the best—and perhaps the only—method available to approximate subjective self-reports of quality of life for persons with profound or multiple developmental disabilities or both (Goode & Hogg, 1994).

When proxy respondents are used, careful consideration must be given to the following questions: Who will serve as proxy? What domains will be assessed? and How can proxy reporting be enhanced? Patrick and Erickson (1993) recommended that proxy reports of highly subjective domains be avoided. In addition, proxy respondents should be asked to rate their perceived accuracy of the information they are providing. Last, these authors recommended that more than one proxy respondent should be used to obtain convergent views on the quality of life of the person being assessed.

THE USE OF DIRECT OBSERVATION

The use of direct observation is an alternative method that may sometimes be desirable when assessing the quality of life of individuals with severe developmental disabilities. This method, however, may have limited value for measuring self-perception in quality of life (Patrick & Erickson, 1993). Furthermore, when direct observation is used, not only is the interpretation of the observation open to bias but so is the representativeness of the observation. That is, observations are best carried out at different times and in various contexts. To avoid these biases, the tools of ethnography, such as participant observation techniques, are often used. Participant observation refers to "research characterized by a period of social interaction between the researcher and the subject, in the milieu of the latter, during which data are unobtrusively and systematically collected" (Taylor & Bogdan, 1981, p. 72). When the assessment of such an ill-defined and subjective concept as quality of life is required, the participant observation approach is probably useful as it provides the means to obtain a detailed in-depth understanding of the everyday lives of individuals.

It is recognized that the two approaches to capturing the subjective elements in quality of life assessment have serious limitations. Although it is clearly inappropriate not to interview individuals who can reliably understand and communicate their own perceptions of the quality of their lives, it is, however, just as inappropriate not to develop and use alternative approaches for those with more severe disabilities. To do nothing because of uncertainty will not advance our understanding.

Our conceptual approach to quality of life assessment, set out in QUOLIS, relies on the use of proxy respondents and participant observation techniques as the best possible way to measure the quality of life for individuals with severe developmental disabilities. QUOLIS was developed for use with people for whom self-reporting was not possible and with the intention of capturing subjective elements of quality of life that could be accurately provided by proxies.

The Quality of Life Interview Schedule (QUOLIS)

In developing QUOLIS, we adopted the use of terms such as *impairment, disability, handicap, habilitation,* and *equalization of opportunities* that are commonly used and understood in health promotion and rehabilitation (United Nations, 1983). We also recognized the importance of providing persons with disabilities their chosen levels of assistance (i.e., support) if their lives were to approach what they might have been without their disabilities. This thinking is in keeping with the recent definition of mental retardation formulated by the American Association on Mental Retardation (Luckasson et al., 1992; Ruedrich, 1994).

Elements of qualitative research are combined with quantitative methods in an interview involving two or more persons who know the person with disabilities—the proxy respondents. These respondents are typically a family member or a friend, and a paid caregiver.

ACCOMMODATING PEOPLE WITH SEVERE DISABILITIES

When one is faced with assessing quality of life of a person whose disabilities preclude direct participation, two key considerations are operative: the need to ensure optimal input by those who know the individual well and the need to consider the effect of any additional disabilities that accompany the intellectual impairment.

To ensure optimal input, the assessor needs to create a context in which those who know the individual well (proxy respondents) can comfortably and comprehensively provide the data that will give the best possible picture.

It has been our experience that family members, friends, and paid staff are very able to empathize and communicate on behalf of people with disabilities.

It is easy to underestimate the effect of the additional disabilities and congenital anomalies that so often coexist with severe intellectual impairment. Although there may be recognizable patterns, each individual is truly unique. Hence the assessment includes a review of the various supports relevant to each disability or congenital defect. The so-called *inverse care law* (i.e., the less you have, the less you get) draws our attention to the extreme importance of all the problems faced by individuals, not just those of interest to assessors or proxy respondents participating in the quality of life assessment.

ASSESSMENT PROCEDURES

The QUOLIS Interviewer

Interviewers are people with good interviewing skills and a sound knowledge of the system of supports for individuals with disabilities. Prior to conducting QUOLIS interviews, they participate in a 1½-day training session. Topics covered include the nature of quality of life, key issues in defining quality of life, approaches to quality of life in the field of developmental disabilities, main features of QUOLIS, QUOLIS indicator statements, and the QUOLIS process. A significant proportion of the training is spent discussing and role playing.

The QUOLIS Interview

The individual's personal characteristics, such as energy level, sociability, and reactivity to stress, as well as recent life events, are reviewed before the discussion shifts to the quality of life assessment (see Table 19.1).

During a semistructured interview, the proxies are asked to recall, from their direct observations and experiences, their perceptions of 72 quality of life indicators. These 72 indicators are grouped into 12 life domains: health services, family guardianship, income maintenance, education-employment, housing and safety, transportation, social-recreational, religious-cultural, case management, advocacy, counseling, and aesthetics.

The interviewer rates each indicator according to four dimensions (see Table 19.2).

The first dimension, *support,* is rated as either available or not available; the second and third dimensions, *access* and *participation,* are rated on 7-point scales (*nil, minimal, poor, ?, moderate, good, optimal*); and the fourth dimension, *contentment,* is also rated on a 7-point scale (*terrible, unhappy, mostly*

TABLE 19.1 Categories of Information Discussed Prior to QUOLIS Interview

Category	Sample Items
Communication	Modes of communication used by the individual
	The individual's effectiveness at expressive communication with familiar and unfamiliar partners
	Ways the individual expresses contentment and discontentment
Disabilities	Level of disability
	Presence and severity of cerebral palsy
	Presence and correction of a visual impairment
Personal characteristics	Energy level
	Sociability
	Reactivity to stress
	Special interests
	Personal goals and aspirations
Recent life events	Death of a significant other
(occurrence and impact)	Changes in daily activities and routines
	New relationships
	Graduation, employment, promotion
	Significant family event

dissatisfied, mixed, mostly satisfied, pleased, delighted). Overall scores can be obtained for each of these four dimensions and dimension scores can be obtained for each of the 12 domains. These summary scores combined with narrative responses obtained during the interview are used by the interviewer to summarize the quality of life of the person being assessed.

The process is further individualized through the use of supplementary indicators for individuals with seven additional types of disabilities: epilepsy, cerebral palsy, hearing impairment, visual impairment, psychiatric disorder, communication disorder, and chronic illness (see Figure 19.1 for a summary).

Psychometric Properties

On the contentment scale, correlation coefficient ranges were .79 to .99 for intrarater agreement and .48 to .95 for interrater agreement (Ouellette-Kuntz, 1989, 1990). Further investigation of the validity and reliability of the QUOLIS scales is currently under way, using 41 QUOLIS interviews.

TABLE 19.2 Dimensions Assessed in QUOLIS

Dimension	Definition	Example
Support	A form of assistance or an opportunity provided to a person; it may or may not be present in a given community	An academic program, counseling, or personal assistance
Access	The degree to which the individual can make use of the support	A residential program is available but access is minimal because there are no vacancies at present.
Participation	The actual use of the support by the individual	Participation is minimal when the individual does not participate regularly in bowling because it conflicts with a favorite television program.
Contentment	The degree of satisfaction apparently experienced by the individual in relation to the particular support	Contentment is "mostly dissatisfied" when an adult likes the group home but misses friends from the institution and wishes to return.

RELEVANCE

Ackoff (1976) claimed that we cannot validly measure quality of life because we lack the measure itself and contended that participative planning should be viewed as an alternative to the quantification of quality of life by those whose objective is to design, plan for, and develop a society in which the quality of life of others is to be improved. Our work developing QUOLIS has convinced us that this tool offers a good method of assessing quality of life of individuals with severe developmental disabilities. QUOLIS asks family members, friends, and caregivers to watch and listen to the communication of contentment and discontentment of the individual with a severe developmental disability and to share their perceptions in the assessment of quality of life. A parent of a young woman with a severe developmental disability described the parents' desire to assist and the subtle indicators that are so important:

> The signs may be primitive but they are there—a welcoming sound; the beginning of a smile; flickering eyelashes; crying. . . . I think that, too often, in cases of handicapped adults, because they do not speak our language, we not only misinterpret their communications, we totally ignore them. (Paproski, 1988, pp. 8-9)

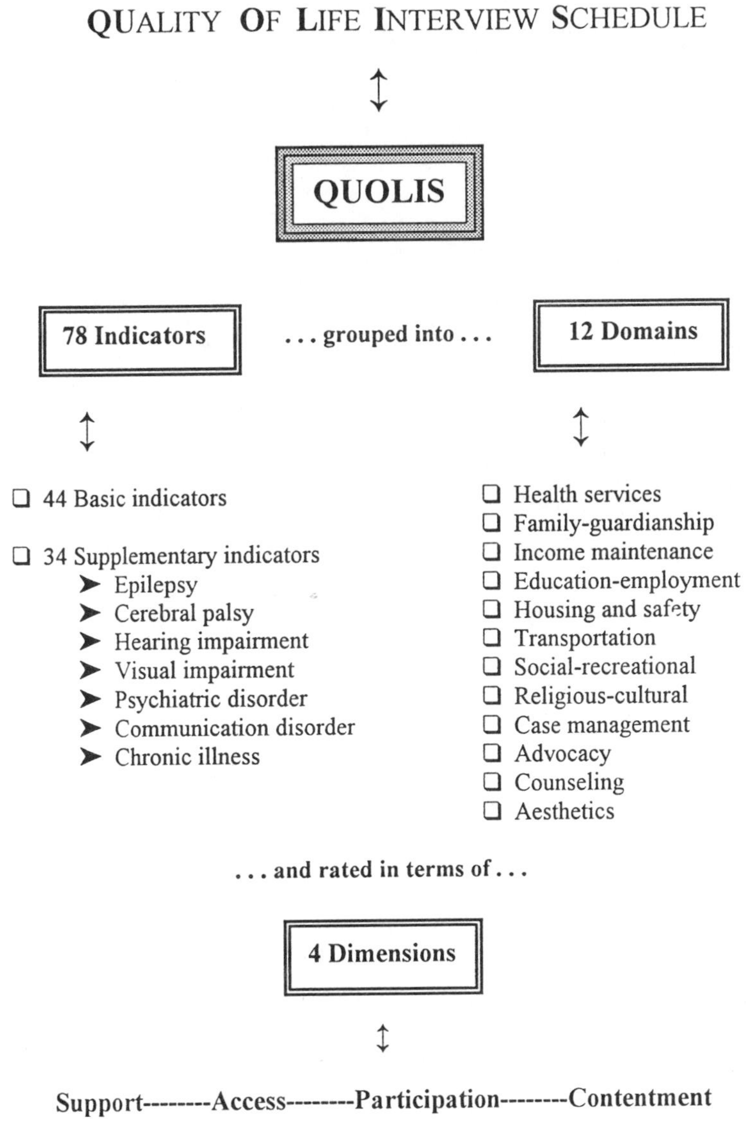

QUALITY OF LIFE INTERVIEW SCHEDULE

↕

QUOLIS

| **78 Indicators** | . . . grouped into . . . | **12 Domains** |

↕   ↕

❑ 44 Basic indicators

❑ 34 Supplementary indicators
   ➤ Epilepsy
   ➤ Cerebral palsy
   ➤ Hearing impairment
   ➤ Visual impairment
   ➤ Psychiatric disorder
   ➤ Communication disorder
   ➤ Chronic illness

❑ Health services
❑ Family-guardianship
❑ Income maintenance
❑ Education-employment
❑ Housing and safety
❑ Transportation
❑ Social-recreational
❑ Religious-cultural
❑ Case management
❑ Advocacy
❑ Counseling
❑ Aesthetics

. . . and rated in terms of . . .

4 Dimensions

↕

Support--------Access--------Participation--------Contentment

Figure 19.1. Overview of QUOLIS: Indicators, Domains, and Dimensions

Implications for Service Provision,
Policy Development, and Research

Because QUOLIS provides a listing of needed supports, the degree to which these are provided, and the contentment level with the provision, it can be helpful in direct planning for individuals and groups. It can also be used to inform professionals on support needs of individuals with severe intellectual disabilities. Also, QUOLIS has a role to play in research endeavors, such as the evaluation of shifts in public policy. In particular, because a significant number of those who still live in institutions are people with severe disabilities, QUOLIS offers an approach to evaluating the effect of deinstitutionalization on their quality of life.

Quality of life considerations are becoming central in service provision, policy development, and research in the field of developmental disabilities. The fact that the American Association on Mental Retardation has added a support element in its definition and classification system for mental retardation (Luckasson et al., 1992) reflects the recognition that support is central to the lives of persons with disabilities. QUOLIS goes a step further in postulating that support is integral to the quality of life of persons with severe or profound developmental disabilities.

Conclusion

Ackoff (1976) claimed that "the growing preoccupation with quality of life is evidence of the maturation of society along a very important and previously slighted dimension of progress" (p. 289). Such progress must not leave behind those members of society who are the most vulnerable—those who cannot speak for themselves—because of our reluctance to quantify their quality of life. Discussions and reviews of quality of life, including terms such as *choice, opportunity,* and *satisfaction,* must occur among the caregivers, friends, and families of individuals who cannot discuss these themselves.

Governments and society in general must not ignore their roles in fostering enhanced quality of life among those with severe disabilities through the provision of support. In his ethical essay on quality of life, Michael Bach (1994) wrote: "The level of quality of life depends . . . on the degree to which the conditions necessary for a person . . . to develop and realize life plans are distributed to them in ways that accord with principles of social justice and just distribution" (p. 139).

20

A Parent's Perspective

Quality of Life in Families
With a Member With Disabilities

Eva R. McPhail

Quality of life is a contemporary term used to explain, examine, and evaluate the conscious events that make up an individual's life. A number of conceptualizations have emerged in recent years that attempt to clarify what we mean by quality of life and to facilitate the identification of indicators that may measure it (e.g., Brown, Bayer, & MacFarlane, 1988; Goode, 1990b; Parmenter, 1988; Woodill, Renwick, Brown, & Raphael, 1994).

With few exceptions (e.g., Isaacs, Percival, Gombay, & Perlman, 1994; Schalock, 1990b), the literature has not dealt significantly with the effect of a child with disabilities on the quality of life of a family. Similarly, it has not documented in any substantive way how the family may contribute to the quality of life of a child with disabilities. Furthermore, the effect of institutionalization of a child with disabilities on the quality of life of the family has not been documented in a sequential way—that is, before, during, and after institutionalization. The purpose of this chapter is, first, to give an account of my own family's story with a view to addressing the quality of life of a

family that has a child with disabilities and second, to suggest some implications of our story for research, policy development, and service practice
in health promotion and rehabilitation.

Paul's Story

Paul is now a healthy 25-year-old young man. Although he has no formal
mode of communication and uses a wheelchair, Paul has an excellent range
of motion and is physically strong. He has good hearing, a keen sense of
smell, definite taste preferences, and the ability to differentiate between hot
and cold. Paul enjoys regular visits with his family, consisting of a father,
mother, older sister, twin brother, younger brother, a brother-in-law, and two
grandmothers.

To his family, though, Paul is a medical miracle. He was the firstborn of
twins, but was born 6 weeks prematurely and weighed only 4 pounds. Even
at the time of his birth, he was given only a 50% chance of living. At 2 weeks
of age, he suffered a petit mal seizure, and doctors discovered he had
contracted meningitis. At best, they considered that Paul now had only about
a 30% chance to survive. He survived. At age 3, the neurosurgeon's best
opinion was that Paul might live for 3 months. He lived.

Paul's early history was fragmented by numerous medical crises. After he
was born, he was isolated in a hospital for 3 months, fed and medicated
intravenously. Family members were allowed to view him only through a
glass wall at specified times. My overriding fear as a young mother was that
my child might die without ever being held or cuddled by a loved one. My
husband and I felt a total loss of control over our child's life and a true
absence of power to change or ameliorate the medical situation. I felt that
the medical community had condemned my child. They were forcing the
family to withdraw from any meaningful relationship with Paul through their
inflexible rules and routines.

At 4 months of age, Paul underwent his first brain operation. The meningitis had closed all drainage tubes and circulation tubes joining the lobes of
his brain. He had a shunt and pump placed in his brain that drained excess
fluid into his body cavity. We brought him home from the hospital, but the
shunt malfunctioned. This was the first in a series of bizarre medical problems. From age 4 months to age 3.5 years, Paul underwent 39 further brain
operations to correct malfunctioning shunts, pumps, and blocked tubes. Each
operation clearly caused more brain damage. At this stage, the neurosurgeon
decided he really could do nothing further to help Paul. He explained that
without medical intervention, Paul would quietly pass away in a matter of

weeks and this was most appropriate, considering all the medical problems. To facilitate a final separation, the doctor suggested placing Paul in a chronic care facility and referred our names to a clinic for support services.

The regional center for the mentally retarded contacted us. Their social worker and public health nurse encouraged us to make a quick, easy decision to place our son in a nursing home, on the basis of the medical reports. I could not make this decision without a great deal of soul-searching. As a support for Paul, a physiotherapist came weekly to teach me some activities to help him. We were able to enroll Paul in weekly swimming lessons, which he loved.

After months of agonizing over a decision, I finally agreed to have Paul's name referred for placement. When informed that Paul's name would be placed on a waiting list for assignment to one of 11 chronic care homes, we were horrified. We were informed that the waiting list was several hundred names long and we should be prepared to wait up to 2 years for placement to occur. Paul was placed at the regional center for 2 months, then moved to a nursing home.

Throughout the many illnesses and this placement process, we, as parents, felt we had very little control over any of the decisions. The medical professionals ignored us. We were treated as a nuisance and were thought to be of no benefit to the health and well-being of our son. Never did we feel we were part of a team working in the best interest of our child.

This was a period of expanding government-sponsored social services, and the impression seemed to deepen that we were incompetent parents. Certainly we had no beneficial ideas as to what was best for Paul, let alone for his family. I was regarded as stubborn and uncooperative because I refused to make a life decision for my child. Even though the social worker knew our family was under stress with one critically ill child and raising two other children, she used every ploy possible to force a decision. The social worker once said, "Your child is not the problem, . . . you are the problem."

The first placement home for Paul was terrible. The building was small, cramped, overcrowded, and smelly. The residents were all bedridden. Some residents were extremely ill, and none was expected to live long. The home was 2 hours from ours. Again, we felt we had no alternatives to placing our child in this location. We were very unhappy and totally depressed after every visit to the place. The visiting was almost worse than never seeing our son again. But fortunately, we were able to locate a children's home close to our native town to which we moved Paul.

This move seemed to herald a time of peace and happiness for all of us. Paul's health started to improve. The home was large and bright and airy. We saw few terminally ill children. The children seemed happy, clean, and well cared for. The staff appeared happy and very willing to discuss daily experiences about Paul. They treated Paul as a normal little boy. Many of the staff loved him, as if he were their own child, and welcomed visits from us at any time. The staff even had birthday parties for the children. Volunteers from the community spent hours taking the children for walks or providing entertainment and musical events. They made special efforts to include the children in local parades, fairs, and other community events. Paul was healthy, active, and happy. He was able to scoot around the home in his walker. We took him for walks and car rides. We took him to visit the grandparents. We hoped Paul would always be able to live at this home.

In 1981, the government allocated funds to provide special programs for children in homes for special care. Again, we had to make a decision regarding Paul's life and the quality of it. As the years away from normal home experiences passed, Paul showed many changes—not all positive. At 12 years old, he had become sober and serious. He spent most of his days in his wheelchair. Although he still liked people to notice him, he was often moody, grumpy, and withdrawn. He began to self-stimulate, shaking and biting his hand, especially when he was upset. His vision appeared less acute, and he rarely concentrated on a face or an object. He seemed content with minimal attention. I felt his greatest frustration was the lack of freedom and mobility. My husband and I agreed to Paul's involvement in the new program.

The program personnel were willing and eager to support any suggestions we made for activities for Paul. They seemed convinced that Paul's life would change dramatically with a program for him. The program therapist determined that Paul had a range of thought processes, that he was able to change his behavior to cope with new and different situations, and that he was aware of changes in routine. He especially noticed male voices and he behaved differently with male caregivers.

The next 3 years saw many changes taking place in Paul's life and ours. Paul once again became an active, happy boy. He learned to feed himself independently. His grandmothers were encouraged to take an active role in Paul's life, such as taking him on weekly swimming jaunts. He went to various community activities. He became more alert and involved in his environment. He responded instantly to his spoken name and began to track people and objects accurately with his eyes. He began to tease his caregivers. He actively involved others in his life by reaching out and grabbing them and often not letting go without a real struggle.

This positive experience enhanced the well-being of the family. We were informed regularly of new programs, activities, and changes in routines. We were encouraged to attend planning sessions. At each step of this new involvement, the program personnel made the parents and family members feel that they were important in the life and well-being of their children with disabilities. Additional changes in government programs included the establishment of a residents' council in which we became involved. It was helpful to meet other parents with children in circumstances similar to our own. We gained much support and encouragement from this shared activity.

In 1985, school boards in our region took responsibility for children with disabilities. Their approach was a stark contrast to the program that we were experiencing. They assessed the children, then began to develop programs for them without informing the parents. The school staff was inexperienced with exceptional students, and for months there were almost no supplies. The staff discouraged parents from involvement with their child during school hours. Because their expectations appeared to be so different from my own, my anger and frustration provoked me into becoming a more assertive advocate for my parental rights and the rights of my child.

In 1986, the government announced an initiative to close all homes for special care for children. The announcement spurred my husband and me to encourage other parents and professional supporters to develop a nonprofit organization to serve youngsters with disabilities on a 24-hour basis. The organization would provide residences and day programs within the community. The corporate policy was (a) to empower parents to take control of their child's life and (b) to provide the child with opportunities to develop skills and talents similar to other young people in the community. The greatest challenge for the organization appeared to be the enlightenment of the community in which these young people would reside. We believed these young people could become valued, functioning members of their community, with the appropriate supports.

In 1989, at the age of 19 years, Paul moved to the suburban home that he shares with three other peers. None communicates through spoken words, and all use wheelchairs. Support workers provide 24-hour care. Paul attended a local high school for 2 years and continues to attend summer camp and Saturday literacy classes.

Paul appears happy, healthy, and interested in his world. His behavior changed with this move. He relishes outings in his neighborhood, trips to local malls, swimming, church, sports activities, celebrations, and outings to his family's home. He continues to show differential preferences for care workers, teachers, and family members. Paul is acutely attuned to his father's voice and touch. He actively seeks ways to involve others in his leisure activities and thoroughly enjoys fun times. He continues to learn.

Paul's Family

Changes have occurred for Paul's family and parents as well. We all look forward with pleasure to shared visits with Paul. His siblings are now able to help care for him. They love to tease him and teach him new tricks. His sister has graduated as a teacher and expects to teach and counsel exceptional students. For the past several years, Paul's youngest brother has worked as a summer camp counselor with young people with disabilities.

The stresses involved in caring for and about Paul had some strong effects on the family. Our idea of building a normal family life through shared activities quickly evaporated. The constant, continual physical and emotional strain prevented us from activities such as holidays and camping. Support for the rest of our family was lessened, as there simply was not enough time to go around. My husband and I were able to continue our careers and provide adequately for the financial well-being of the family only with great stress.

How one fits with other people and the environment may be the most critical of the components of quality of life for families that include a member with a disability (see Renwick & Brown, Chapter 7, this volume). The family constantly grieves its loss. Paul was often absent from the family for extended periods of time, due to medical procedures. When he was at home, family members gave exceptional amounts of time, energy, and money to provide for him, sometimes making others feel ignored or undervalued in the process. Social and emotional acceptance by family and friends was reduced due to the continual physical and medical demands placed on the family. Regular inclusion in extended family functions was often forfeited due to emergency situations. Feelings of isolation occurred because there seemed to be little understanding by others of the physical and emotional strain on the nuclear family. Isolation from neighbors and friends due to lack of understanding is inevitable. Natural supports that might otherwise have developed with community, church, and schools did not materialize. For me, the most important resource was the constant support of my spouse.

Social growth and sometimes educational growth for other children and the parents is limited by the physical realities of caring for a child with disabilities. Who has time or energy to ensure that another child in the family attends hockey practices or piano lessons? Private time alone for parents is next to impossible. Little spontaneity in family action is possible because organized, scheduled routines are essential for the adequate functioning of the total unit. Parents and siblings continually question their own ability and vision and continually search for normalcy.

What one does and wants is similar in families with members who have a disability, as in all other families. Our family has the same aspirations for happy, fulfilled lives as other families do. Unfortunately, many of the hopes and dreams for growth and development, not only for Paul but also for other family members, seem jaded. Inability to function successfully in one area of life affects significantly an individual's perceived ability to function successfully in other areas. Perceived lack of success in adequately caring for a child discourages many family members from searching for growth in other areas of life, thus limiting the potential of the family and its individual members.

How has Paul's twin handled all the changes? Renzulli and McGreevy (1986) claimed that the closest and most fascinating bond that exists among human beings is that shared by twins. Paul's twin seemed to develop normally, although the unexpected hospitalizations and the other disruptions affected him deeply. He did experience some difficulty starting school, making a few friends but tending mostly to prefer his own company. Perhaps this was because Paul was placed in the nursing home the year his twin was in grade one.

We are unsure of the effects on Paul's twin. He experienced difficulty learning to read and difficulty in making and keeping friends. He tends to be shy and timid. He reads voraciously and is a superb artist. During his last year in high school, he worked diligently to bring Paul back to his home community, even though he was experiencing social and emotional distress. Counseling was requested from the school, but none was available.

Now, when he is asked how he feels about Paul, his twin has no real answer. He says he is sad that Paul is disabled. He says he doesn't know what it is like not to be a twin. He says he wishes Paul was normal, because then he would always have his own best friend.

The Present

The family still feels some regret that Paul is not included more frequently and regularly in our family life. Still, we have a measure of control over his location, space, activities, and well-being. We are included in planning sessions for Paul and have access to him at all times. Our presence adds to Paul's life, and Paul gives the family one reason for being. In discussions with family members, it was agreed that our vision of family has only been enhanced by the inclusion of Paul.

My vision for Paul has grown and expanded because of the renewed personal involvement. My enthusiasm for change, however, has been jaded by the reality of Paul's situation. He has gained entry into his community but has he really become a vital, valued, functioning member of it? I am happy that Paul is located close to our home so that I can visit with him frequently and regularly, but I continue to worry about his daily care, safety, and well-being. The rehabilitation doctor says that Paul has great potential to learn and grow and develop but there are no education programs to help him do this. It has been extremely difficult and frustrating to access competent professionals to assess Paul's visual impairment, his psychological potential, or his communication potential. Quality of life, to me, includes the availability of options and opportunities from which to make choices and the freedom to make those choices (see R. Brown, Chapter 18, this volume; Fine, Chapter 24, this volume). This is what is lacking in Paul's life and in our lives. Thus a number of questions continue for me:

What growth opportunities exist for Paul? He does have access to many community services such as malls, churches, health centers, libraries, and recreational centers. Does he have enough opportunities for growth and exploration?

Has Paul really become a valued member of his community? Are his potential skills and abilities acknowledged, enhanced, or supported? Has he developed any self-meaning as a member of his community?

Are Paul's personal needs and desires being met? Are there creative opportunities and a flexible approach to enhance the quality of life for vulnerable citizens within the care system of which he is a part?

Will there be adequate choices for Paul in the future? We are concerned that opportunities still do not exist that will encourage Paul's growth and development to his full potential. We support Edgerton's (1990) view that quality of life is not dependent on the individual availing himself of certain programs or services but on making choices to find satisfaction. But we feel frustrated as there are still almost no opportunities for choice in residential care, day programs, educational programs, recreation, or leisure pursuits.

Suggestions for Improving
Quality of Life of the Family

Families that have a member with a disability have the same needs as all other families and should be assessed in the same way. As Paul's story illustrates, disability brings something of extra quality to a family but detracts from its quality in other ways. We view Paul's effect on our lives as positive and enriching. Involvement with him has given the family a vision of the tremendous potential inherent in every individual, a sense of satisfaction in helping others, a sense of competency in dealing with dilemmas, and increased knowledge and awareness. Like other parents and families who have children with disabilities (Abbott & Meredith, 1986), we found that we developed additional personal and family strengths as a result of our experiences. But there is no doubt that we encountered frustration along the way and continue to do so. There are a number of things that could lessen the negative effect of disability in a family such as ours, enabling the family to take more control in effecting positive change, and thus help to enhance its overall quality of life:

Continuous in-home health care support would have alleviated many of the physical and emotional difficulties. It would have facilitated a more normal acceptance of Paul and allowed time and energy for us to deal more effectively with the well-being of Paul's siblings.

Inclusion of parents in decisions about Paul's medical care, and later his residential care, would have alleviated some of the parental feelings of loss of control, loss of esteem, and frustration. Parental feelings of anger, remorse, guilt, and extreme loss may have been lessened by a better understanding of the medical opinions and options for support to Paul and our family.

Individualized supportive health, medical, and rehabilitative services that valued and included the parents and siblings as full participants in the child's life would have made the family feel valued and competent as a whole unit.

Inclusion of the child with disabilities, parents, and siblings in true life experiences would have encouraged and enhanced our family's perception of competency and well-being.

Inclusion in a regular school setting would have encouraged Paul's growth and the growth and development of the family's vision for Paul. The constant changes during Paul's childhood not only frustrated the family but clearly demonstrated to the family the devaluation a system places on an exceptional child and his family.

Implications for Research

Quality of life for children and young adults with disabilities appears to be highly dependent on their families. Interventions to promote quality of life, therefore, need to focus on helping the family cope with the ordinary and special needs of children with disabilities. Research in health promotion and rehabilitation should focus on evaluating and establishing exemplary practices of collaborative support for families. Such research may well verify Crutcher's (1990) suggestion that society should provide options and opportunities for growth.

Additional study is still required on exemplary practices in moving individuals from institutions back to communities and on identifying successful efforts to accommodate and include these vulnerable citizens within communities. Such study needs to focus particularly on the roles that families do or could play.

Last, the role of quality of life measures and assessments needs to be evaluated concerning their ability to effect positive change in the quality of life of children and adults with disabilities. It may be that they herald a renewed vision of family support in the lives of individuals with disabilities.

Implications for Policy Development and Service Provision

Families of children with disabilities face extraordinary challenges in raising their children, including (a) implementing specialized care routines, (b) frequent terms of hospitalization, (c) frequent medical consultations, (d) excessive time and energy expenditure to locate needed services, (e) financial and temporal demands to deal with medical and rehabilitative equipment and services, (f) exclusion of the family by professionals in decisions regarding their child, and (g) lack of time to devote to other children and spouse or to meet their own needs. The issues raised by the experiences of our family may not be typical of all families but all are shared to some degree depending on a number of factors, such as family structure and nature of the disability.

The quality of life of both the individual with disabilities and the family supporting that individual can be significantly enhanced by appropriate, coordinated, and meaningful rehabilitative services. A renewed vision and implementation of comprehensive health and social services determined by a health promotion focus can only benefit families and vulnerable individuals. In doing so, service providers and policy developers must discover and facilitate ways to value and include families in services for individuals with a disability. The professionals must recognize and support parents in strengthening informal or natural family networks as well as provide flexible family-specific public services. Services must promote the well-being of the total family and the integration of the family into the fiber of the community. Services must be comprehensive, coordinated, readily available, and equitable to all families wherever they live. Professionals must be sensitive and accountable for the formation of policy that encourages society to provide options and opportunities for choices. Policy developers and service providers must be encouraged to become partners with families to help create individual and exemplary services for individuals with disabilities, and, in doing so, to improve quality of life for vulnerable individuals.

The quality of life for families that have a member with a disability has not been fully acknowledged or studied. Rather, the focus on quality of life has been at the level of the individual or group of individuals. In health promotion and rehabilitation, a quality of life focus should prove useful because there needs to be continuing study, discussion, and evaluation to establish how efforts that effect change relate to improving the quality of life of families with members having a disability.

21

Quality of Life of Older Adults

*Toward the Optimization
of the Aging Process*

Dennis Raphael

Quality of life research has tremendous potential for optimizing the aging process and improving the health status of older adults. The health status of older adults has particular importance considering recent demographic trends of increases in the number of older adults and the difficulty the government faces in meeting associated increases in health care costs. This chapter provides a rationale for focusing on quality of life as an important component of health promotion and rehabilitation efforts. Recent research in this area is reviewed, and the implications for health promotion and rehabilitation efforts are drawn. Results from an application of a new approach for assessing quality of life among older adults is presented, and again the implications for health promotion and rehabilitation efforts are drawn.

The Increasing Importance of
Older Adults in North American Society

Older adults make greater use of health care resources through greater numbers of physician office visits, prescriptions and over-the-counter medication, and hospital visits (Lubitz & Prihooda, 1983; Ministry of Health, 1991; Soldo & Manton, 1985; Waldo & Lazenby, 1984). In 1981, Canadian seniors, themselves 9.7% of the population, accounted for approximately 20% to 25% of total care expenditure (Fletcher, 1986). By 1993, the Ontario government (Ontario is the largest province in Canada) estimated that 40% of its health care budget was being spent on 12% of its population, those over age 65 (Government of Ontario, 1993). Although much of this spending reflects the reality that incidence of illness and disability is associated with aging (Havlik, Liu, & Kovar, 1987), there is also evidence that a significant proportion of health care use may result from a lack of emphasis on disease prevention and health promotion (Kaplan & Hahn, 1989) and inadequate primary care (Senior Citizen's Consumers' Alliance on Long-Term Care [Senior Citizen's], 1992). For example, estimates are that between 5% and 15% of seniors entering hospitals in Ontario are admitted with a drug problem—the direct consequence of either too many drugs, wrong dosages, or the failure of patients to take medicines properly. An official responsible for Ontario's drug benefit program stated, "Patients are often prescribed drugs they don't need, or are given new, expensive drugs that don't work any better than older, cheaper ones. The result is that seniors are being drugged silly" (Senior Citizen's, 1992, p. 29).

In Ontario, as in the rest of North America, only a very small percentage of health care dollars is allocated to health promotion and disease prevention activities, despite estimates that up to 50% of the effects of aging can be obviated by health-promotive behaviors (O'Brien & Vertinsky, 1991). The need to identify means of enhancing seniors' functioning outside the traditional health care system attains even greater importance in light of recent demographic trends. Statistics Canada reports that whereas those 65 years or older constituted 11.6% of the 1991 population (Desjardins, 1993), this proportion will increase to 12.9% in 2001, 14.6% in 2011, 18.6% in 2021, and 22.7% in 2031. The implications of this demographic shift for health care are starkly presented by Ontario government estimates that current health care spending of $17 billion will balloon to $34 billion by the year 2000 if recent spending increases continue (Government of Ontario, 1993). In view of these alarming projections, there is a need to examine how the functioning and health of seniors can be improved and whether health promotion activities, including a focus on quality of life issues, can be the vehicle for these improvements.

Quality of Life and
Seniors' Functioning

The model of aging developed by Baltes and Baltes (1990a) provides a useful framework for understanding the aging process and how quality of life factors can affect it. Their approach is valuable for three reasons: (a) The model was influential in outlining the potentialities of the later years in contrast to the prevailing decline models (Baltes, 1968, 1973; Baltes, Reese, & Lipsett, 1980; Baltes, Reese, & Nesselroad, 1977; Baltes & Schaie, 1976); (b) the research base of the model is founded on methodologically rigorous studies; and (c) the model has served as a useful heuristic for numerous examinations of the potentialities of late adulthood and the effects of interventions (Baltes & Baltes, 1986). Baltes and Baltes (1990a) outline a number of propositions concerning aging. The key ones are that (a) there are differences between normal, optimal, and sick aging; (b) much latent reserve exists among most seniors; and (c) knowledge-based pragmatics can offset age-related decline in cognitive mechanics.

Support for these propositions is seen in training and intervention studies that show that seniors possess reserve capacities (Baltes & Baltes, 1990b) that can be drawn on to enhance functioning. When provided with appropriate intervention, training, or stimulation, "average" seniors can improve their memory functioning (Kliegl, Smith, & Baltes, 1989), learn to function more independently (Baltes & Wahl, 1987), or increase their capacity for new learning (Baltes, 1987; Charness, 1985; Dixon & Baltes, 1986; Rybash, Hoyer, & Rodin, 1986). The recent Baltes and Baltes volume (1990b) summarizes evidence for the distinction between types of aging, availability of reserve (which contributes to the difference between average and optimal functioning), and the effects of psychologically oriented training and interventions on general cognitive functioning (Schaie, 1990), memory skills (Backman, Mamtyla, & Herlitz, 1990), exercise (Ericsson, 1990), and personal control (Brandtstadter & Baltes-Gotz, 1990; Lachman, 1986). Particularly important is the work that indicates that minimal interventions focused on enhancing control perceptions may profoundly affect rates of mortality and morbidity even among institutionalized seniors (Baltes & Reisenzein, 1986; Rodin, 1986a, 1986b; White & Janson, 1986).

Within this framework, why should health promoters and rehabilitation workers focus on quality of life issues? There appear to be at least four somewhat overlapping reasons: (a) quality of life may be a determinant of the form that aging takes for a particular individual, (b) improved quality of life may be a desired goal of health promotion activities, (c) quality of life can serve as an indicator of needs, and (d) quality of life provides a focus for the role of environments within health promotion and rehabilitation efforts.

QUALITY OF LIFE AS
A DETERMINANT OF HEALTH

A body of research supports the distinction between normal, optimal, and sick or pathological aging (Rowe & Kahn, 1987; Whitbourne, 1985). *Normal aging* is the average process in any given society. *Optimal aging* occurs under development-enhancing and age-friendly environmental conditions. *Sick* or *pathological aging* is characterized by medical etiology and illness. Support for this distinction comes from demographic studies of lifestyle and health relationships (Berkman & Breslow, 1983; Kaplan & Hahn, 1989) and of social support and health (Berkman & Smye, 1979; Cohen & Smye, 1985), and studies of cognitive functioning across the age span (Schaie, 1990). There are clearly differences among older adults in levels of functioning in the absence of medical pathology. These differences appear to result from contrasts in lifestyle, social supports, socioeconomic status, and other environmental factors. Although normally termed *social determinants of health,* these extraindividual factors are categorized as quality of life components by a variety of writers (Green & Kreuter, 1991; Raphael, Brown, Renwick, & Rootman, 1994b). These descriptive studies suggest that seniors' levels of functioning associated with normal or average aging in Western countries may be well below achievable levels and that quality of life components are essential contributors to these differences. Health promoters and rehabilitation workers attempting to increase control by individuals over their health and its determinants cannot ignore quality of life issues.

QUALITY OF LIFE AS A HEALTH PROMOTION
AND REHABILITATION OUTCOME

Defining health as a resource for living rather than merely the absence of disease (Epp, 1986; World Health Organization, 1986) suggests that quality of life could be an outcome of health promotion and rehabilitation efforts. And it does appear that many of the goals and objectives of identified health promotion programs for older adults involve quality of life issues. For example, the Mandatory Programs for Healthy Elderly put out by the Ontario Ministry of Health (Ministry of Health, 1991) calls for public health departments to (a) focus on health promotion and disease prevention, (b) enhance coping, (c) promote self-care, (d) facilitate empowerment and promote independence, (e) create positive social environments, and (f) plan healthy physical environments. Green and Kreuter (1991) argue that quality of life issues are the ultimate outcomes of health education and health promotion interventions. In addition, health care providers and rehabilitation workers are increasingly using quality of life indicators to evaluate the effect of their interventions. Health-related quality of life is an important area and has the potential to improve the efficacy of health care and rehabilitation efforts.

QUALITY OF LIFE AS AN INDICATOR OF NEED

Another important aspect of quality of life work is the extent to which it causes policy makers, health promoters and providers, and consumers themselves to reflect on the needs of older adults. Time is rarely taken to consider the importance of various issues and consider society's responsibilities to provide a quality life for all of its citizens. The increasing focus of a range of health professionals on quality of life issues directs attention to areas of service provision and social and health policy reform.

QUALITY OF LIFE AND THE ROLE OF ENVIRONMENTS

A quality of life focus directs attention to environments. Many aspects of life quality are concerned with environmental and societal factors in addition to personal characteristics, such as attitudes, beliefs, and behaviors. Quality of life reflects individuals' perceptions of and responses to their environments, thereby directing attention to the effect of government policies and services and other institutions on individuals' quality of life. In this way, a quality of life focus puts a human face on the determinants of health literature. Interestingly, the questions raised by such a focus on determinants of health parallel many of the issues current in the health promotion area. Should promotion efforts be directed toward individuals, communities, or social policy? Essentially, a quality of life focus expands the field of vision of health promoters beyond that of physical, mental, and social health to a concern with the individual within their immediate and more distant environments.

Quality of Life Among Older Adults

The recent volume *The Concept and Measurement of Quality of Life in the Frail Elderly* (Birren, Lubben, Rowe, & Deutchman, 1991) focuses specifically on quality of life issues among older adults. As is often the case in quality of life research, many authors direct their attention to providing operational definitions of quality of life rather than providing a conceptual basis for their measures. The most developed definition of quality of life among seniors was provided by Lawton (1991): "Quality of life is the multidimensional evaluation, by both intrapersonal and social-normative criteria, of the person-environment system of an individual in time past, current, and anticipated" (p. 6).

Lawton's definition calls for both objective and subjective evaluations. The criteria against which judgments of quality of life are to be made include both personal perceptions of satisfaction and observer judgments based on normative criteria. Lawton (1991) sees the content domains of "the good life" as behavioral competence, perceived quality of life, objective environment, and psychological well-being. By no means is Lawton's conceptualization of quality of life among the elderly the only one. Arnold (1991) summarizes the range of available conceptualizations of quality of life among the elderly and concludes that a majority of researchers appear to agree that any definition of quality of life should consider physical functioning and symptoms, emotional functioning and behavioral dysfunctioning, intellectual and cognitive functioning, social functioning and the existence of a supportive network, life satisfaction, health perceptions, economic status, ability to pursue interests and recreations, sexual functioning, and energy and vitality.

Arnold (1991) argues that because "there is no absolute theoretical model of what constitutes quality of life, measures must approximate our understanding of the elements of a very abstract concept" (p. 58). She then summarizes a number of measures, most of which are predominantly health based. A review of these conceptions of quality of life suggests that each was limited in either focusing solely on seniors, the specific assumptions concerning quality of life, or the definitions of the domains of quality of life. It has been argued that quality of life conceptualizations should be guided by the following principles (Raphael et al., 1994b): The primary dimensions of quality of life should be the same for all people—seniors and nonseniors and those with or without illness or disabilities. Second, quality of life should take into account the person as well as the environments in which he or she lives. And third, quality of life should be holistic in nature, considering all aspects of a person's life, such as physical, psychological, spiritual, and social dimensions.

The Centre for Health Promotion
Approach Toward Quality of Life

Researchers at the Centre for Health Promotion, University of Toronto, developed a conceptual model for assessing quality of life (see the Renwick & Brown chapter, this volume). The model was developed to be applicable to all individuals, and quality of life was defined as "the degree to which the person enjoys the important possibilities of his or her life." The definition, simplified to "How good is your life for you?" focuses on the important possibilities that exist in the three spheres of *being, belonging,* and *becoming.* The applicability of the model's concepts is examined for relevancy for a population, instruments are then defined, and collection of data is carried out.

APPLICATION OF THE
MODEL TO OLDER ADULTS

The North York Community Health Promotion Research Unit (NYCHPRU) is a joint project of the Centre for Health Promotion, University of Toronto, and the North York Public Health Department. North York is one of six cities composing Metropolitan Toronto in the Province of Ontario, Canada. The mission of NYCHPRU's five working groups is to undertake innovative research on community health promotion. The Health Promotion and the Elderly Group consists of university researchers, public health department staff, community service agency staff, and community members. The group has been studying quality of life issues among seniors living in the community: first, among those requiring few supports and also seniors considered frail—that is, either in need of services or at significant risk for requiring services in the near future. The members of the group reviewed the Centre for Health Promotion quality of life model as a basis for assessing quality of life and developed a self-administered Quality of Life Profile: Seniors Version (QOLPSV).

INSTRUMENT DEVELOPMENT
AND DESCRIPTION

Development of the QOLPSV began with a series of 12 group meetings with close to 120 seniors. Seniors living in the community were approached in a range of settings and asked, "What does the term *quality of life* mean to you?" They were also asked, "What are some areas of concern to seniors?" This elicited information that seniors may not have initially considered to be related to quality of life. These comments were collected, reviewed, and developed into instrument items. Although all of the significant contributions made by seniors were included (determined by the extent to which these issues were raised across the 12 groups), some areas not mentioned by seniors were added by service providers (e.g., foot care), and others were suggested by the literature on aging (e.g., vision and hearing issues).

The draft instrument was then reviewed again by members of the working group. It also benefited from review of the instrument by Ontario Ministry of Health and Health Canada staff associated with our project. The instrument was then piloted by having two groups of 12 seniors complete the questionnaires. Additional modifications were made on the basis of their comments and then on comments made by an additional group of representatives from each of the initial 12 groups. Approximately half of the items appear specific to seniors' issues and the other half are generic issues relevant to all individuals. The QOLPSV, therefore, has an especially strong emphasis on content validity, with criterion and construct validations (to follow).

QOLPSV: DESCRIPTION AND CONTENT

The QOLPSV consists of 111 items encompassing quality of life issues. There are 12 items in each of the first six subdomains and 13 items in the last three. The respondent provides both *Importance* and *Satisfaction* ratings for each item. Table 21.1 provides two items from each subdomain. For each item, the individual is asked to answer these questions: "How important is this to me in my life?" (from *extremely important* to *not at all important*) and "How satisfied am I with this part of my life?" (from *extremely satisfied* to *not at all satisfied*). The respondent then indicates the amount of control (from *almost total control* to *almost no control*) and opportunities for improving or maintaining control (from *a great many* to *almost none*) that he or she perceives in the broad nine subdomains (e.g., my physical health, my thoughts and feelings, where I am living or will be living, being able to use what my community has to offer, etc.).

Quality of Life Survey

Once developed, the QOLPSV was used to survey a group of seniors. The purpose of the survey was to (a) examine the internal consistency of the QOLPSV, (b) evaluate its concurrent validity, (c) examine correlates of QOLPSV scores through administration of a demographic questionnaire, and (d) examine the levels of importance and satisfaction of various issues to seniors.

TABLE 21.1 Examples of Items in the Quality of Life Profile: Seniors Version

Domain	Item (Each Rated for Importance and Satisfaction)
Physical being	Being physically able to get around my home-neighborhood
	Good nutrition and eating the right foods
Psychological being	Being able to have clear thoughts
	Coping with what life brings
Spiritual being	Feeling that my life is accomplishing something
	Participating in religious or spiritual activities
Physical belonging	Having a space for privacy
	Living in a place especially equipped for seniors
Social belonging	Being able to count on family members for help
	Having neighbors I can turn to
Community belonging	Being able to get dental services
	Going to places in my neighborhood (stores, etc.)
Practical becoming	The caring I do for a spouse or other adult
	Doing work around my home (cleaning, cooking, etc.)
Leisure becoming	Having hobbies (gardening, knitting, painting, etc.)
	Participating in organized recreation activities
Growth becoming	Improving or keeping up my thinking and memory skills
	Adjusting to changes in my personal life

INSTRUMENTS

The instruments included the QOLPSV, a demographics questionnaire, and four widely used and demonstrably reliable and valid instruments: the Life Satisfaction Scale (Neugarten, Havighurst, & Tobin, 1961), Memorial University of Newfoundland Scale of Happiness (Kozma, Stones, & McNeil, 1991), Social Health Battery (Donald & Ware, 1984), and activity items taken from a national study of seniors (National Council on the Aging, 1975). Matrix sampling was used and each participating senior completed only one validation instrument in addition to the QOLPSV and the demographics questionnaire.

SELECTING PARTICIPANTS AND SITES

Study participants consisted of participants in the North York Public Health Department's Healthful Living Program for seniors. This program is a community-based outreach and takes place in churches, senior housing, senior centers, housing projects, libraries, and other places. Although not a random sample of seniors in North York, the participants represented a wide range of seniors currently involved in public health activities. Administration, which involved self-reporting through group paper-and-pencil completion of the QOLPSV, one validation instrument, and the demographics questionnaire, was carried out by 15 public health nurses to 15 groups consisting of, on average, 20 seniors. A total of 205 usable data sets were received (67% voluntary participation and response rate). Administration took 60 minutes.

Participant Characteristics. Average age of the respondents was 73 years (*SD* = 6.97), and of the 199 providing gender information, 46 (23%) were male and 153 (77%) were female. Marital status was as follows: married, 44%; widowed, 42%; never married, 6%; separated, 3%; and divorced, 8%. About 40% had not graduated high school, whereas 34% had at least some college or university education. Ten percent indicated incomes of less than $6,000, whereas 14% reported annual incomes of $50,000 or higher. Except for underrepresentation of seniors reporting poor health, the sample was similar in self-reported health status to the national sample studied in Canada's 1990 Health Promotion Survey (Penning & Chappell, 1993) (Table 21.2).

RESULTS

The mean scores and associated standard deviations for importance, satisfaction, and basic quality of life scores for the nine subdomains are presented in Table 21.3. Mean scores for importance and satisfaction could range from 1 (*not at all important* or *not at all satisfied*) to 5 (*extremely important* or *extremely satisfied*). For all the means provided in the table, missing item responses were dealt with by substituting the person's mean subdomain score for answered items. Individual item results (not tabled) are based only on valid responses.

Importance Scores

Seniors rated the *being* domain, more specifically, the *physical being* and *psychological being* subdomains, as being more important than the *belonging* and *becoming* domains. Overall, all areas were rated toward the more rather than the less important pole (all > 3.0). Perusal of the item means indicated the seniors as a group rated as most important (> 4.50 on the 1-5 scale) the following items (when *n* < 180, the *n* is provided): physical being:

TABLE 21.2 Distribution of Self-Reported Health Compared With National
Sample of 65+ Seniors (in percentages)

Health Status	Study Sample	National Sample
Excellent	15	16
Very good	30	28
Good	29	30
Fair	22	19
Poor	4	7

(a) being physically able to get around my home-neighborhood (4.70), (b) being physically able to see and hear (4.80), (c) maintaining my personal hygiene (4.64), and (d) my overall physical health (4.65); psychological being: (a) being free of mental illness (4.7) and (b) being able to have clear thoughts (4.5); physical belonging: (a) living in a safe place (4.6) and (b) living in Canada (4.52); community belonging: (a) being able to get medical services (4.58) and (b) having transportation that allows me to get where I want to be (4.5). No becoming items were rated above 4.5.

Satisfaction Scores

Seniors rated their satisfaction with belonging items slightly higher than being items and somewhat higher than becoming items. Seniors were especially satisfied with physical belonging items. Items rated as > 4.0 (rather than < 4.5) were physical being: maintaining my personal hygiene (4.22); psychological being: being free of mental illness (4.13); physical belonging: (a) my living in a safe place (4.03), (b) my having a space for privacy (4.08), (c) my having enough room for myself (4.06), (d) my having my own personal things (4.20), (e) my living in a comfortable place (4.23), and (f) my living in Canada (4.50); social belonging: (a) my having a spouse or special person (4.0) ($n = 127$) and (b) my not being a burden to people in my family (4.11); and community belonging: my ability to get medical services (4.02). No becoming items were at the 4.0 or higher level.

Quality of Life Scores

Satisfaction ratings are weighted by the importance ascribed to each subdomain by the person to produce basic quality of life scores. Basic quality of life scores can range from −3.33 (*not at all satisfied with extremely important issues*) to 3.33 (*extremely satisfied with very important issues*). Although basic quality of life scores above 0 can be seen as reflecting

TABLE 21.3 Importance, Satisfaction, and Basic Quality of Life Scores for the Nine Subdomains of the Quality of Life Profile: Seniors Version (QOLPSV)

Quality of Life Domain	Importance		Satisfaction		Basic Quality of Life	
	M	SD	M	SD	M	SD
Physical being	4.43	.52	3.71	.79	1.11	1.23
Psychological being	4.35	.56	3.78	.76	1.10	1.23
Spiritual being	4.05	.62	3.67	.70	1.06	1.07
All being items	4.28	.50	3.69	.69	1.08	1.07
Physical belonging	4.22	.57	4.02	.67	1.55	1.06
Social belonging	3.87	.68	3.66	.71	1.04	1.05
Community belonging	4.07	.63	3.65	.75	.99	1.14
All belonging items	4.06	.55	3.80	.66	1.19	1.00
Practical becoming	3.39	.72	3.51	.76	.84	1.03
Leisure becoming	3.52	.75	3.41	.82	.74	1.07
Growth becoming	3.92	.69	3.45	.75	.76	1.11
All becoming items	3.62	.62	3.46	.70	.77	.98
All items	4.00	.50	3.64	.63	.97	.94

positive quality of life and scores below 0 as representing negative quality of life, the absolute meaning of score levels is an area of continuing investigation. These tentative labels have been suggested: *model* or *exemplary*, >1.50; *very acceptable*, .51 to 1.50; *adequate* −.50 to +.50; *problematic*, −.51 to −1.50; and *very problematic*, <−1.50. Further validation work with larger samples will lead to clearer definition of the score meanings.

Quality of life scores closely parallel the findings seen for satisfaction scores. Seniors' quality of life scores were highest in the physical belonging area and lowest for the leisure becoming domain. Items that were rated especially high (>1.5 on the −3.33 to 3.33 scale) were physical being: (a) my maintaining of my personal hygiene (1.94) and (b) my being free of mental illness (1.82); physical belonging: (a) my making of my own household decisions (1.55), (b) my living in a safe place (1.65), (c) my space for privacy (1.69), (d) my having enough room for myself (1.62), (e) my own personal things (1.83), (f) how comfortable my place is (1.86), and (g) living in Canada (2.40). Social belonging items rated especially high for quality of life were (a) my spouse or special person (1.70; $n = 123$), (b) my grandchildren (1.53; n = 139), and (c) my not being a burden (1.68). The community belonging item, the medical services I receive, (1.63) was also rated high. No practical becoming, leisure becoming, or growth becoming ratings were especially high.

Items rated lower for quality of life (<.75) were physical being: (a) having enough energy (.68) and (b) having healthy feet (.58); psychological being: (a) being free of worry, stress, and sadness (.41) and (b) being able to remember things (.69). For spiritual being: my feeling that my life is accomplishing something (.59); social belonging: (a) having acquaintances (.69), (b) neighbors I can turn to (.37), (c) sexual intimacy (.3; answered by 97 persons); community belonging: (a) feeling government is understanding of my needs (.34), (b) having enough money to live comfortably (.42), and (c) having events in my community to go to (.58). All of the becoming items were rated lower than .75 except (a) the caring I do for a spouse (n = 123), (b) the pet I have (n = 49), (c) doing things around my home, (d) doing things to take care of myself, (e) going to appointments, (f) shopping, (g) traveling and taking trips, (h) indoor activities, (i) holiday activities, (j) accepting I am getting older, (k) adjusting to personal changes, (l) trying new things, and (m) sharing ideas.

Control and Opportunities

Seniors showed the greatest extent of control (on a scale from 1 to 5) for psychological being (3.96), social belonging (4.03), and practical becoming (4.00). Least control was seen in physical being (3.65) and community belonging (3.66). Seniors perceived more opportunities in the physical belonging (3.81), psychological being (3.61), and spiritual being (3.59) areas.

Reliability and Validity of the QOLPSV

All domain and subdomain importance, satisfaction, and quality of life indicators showed high internal consistency (Cronbach's alpha > .90). Patterns of correlations with the four additional measures of functioning (Life Satisfaction Scale, Memorial University of Newfoundland Scale of Happiness, Social Health Battery, and activity items [National Council on the Aging]) provided direct evidence of criterion validity (see Table 21.4). The especially high correlations of the NCA with leisure becoming and the consistent correlations of the other general indicators of well-being with our quality of life instrumentation provide beginning evidence of construct validity.

TABLE 21.4 Correlation of Quality of Life Profile: Seniors Version (QOLPSV)
Domain Quality of Life Scores With the Four Validation Measures

Quality of Domain	Life Satisfaction Scale	*Validation Measures*		
		Memorial University of Newfoundland Scale of Happiness	Social Health Battery	Life Activity Items (NCA)
Being				
Physical	.19	.15	.45**	.22
Psychological	.26*	.46*	.47**	.11
Spiritual	.22	.44**	.46**	.27
Belonging				
Physical	.20	.49*	.55***	.38*
Social	.37*	.59***	.57***	.39*
Community	.34*	.62***	.62***	.18
Becoming				
Practical	.30*	.39*	.52***	.36*
Leisure	.36**	.36*	.52***	.62***
Growth	.29*	.47**	.30*	.41**

$*p < .05; **p < .01; ***p < .001.$

DEMOGRAPHIC CHARACTERISTICS
ASSOCIATED WITH QUALITY OF LIFE SCORES

Education and income were not related to any domain or subdomain quality of life. Age was related only to physical being and even then at a barely significant ($r = -.16, p < .05$) level. Health status, however, was related to all domain and subdomain quality of life scores ($p < .001$). It was most highly related to physical being (.57) and less related to social belonging (.37), physical belonging (.38), practical becoming (.38), and spiritual being (.39). All other relationships were in the .40 to .49 range, and overall quality of life correlated .50 with health status. Composite scores of control and opportunities scores showed strong significant ($p < .001$) correlations (>.60 and >.50, respectively) with quality of life domain scores, highlighting the importance of these issues for seniors' lives.

Discussion

POSSIBLE LIMITATIONS AND CAUTIONS

The validation survey of the QOLPSV described here involved seniors currently living in the community who were involved with health promotion activities. These seniors are an important segment of the seniors population, and many health promotion workers direct their energies toward this group. Other seniors, especially those who are isolated and unknown to service providers, are a continuing concern of health personnel, and means of assessing their quality of life must be developed. Collection of quality of life scores describing seniors either unwilling or unable to participate in the group activities from which these data were collected would complement these findings and clarify the usefulness of the QOLPSV for working with these other seniors.

Development of Short and Brief Versions of the QOLPSV

The results of the study were promising, but one concern was the length of the questionnaire. With the use of content validity considerations, short (54-item) and brief (27-item) versions of the QOLPSV were developed. Psychometric validation of these instruments has been carried out, and both appear to serve as adequate proxies when quicker assessments of quality of life are needed. These instruments may be especially useful for screening and research purposes with a range of populations of seniors. Although, to date, seniors have completed paper-and-pencil instruments, the QOLPSV could be administered using an interview format, either face-to-face or using a telephone survey.

Implications for Health Promotion Practice

Because our work is carried out closely with public health professionals, most of our thinking concerning implications is within this sphere, though these should be appropriate to other health promoters in a range of venues. One application of a quality of life assessment is to use it directly in determining health and service needs. For example, in the case of the present administration, the low scores reported for the areas of practical, leisure, and growth becoming and specific items related to purpose and meaning, social relationships, and community involvement outline priority areas among these respondents that could be addressed in the Healthy Elderly Groups or similar groups conducted by public health departments or other health promoters. On the other hand, the relatively high scores of other items (e.g., personal safety or maintaining personal hygiene) suggest that although these areas should probably not be ignored by public health professionals, there is probably less need for focus.

Another application of the QOLPSV is to use it as a means of evaluating the effect of programs. If one of the goals of public health or health promotion programs is to improve quality of life of seniors to whom its programs are directed, the measure should be an appropriate and important way to evaluate whether these programs have made a difference in people's lives. Our working group has also suggested (Raphael & McClelland, 1994) that in addition to these applications, the QOLPSV could be used for informal assessment of seniors' health promotion needs through discussion and review by seniors and health promoters of the content in the QOLPSV, applying the QOLPSV for probability surveys of seniors within a particular area or jurisdiction, and community development activities where review and discussion or even application of the QOLPSV by seniors to seniors could serve to energize seniors within their communities. The final health promotion application is to use the results of quality of life assessments to advocate government directly to develop health-promoting social and health policies.

Implications for
Rehabilitation Practice

The quality of life of those likely to receive rehabilitation services remains a priority of health care providers, however, and identification and evaluation of the components of quality of life of such people is an essential part of any service delivery effort. The ultimate evaluation of any rehabilitation effort should therefore take into account the quality of life of the consumer. Although quality of life is just one component of the entire complex of system review (i.e., quality assurance, systems audit, and program effectiveness evaluation), the focus on quality of life of the consumer assures it an essential role. Our findings that self-reported health status is related to quality of life suggest the important effects that rehabilitation efforts may have on seniors' well-being.

Conclusion

The health and health care needs of the elderly are assuming increasingly greater importance. Demographic trends, decreases in mortality from previously deadly diseases, and important improvements in treatments such as cardiovascular disease are contributing to significantly higher numbers of elderly people. Increasing demand for services has arisen, unfortunately, at a time when fiscal responsibility is an important consideration. Service providers and government funders must rationalize service provision and be cost effective while, at the same time, providing quality services to ever-increasing numbers of elderly people. Long-term care of the elderly and long-term care reform are important focuses of health professionals in North America (Koff, 1988).

Quality of life assessment is also consistent with recent developments in health promotion and rehabilitation efforts. Quality of life is an obvious determinant of health among seniors and may well be a key factor in differentiating between pathological, normal, and optimal functioning among seniors. If this is the case, the assessment and focus on quality of life is a fertile area for public health planning and practice. And because rehabilitation efforts usually occur when the individual is in a health-related crisis, enhancing quality of life should be an essential component of these efforts. The goal of the working group was to develop a new approach to assessing the quality of life of seniors living in the community. The model and associated instrumentation should be useful in the ongoing study of the quality of life of seniors living in the community, and may be especially useful for health promoters and rehabilitation workers.

22

Quality of Life and
Adolescent Health

Dennis Raphael

Interest in adolescence has been noticeable since antiquity (Kiell, 1964), yet the scientific study of adolescence began only during the early part of this century (Conger, 1991; Petersen, 1988). The actual amount of research with adolescents has been described as meager with most carried out by social scientists examining normal adolescent development (Petersen, 1988; Takanishi, 1993a). This omission is now being rectified and research into adolescent development is now an active area of inquiry (Horowitz, 1989; Takanishi, 1993b; Zaslow & Takanishi, 1993).

Adolescent health has also become an increasingly important focus for government health officials, social policy analysts, and behavioral researchers (Dryfoos, 1990; Millstein & Litt, 1990; Millstein, Petersen, & Nightingale, 1993; Zaslow & Takanishi, 1993). One reason for this is the realization that in contrast to other age groups, mortality and morbidity rates for 10- to 25-year-olds in Western countries have been increasing over the past few decades (Hurrelman & Losel, 1990). Most recently, the U.S. Office

307

of Technology Assessment (OTA) (1991) compiled three large volumes summarizing all recent empirical work bearing on adolescent health, and the Carnegie Council on Adolescent Development released a number of reports on the same issue (Carnegie Council, 1989, 1992; Feldman & Elliot, 1990). In the United States, the increasing emphasis on adolescent health appears related to growing evidence of adolescent involvement in societally unsettling activities:

> In the 1990's the state of adolescent health in America reached crisis proportions: large numbers of 10- to 15-year-olds suffer from depression that may lead to suicide; they jeopardize their future by abusing illegal drugs and alcohol, and by smoking; they engage in premature, unprotected sexual activity; they are victims or perpetrators of violence; they lack proper nutrition and exercise. Their glaring need for health services is largely ignored. (Carnegie Council, 1992, p. 21)

In Canada, the increasing interest in adolescent health is related more to the maturing of health promotion perspectives (Pederson, O'Neill, & Rootman, 1994) and awareness of the importance of developing health-promoting attitudes and habits during adolescence:

> Adolescence offers unique opportunities for investment in health and well-being. First, good mental and physical health enables young people to make the most of these precious years, which provide the foundation for adult life. Second, the lifestyle patterns adopted in youth often continue into adulthood and thereby influence long-term prospects for health and the risk of chronic disease. Finally, while the death rate among young people is low, most of these deaths are preventable. (Schabas, 1992, p. 1)

Behavioral researchers have been moving away from a focus on the study of single problems, such as smoking, drinking, or sexual behavior, and toward examining clusters of problem behaviors and identifying means of promoting general health and coping (Elliot, 1993; Hurrelman & Losel, 1990; Takanishi, 1993b). These reflections on and investigations of adolescent health have only recently been organized within health promotion perspectives (Millstein et al., 1993; OTA, 1991). In addition, with the exception of Lindstrom's (1994) quality of life work of children in the Nordic countries, adolescent health research has not been presented within a quality of life conceptualization. In this chapter, the value of a quality of life perspective for examining aspects of adolescent health is considered.

Conceptualizing Adolescent Health

Four perspectives on adolescent health are in the literature: transition to adulthood, coping and well-being, absence of mortality and morbidity, and healthy lifestyles-avoidance of risk behaviors.

HEALTHY ADOLESCENCE
AS SUCCESSFUL TRANSITION

The developmental task approach identifies tasks that allow advancement to higher levels of development (Havighurst, 1953). Nine were initially outlined, each of which required the acquisition of certain skills, knowledge, functions, and attitudes. Although developmental tasks probably vary between historical times and places (Conger, 1991), achieving independence, adjusting to sexual maturation, establishing cooperative relationships with peers, preparing for a meaningful vocation, and achieving a core set of basic beliefs and values appear basic (Feldman & Elliot, 1990). The developmental task approach has been influential in the adolescent literature, and most compendiums and textbooks on adolescence are organized around these themes (e.g., Conger, 1991; Petersen, 1988).

HEALTHY ADOLESCENCE AS
A STATE OF COPING AND WELL-BEING

It is also important to focus on adolescence as important in itself. Put simply, we want adolescents, as we do all citizens, to be happy and adjusted. An extensive body of research has examined adolescent coping and its antecedents, including child-rearing practices, parents and peers, employment and unemployment, and school failure (Conger, 1991; Hurrelman & Losel, 1990). Coping is especially important during adolescence because the period is one of rapid change in both the personal sphere, involving the onset of puberty and specific cognitive abilities, and the social sphere, involving shifting responsibilities and changing school milieus (OTA, 1991).

HEALTHY ADOLESCENCE AS
ABSENCE OF PHYSICAL AND MENTAL ILLNESS

Traditional definitions of health focus on illness and direct attention to mortality and morbidity indicators. Although available data suggest that adolescents represent a relatively healthy segment of the population, recent analyses in North America (Carnegie Council, 1992; Ontario Children's Health Study [OCHS], 1989; OTA, 1991) have outlined significant incidence of physical and mental disorders and correlates of these disorders.

HEALTHY ADOLESCENCE AS HEALTHY BEHAVIORS

Expanded definitions of physical and mental health include developing health-enhancing behaviors and avoiding risk behaviors. Seven major health issues for young people have been identified: tobacco use, alcohol use, road safety, healthy sexuality, physical activity, nutrition and healthy weight, and suicide and mental health (Schabas, 1992; U.S. Department of Health and Human Services, 1991). These four definitions inform the range of research focused on adolescents.

What Do We Know About Adolescent Health?

DEVELOPMENTAL TASKS

Research into adolescent development usually focuses on the psychological processes associated with achieving independence, adjusting to maturation, establishing peer relationships, and preparing for a meaningful vocation (Conger, 1991; OTA, 1991). This research tradition examines the effects of class, gender, culture, family practices and attitudes, education, chronic illness, and societal factors, such as unemployment, on these outcomes. These concepts are not explicitly assessed in broad-based surveys of adolescents, and it is difficult to estimate proportions of adolescents mastering them. Yet inferences can be drawn from a variety of sources.

For example, in the case of vocational preparation, such surveys of academic achievement as the recent *International Assessment of Educational Progress* paint a frightening picture of U.S. students' science and mathematics knowledge and skills (Lapoint, Askew, & Mead, 1992; Lapoint, Mead, & Askew, 1992). Similar concerns of lack of vocational preparation have been raised in Canada (Coalition for Education Reform, 1994). Inferences concerning mastery of other developmental tasks can be drawn from data on teenage pregnancy, delinquency, violence, and other problem behaviors (Carnegie Council, 1992; OTA, 1991; Schabas, 1992). None of these data are especially encouraging.

The contribution of the developmental task literature is the explication of the processes by which tasks are attained. Much is known, for example, about adolescents who successfully achieve independence (Elder, 1980), adjust to physical maturation (Brooks-Gunn & Petersen, 1983; Jessor, 1984), show positive peer relations (Hartup, 1983), are interested in future vocations (Conger, 1991), and do well in school (Dornbusch, Ritter, Leiderman, Roberts, & Fraleigh, 1987; Rutter, Maughan, Mortimore, & Ouston, 1979). Not surprisingly, many of the factors associated with success are also related to health and healthy behaviors: higher social status, cultural group, positive family interactions, and supportive societal structures (Conger, 1991; OTA, 1991).

ADOLESCENT COPING

Epidemiological surveys paint a depressing picture of adolescent coping. In North America, about 20% of adolescents have a diagnosable mental disorder and a similar proportion of adolescents report attempting suicide (OCHS, 1989; OTA, 1991; Schabas, 1992). The Carnegie Council (1992) estimates that 25% of 10- to 18-year-olds are at serious risk of being harmed by their own behavior and an additional 25% are at moderate risk—certainly not indicators of successful coping.

PHYSICAL HEALTH AND ILLNESS

Mortality and morbidity statistics among North American adolescents are relatively low compared with other age groups (OTA, 1991; Schabas, 1992). Adolescents "have the lowest number of outpatient visits to office-based physicians per year and are among the least likely to be hospitalized" (OTA, 1991, p. i). About 9 in 10 North American adolescents rate their health as excellent or very good, and almost all parents (97%) report their 10- to 18-year-olds as having good to excellent health. Nonetheless, these self-reports of health status may be deceiving.

The great majority of adolescent deaths are due to preventable causes, such as violence, accidental injury, and suicide (OTA, 1991; Schabas, 1992) and almost 10% of adolescents experience serious chronic physical conditions, such as hay fever (9%), asthma (6%), migraine headaches (3%), and heart disease (2%), to mention just a few. In the United States, many adolescents experience serious chronic acne, and half of female adolescents miss school or work due to menstrual distress. The adverse effects of illness and disability on adolescent functioning are well documented (OTA, 1991).

HEALTHY BEHAVIORS

Nutrition and Fitness

Many adolescents experience nutritional and fitness problems usually involving mineral deficiencies, imbalanced diets, and being overweight or obese (OTA, 1991). Adolescents are also not knowledgeable about this area (Johnson, Johnson, Wang, & Smiciklas-Wright, 1994; Perry-Hunnicut & Newman, 1993). Meredith and Dwyer (1991) provide evidence that adolescents' fitness levels are declining over time with clear health implications.

Risks to Health

Seven major health issues in young people's lives are tobacco use, alcohol use, road safety, healthy sexuality, physical activity, nutrition and healthy weight, and suicide and mental health (Schabas, 1992). The available data on these issues are not encouraging. About 22% of Canadian youth aged 12 to 19 smoke regularly and 50% have consumed alcohol at least once in the past year. Among males who report some drinking, 44% report having 10 or more drinks on at least one occasion in the past year, whereas in the United States, it is reported that 33% of adolescents report ongoing episodes of more than five drinks on an occasion (OTA, 1991). Surveys in the United States indicate significant proportions of adolescents report use of alcohol, cigarettes, marijuana, and cocaine.

Why a Quality of Life Perspective?

Examining adolescent health and its determinants within a well-developed quality of life perspective achieves various aims. First, because quality of life approaches usually consider a broad range of determinants, including both psychological and societal aspects, a quality of life approach should help identify determinants of adolescent health that may not have been considered to date. Second, a quality of life perspective draws attention to determinants of health at a range of levels: specifically, personal factors, such as attitudes and beliefs; community factors, such as family, peers, employment, and schools; structural factors, such as income distribution and educational and employment opportunities. Usually, research into the health of adolescents is limited to only one or two of these levels without considering level interrelationships.

Third, a quality of life approach allows for consideration of multiple perspectives—in this case, the views of adolescents, their parents, service providers, and government analysts, among others concerned with adolescent health. Consideration of the views of adolescents and those close to them helps put a human face on the determinants of health and healthy behavior during adolescence. Last, a quality of life perspective can be linked to health promotion and rehabilitation perspectives suggesting means of promoting positive health and healthy behaviors among adolescents.

DEFINING QUALITY OF LIFE

Two well-developed quality of life conceptualizations guide this analysis of determinants of adolescent health. The first is the quality of life domains of the Centre for Health Promotion, University of Toronto (see the Renwick & Brown chapter, this volume). The model was initially developed to highlight self-perceived aspects of individuals' lives and is useful for examining issues from the perspective of the individual and his or her immediate surroundings. The second conceptualization is Lindstrom's (1994), which considers societal and structural factors related to the quality of life of children.

Quality of Life Analysis

The Centre for Health Promotion framework is used here to examine the personal characteristics of adolescents (*being*), aspects of their immediate environments (*belonging*) and activities (*becoming*), and how they are related to health outcomes.

BEING: PERSONAL VALUES, ATTITUDES, KNOWLEDGE, AND BEHAVIORS

At any point in time, individuals possess a personal repertoire of values, attitudes, knowledge, and behaviors that affect health. Consideration of the specific characteristics predictive of positive health outcomes during adolescence does not preclude analysis of environmental precursors of these skills or abilities and such analyses are considered throughout this section. Three main themes (not necessarily in order of importance) are apparent in the current literature: resiliency and associated factors; general coping abilities, including factors associated with mental health; and factors associated with a range of specific problem behaviors.

Jessor (1993) identifies the following individual protective factors: high intelligence, value on achievement and health, intolerance of deviance, church attendance, and involvement in school and voluntary clubs. He finds a relationship between these factors and problem behaviors, such as illicit drug use, delinquency, drunk driving, unhealthy eating, tobacco use, truancy, dropout, and health or lifestyle compromising outcomes, such as illness, poor social roles, and poor preparation for adulthood. In recent work, Jessor, Donovan, and Costa (1990) found that expectations for academic achievement and intolerant attitude toward deviance were related to involvement in exercise, healthy eating, using seat belts, and adequate sleep.

BELONGING: THE EFFECT
OF ENVIRONMENTS

An attempt to identify parental and familial influences on adolescent health was carried out by the OTA (1991). The definition of health used was broad and integrated aspects of all four of the definitions of health outlined earlier. Table 22.1 provides a summary of the OTA's work.

The *Ontario Child Health Survey* identified a range of environmental factors related to child and adolescent dysfunction among the Ontario population (OCHS, 1989). The following were predictive of psychiatric disorder: family dysfunction, being on welfare, living in subsidized housing, few friends, low income, single-parent family, unemployed parent, mother's low education, and overcrowded housing. These findings suggest that structural factors, including unequal allocation of resources and availability of health-supporting environments, may contribute to adolescent health problems. Policy makers, however, prefer to focus on aspects of environments that can be affected without questioning basic societal assumptions concerning opportunities and distribution of wealth. The OTA (1991) volumes outline a drastic need for recreation and leisure resources, municipal recreation centers, and an increased role for churches and synagogues, among others. Behavioral researchers show a similar limited emphasis and focus on the establishment of social support and communication networks (Bo, 1990; Hopkins & Emler, 1990; Schwarzer & Leppin, 1990).

BECOMING: DAILY ACTIVITIES
AND OPPORTUNITIES FOR GROWTH

Of all of life's periods, adolescence would appear to be the one where daily activities and opportunities for growth and development would be important.

TABLE 22.1 Parental and School Influences on Adolescent Health

Focus	Aspect	Mechanism	Outcomes
Parents	Health values	Modeling	Increased nutrition, fitness
	Behaviors	Open communication	More healthy sexual behavior
	Child-rearing	Promoting autonomy	Better psychological health
	Substance abuse	Modeling, interactions	More substance abuse Attitude transmission
	Lack of knowledge	Communication	Less treatment of illness More misinformation
	Maltreatment	Child abuse	Range of problem behaviors
Schools	Academic policies	Academic emphasis	Higher dropout rate of poorer students
	School size	Large schools	More dropouts, vandalism, violence
	School transitions	Movement into junior high school	Less achievement, especially girls
	Class size	Smaller classes	May improve poor performance
	Teaching policies	Cooperative approach	More positive school outcomes
	Parental involvement	Multiple mechanisms	More positive school outcomes
Discretionary time	Community interest	Develop skills	Better health outcomes
	Leisure activities	Enhance satisfaction	Greater self-efficacy, socialization
	Employment	Socialization	Better societal integration

SOURCE: Adapted from the Office of Technology Assessment (1991).

Adolescent problem behavior is more likely to occur when opportunities for satisfying daily activities are absent, and alienation and risk behavior appear more likely when opportunities are not seen as available for future satisfaction and happiness. Activities and opportunities in four spheres are considered: daily activities, including family relations and leisure; daily school activities; employment; and perception of future opportunities.

Daily Activities

Relatively little work has focused on adolescents' daily activities. Csikszentmihalyi and Larson (1984) found that the largest proportion of time was spent on leisure (40%), followed by maintenance activities, such as chores and errands, eating, transportation, resting, and personal care (31%). Productive activities involving studying, classwork, or jobs consumed 29% of the time. Farley (1979) found that passive leisure activities, such as TV watching, were by far their greatest activities. Schneller (1988) and Selnow and Reynolds (1984) found TV watching to be negatively related to involvement in productive activities, such as social or cultural events or membership in church, school, and musical groups.

The correlation of TV watching with low academic achievement is well known, yet whether TV watching is a cause or outcome of poor achievement is still unclear (Educational Testing Service [ETS], 1986). An interesting study by Hansell and Mechanic (1990) found that U.S. adolescents whose parents showed interest in their activities and reported having dinner with their parents or attending religious services were less likely to drink alcohol, smoke marijuana, and use tobacco. Adolescents whose parents showed interest were also more likely to wear a seat belt, participate in sports, exercise, and eat breakfast. These factors also predicted change over time and were interpreted as involving the participation of adolescents in adult-related behaviors. Involvement in peer activities was related to decreasing health behaviors.

School Activities

Knowledge in this area can be stated simply. Adolescents who do poorly in school are at risk for a range of negative outcomes. These include dropout and unemployment, early pregnancy and childbirth, delinquency, drug abuse, and a range of unhealthy behaviors, such as drinking and smoking (Carnegie Council, 1992; Conger, 1991; OTA, 1991). Adolescents in the nonacademic tracks of secondary schools also smoke and drink more, whether in Poland, Germany (Silbereisen, Schonpflug, & Albrecht, 1990), Canada (Allison, 1992), or the United States (OTA, 1991). Hansell and Mechanic (1990) found poor grades were related to adolescent use of alcohol, marijuana use, smoking, nonuse of seat belts, less involvement in sports and exercise, and not eating breakfast.

A German study (Nordlohne & Hurrelman, 1990) identified poor school performance as a predictor of conflicts with parents leading to poor self-related health status, frequency of health complaints, and use of drugs. In Germany, poor school performance is seen as a predictor of family conflict and poor health. In contrast, in the United States and Canada, it is more common to view family conflict and dissension, itself associated with poverty and unemployment, to be a predictor of poor school performance. In either case, inadequate school performance is a distinctive marker identifying a poor prognosis for current and future adolescent adjustment and health.

Employment Opportunities

A recent review of a decade of studies (Kablaoui & Pautler, 1991) concluded that, generally, youth employment has a positive effect on adolescents still enrolled in school. In the United States, white adolescents were more likely to have these jobs and were therefore more likely to show increased personal responsibility and earning power, development of social skills, improved grades and participation in school-related activities, lower unemployment rates after graduation, and better jobs after graduation (Kablaoui & Pautler, 1991). Steinberg, Fegley, and Dornbusch (1993), however, in a carefully designed longitudinal study of 1,800 U.S. high school students, found that taking a job for more than 20 hours a week was directly related to increased delinquency and drug use, disengagement from school, and diminished self-reliance. These findings suggest that employment up to 20 hours a week has many positive benefits for adolescent development.

Youth unemployment after the completion of school, either through graduation or school dropout, is now one of the greatest social problems in the Western world (Hammarstrom, 1990). A consistent relationship is seen between unemployment and psychological disorders (Graetz, 1993; Tiggeman & Winefield, 1984). Hammarstrom (1990), in an attempt to examine youth unemployment effects on somatic health as well as alcohol and drug consumption, studied a large cohort of Swedish adolescents over a 5-year period. With good statistical and other controls, she found both direct and indirect effects of youth unemployment on psychological symptoms and alcohol consumption.

Perception of Future Opportunities

One study will illustrate the commonsense notion that adolescents who perceive greater opportunities are less likely to engage in risky and unhealthy behavior. Jessor et al. (1990) developed a measure of perceived life chances in the opportunity structure. The measure has 10 items, and three examples are as follows: What are the chances that (a) you will graduate from high school, (b) you will go to college, and (c) you will have a job that pays well? Scores on this measure were related to a health behavior index consisting of exercise, healthful eating, adequacy of sleep, and seat belt use for both black and white U.S. adolescents in middle and secondary schools. Perceived life chances were also related to a socioeconomic index, as were health behaviors. Unfortunately, the relationships of perceived life chances with problem behaviors, such as delinquent behavior, marijuana use, frequency of drunkenness, and sexual intercourse, were not reported. Because the *Health Behavior Index* and problems were correlated, however, it can be assumed that such an association between perceived life chances and problem behaviors exists. The authors stated that "the present findings suggest that the linkage between adolescent health behavior and the larger social environment may be mediated, at least in part, by the perception of life chances in the opportunity structure" (Jessor et al., 1990, p. 39).

Current Recommendations Based on This Work

Most work in the adolescent health area is psychologically oriented with emphasis on individual characteristics and behaviors and immediate environments, with occasional reference to broader social issues. For example, the Carnegie Council (1992) outlined a number of recommendations in *Fateful Choices: Healthy Youth for the 21st Century.* These called for (a) offering at least 2 years of health or life science education, or a combination of the two, for all adolescents; (b) health insurance coverage and access to health care through school-related health services; (c) enlistment of the media to reduce violence, substance abuse, and irresponsible sexual behavior; (d) preparation for the world of work through mentoring, job creation, internships, and apprenticeship programs; (e) education of health care providers and educators concerning adolescence; and (f) establishment of school safety zones, restriction of access to firearms and unregistered firearms, and establishment of youth organizations.

Similar policy options (and associated strategies) were provided in the OTA report (OTA, 1991): (a) Improving adolescents' access to appropriate health and related services (e.g., providing seed money for community-based health centers for adolescents; mandating expansion of Medicaid eligibility for adolescents), (b) taking steps to restructure and invigorate the federal government's efforts to improve adolescent health (e.g., create a new federal agency to undertake broad efforts to improve adolescent health, encourage development of demonstration projects in specific adolescent health areas), and (c) taking steps to improve environments for adolescents (e.g., improving supports to families, limiting adolescent access to firearms). It could be suggested that the recommendations of both the Carnegie Council and the OTA fail to deal with basic issues underlying many of the observed problems associated with adolescence. These issues include inequality of economic resources, marginalization of minority groups, lack of employment opportunities, abundance of illegal firearms, and multibillion dollar industries that promote alcohol use, tobacco use, and junk food consumption among children.

Broader Quality of Life Considerations

Lindstrom's (1994) framework focuses on some of these broader issues (Table 22.2). Without dwelling on the similarities and differences between the Centre for Health Promotion and the Lindstrom models, it is apparent that the Lindstrom model explicitly focuses on important macro-issues related to the allocation of economic resources and the distribution of education, housing, and welfare opportunities. Indeed, Lindstrom specifically outlines the importance of the principle of equity in his analysis.

Lindstrom's work grew out of earlier research using the Physical Quality of Life Index (PQLI) (consisting of infant mortality, life expectancy, and basic literacy rate indicators), which found that the Nordic countries of Sweden, Norway, Iceland, and Denmark ranked 1 to 4, respectively, with Canada 9th and the United States 10th. Comparisons using the National Index of Children's Quality of Life based on children in the labor force, female enrollment in elementary school, and PQLI ranked Iceland, Luxembourg, West Germany, Denmark, and East Germany 1 to 5; the United States was 8th. Lindstrom (1994) applies these types of quality of life dimensions toward an analysis of quality of life among Nordic children. The summary provided here of the global and the external spheres is illustrative of the approach, and readers are urged to obtain the Lindstrom monograph. Similar analyses could be applied to assessing quality of life of adolescents in the United States and Canada.

GLOBAL SPHERE

The Nordic countries exhibit an extremely low infant mortality rate and, because of extensive multistrategic preventive programs, the lowest accident rates in the world (Lindstrom, 1994). These countries immediately ratified the UN Convention of the Rights of the Child in 1990, and Norway and Sweden have Children's Ombudsmen Offices that act independently on both individual and collective children's issues. The other Nordic countries are considering establishing similar offices. In the equity area, Sweden and Norway have the most equal distribution of income among 18 countries of the Organisation for Economic Cooperation and Development (OECD), and progressive taxation rules have led to single parenthood actually related to a net benefit in resources rather than the opposite.

TABLE 22.2 A Quality of Life Model for Children

Spheres	Dimensions	Examples
Global		
	Macro environment	Physical environment
Ecological, societal, and political resources	Culture and human rights	Responsiveness to the Convention on the Rights of Children[a]
	Welfare policies	Welfare distribution
External		
	Work	Parental education, employment, satisfaction
Social and economic resources	Income	Income distribution
	Housing	Housing quality and satisfaction
Interpersonal		
	Family structure and function	Satisfaction with family, lack of negative events
Resources in social relationships and support	Intimate friends	Support from friends, neighbors, and society
	Extended social	
Personal		
	Physical	Growth, activity
Personal resources	Mental	Self-esteem and mood
	Spiritual	Meaning of life

SOURCE: Reprinted with permission from Lindstrom (1994).
a. As this chapter was being completed, Canada released its first report on the Convention of the Rights of the Child (Government of Canada, 1994).

EXTERNAL SPHERE

Materially, most Nordic families are provided for, and significant investment occurs in paid maternity and paternity leave, day care services, and paid sick leave due to illness of children. Education levels are systematically increasing, and differences in education between men and women have virtually disappeared. There is also an increasing mix in marriages between members of differing social classes. Employment rates among women are the highest in the world, and work satisfaction is high. Although income and costs vary between Nordic countries, differences in family incomes are "partly compensated by the welfare state in the form of cash transfers, tax reduction and support for housing" (Lindstrom, 1994, p. 71). Single parent-hood is not an economic problem, as is the case in North America. A majority of the population live in detached housing, and generally, small-scale hous-ing is the preferred standard.

The importance of Lindstrom's model is its consideration of macrolevel societal aspects of quality of life. These analyses are rarely done within the United States and only occasionally in Canada. In addition, Lindstrom's empirical work, consisting of extensive surveys of parents and their chil-dren, focuses on the external, interpersonal, and personal spheres and uses a combination of objective measures of immediate environments and subjective measures of satisfaction. These provide a rich source of ideas for considering the quality of life of children and adolescents (Lindstrom & Eriksson, 1993a, 1993b).

Lindstrom tends not to consider the direct causal links between quality of life measures and children's health as conventionally defined (although he points out that equity in economic resource allocation is the best predictor of low infant mortality rates among the 18 OECD countries). He sees his model as a means of assessing health as a resource for daily living. He sees quality of life itself serving as an indicator of healthy functioning: "The potential of the quality of life concept lies in its basically positive meaning and interdisciplinary acceptance. This can be used to develop health into a resource concept, as is the intention of the WHO [World Health Organiza-tion] *Health for All Strategy*" (Lindstrom, 1992, p. 305).

The Adolescent Quality of Life Project

"One piece still missing is the direct dialogue with the children" (Lindstrom, 1994, p. 7). The Centre for Health Promotion in cooperation with the School of Nursing, Laurentian University, Sudbury, Ontario, Can-ada, has identified quality of life issues through direct dialogue with adolescents. Based on focus groups with Ontario adolescents, the literature on adolescent concerns (Weiler, Sliepcevich, & Sarvela, 1993, 1994), and the quality of life framework presented earlier, a 54-item Quality of Life Profile: Adolescents' Version was developed (Raphael, Rukholm, Brown, & Bailey, 1995) and validated in the spring of 1995. Scores were related to adolescent smoking and drinking and adolescent perceptions of their current happiness and future opportunities. The results should help com-plete the adolescent quality of life picture. Table 22.3 presents some sample items.

TABLE 22.3 Examples of Items in the Quality of Life Profile: Adolescent Version

Domain	Item
Physical being	My appearance—how I look
	Making healthy choices (re: alcohol, drugs, smoking)
Psychological being	Being independent
	Knowing where I am going
Spiritual being	Having hope for the future
	Feeling that life has meaning
Physical belonging	The earth and its environment
	Feeling safe when I go out (school, neighborhood)
Social belonging	Being appreciated by others
	The friends I have
Community belonging	Being able to access medical-social services on my own
	Having things to do in my community in my spare time
Practical becoming	Looking after myself and my appearance
	The work I do at a job while still a student
Leisure becoming	Participating in sports and recreation activities
	Visiting and spending time with others
Growth becoming	Planning for a job or career
	Solving my problems

NOTE: Each item is rated for importance and satisfaction.

Implications for Health Promotion Practice

The content of this review suggests that health promotion work with adolescents should consider the complex of factors that affect adolescent health and health behavior. As noted earlier, recommendations pertaining to adolescent health frequently focus on individual and family factors and to immediate environments, such as neighborhoods. These are indeed important considerations, and there is surely need for action on a number of these fronts. Adolescents need to be provided with information about health risks, and families need to be supported. Similarly, adolescents should be provided with opportunities for improving leisure and daily activities and for engaging with growth-enhancing environments, be these environments schools, workplaces, or neighborhoods.

But this review also suggests that there are many structural and societal factors that serve to affect adolescent health. These factors may not normally fall within the purview of traditional health and health promotion services but will include economic resource allocation, providing opportunities for fuller employment, and developing health-enhancing social and health policies. This broader view of health determinants directs attention to these distal factors that affect health and well-being. These factors may well be the most difficult to change but may, in the long run, show the greatest promise for enhancing the health and well-being of adolescents.

Implications for Rehabilitation Practice

This review of quality of life considerations has outlined specific areas of concern to adolescents, and these concerns may be especially important to adolescents who are ill or who have disabilities. These latter adolescents may be especially susceptible to stresses related to coping and mastering developmental tasks. Adolescence is a relatively compact period lasting less than a decade, and within this period, it is expected that adolescents will master a wide range of developmental tasks. Adolescence is a difficult period for many well or able adolescents, so it can be expected that it may be even more difficult for adolescents involved in rehabilitation activities.

The complex nature of the period and the apparent effect of a range of factors on adolescent coping and adjustment requires that rehabilitation workers pay appropriate attention to the effect of an illness or disability on the adolescent's quality of life. Because an adolescent's quality of life may have a direct effect on health and well-being, quality of life should be a central concern. The manner in which this concern may manifest itself in practice is through a focus on the adolescent's personal adjustment, examination of his or her attitudes and beliefs concerning the illness or disability, and examination of the adolescent's immediate familial and school environments. And as has been noted, there are certainly societal and structural factors that may affect the adolescent's immediate life situation (e.g., availability of services, school opportunities, transportation) or the adolescent's future (e.g., employment opportunities, special supports, and so on). In either scenario, the quality of life of the adolescent in rehabilitation needs to be considered as a central focus of service efforts.

Summary and Conclusions

Quality of life seems implicated in a wide range of adolescent health outcomes and health-related behaviors. A quality of life framework provides a unifying framework for bringing together a variety of factors implicated as either promoting or inhibiting health among adolescents. Most work has focused on adolescent personal characteristics and their immediate social environments as predictors of health status and healthy functioning. Within this framework, the development of personal interventions and neighborhood programs have been recommended. For a broader analysis, Lindstrom's work identified important aspects of cultural values and economic resource allocations.

Recent work focused on the final missing part of the quality of life picture, the direct perceptions of adolescents, was mentioned. A significant body of knowledge is accumulating concerning factors related to adolescent health, and a quality of life emphasis draws attention to the need for analysis at a range of levels: individual, community, and societal. The challenge for policy makers and health providers is to translate these findings into social policies, neighborhood interventions, and adolescent-focused approaches that will support health-enhancing environments for adolescents.

PART

IV

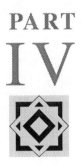

C: MAJOR LIFE ACTIVITIES

23

Work, Employment, and Mental Health

Implications for Quality of Life

Martin Shain

◆ This chapter is devoted to a consideration of the relationship between work and mental health. There will be a concentration on the work arrangement known as *employment*. The assumption here is that sound mental health is a prerequisite for quality of life (as defined in this volume). The writer's perspective is that work in our society is an important influence on mental health and that we need to augment health-promoting aspects of work and to diminish health-defeating aspects. We know more than enough about work and its effect on mental health to achieve this objective given the necessary political will to do so.

To develop the argument, we need to begin with practical definitions of the terms *work* and *mental health*. My intent is to focus on one particular work setting—namely, the employment relationship, but in passing, I will comment on other situations in which work is to provide context.

Practical Definitions

WORK

For purposes of this discussion, *work* is defined in its broadest sense as the process of applying human energy—be it mental, physical, or both—to the generation of material or immaterial products or outcomes. This broad definition allows us to regard as work the raising of children, the raising of grain, developing a concept, mowing a lawn, assembling an automobile, the performance of a concerto, pushing a wheelbarrow, and building a wall or climbing one. As such, it incorporates what might be considered leisure pursuits in some settings and forced labor in others. It does not, in itself, indicate whether energy is expended for the benefit of the performer or on behalf of another. It says nothing about reward or remuneration. It is mute on the subject of direction and governance. It implies nothing about whether the product or outcome is valued or even perceived by anyone other than the performer.

Within the broad spectrum of activities that can be defined as work, those performed in the context of the specific relationship known as employment represent a relatively narrow band. Yet in our society, there is a tendency to think of work and employment as almost synonymous. This has implications in terms of mental health both for those who function within such relation-ships and for those who do not. "Having work" seems to be very important to those who have it or want it, whereas "not having work," in the sense of employment or receiving remuneration for energy expended, is often seen in a negative light. This phenomenon can be partly explained by reference to the mental health benefits often perceived to be associated with employment. But the development of this point awaits a practical definition of mental health.

MENTAL HEALTH

Even though it is vast and full of contradictions on many points, the literature on mental health can be found to support a general definition of this elusive state. It is a state in which the individual has (a) a capacity for joy and happiness; (b) a sense of self-worth, confidence, and efficacy; (c) a sense of personal identity and meaning; (d) a sense of belonging to a meaningful and supportive group; and (e) the motivation to be involved in the maintenance of a social order. It also emphasizes that the individual experiences freedom from chronic symptoms of distress, including excessive anxiety and depression; periods of relative peace of mind and calmness; and freedom from chronic feelings of hostility and anger.

In this definition, mental health is seen as far more than the absence of symptoms: The active presence of thoughts and feelings equip the individual to function successfully in society. Central to this cognitive, conative, and emotional state is a sense of autonomy: the sense that one exists as a unique and valuable entity who enjoys freedom of thought and action as constrained only by the liberties of others and who may and does choose to live among others according to a social compact to which he or she is a free and consenting partner. The working definition given here is consistent with Health and Welfare Canada's (1988), which states that

> mental health is the capacity of the individual, the group and the environment to interact with one another in ways that promote subjective wellbeing, the optimal development and use of mental abilities (cognitive, affective and relational), the achievement of individual and collective goals consistent with justice and the attainment and preservation of conditions of fundamental equality. (p. 7)

Optimal mental health, then, requires that individuals be actively autonomous—that they possess and exercise the fundamental freedom to influence what happens around them and to them. In this sense, mental health can be acquired only in supportive social and political climates. There is, therefore, an intimate relationship between the requirements for the mental health of individuals and the requirements for a democratic society. For instance, conditions of political freedom and equality as prerequisites for sound mental health are prescribed in the Health and Welfare Canada (1988) definition previously noted. True autonomy can be gained only by negotiation and intercourse with others so that one may locate oneself in reference to them in social, economic, and political space. Consequently, the political conditions that facilitate such negotiation and intercourse and that guarantee a basic individual right to participate must prevail as prerequisites to sound mental health (Emery, 1989). Yet these political conditions are unlikely to come about unless they are created by members of society who already enjoy sound mental health. So mental health and true autonomy are both antecedents and consequences of a democratic society. This inevitable reciprocity highlights the essential tension between conditions of the mind and conditions of society. This assertion can be found in various forms in accounts of factors that influence a healthy democracy. The works of Cole (1919) and Pateman (1970) are particularly informative in this regard.

It is clear from the foregoing that mental health seen in this manner is in many ways a product of relationships with others even though it also helps to shape relationships with others. For example, I am in some measure better or worse off emotionally simply as a result of talking to or dealing with you. But I also accrue the net gain or loss from dozens of such transactions during the course of a day, a month, or a year. Much of the research conducted on the relationship between psychosocial conditions and mental health is in some way allied to this notion of wellness as a product of human transactions. Furthermore, both physical and mental health can be considered, in some measure, as products of relationships or transactions with others (see reviews by Alonzo, 1985; Mechanic, 1986; Stokols, 1992).

Seen in the ways just described, mental health is clearly an essential component of a life worth living. It is doubtful whether any but a few would define a life characterized by joylessness, low self-esteem, powerlessness, isolation, depression, and relentless agitation as a satisfactory life. Consequently, it may be said without sophistry that factors contributing to sound mental health, by definition, augment the quality of life. It is important to keep in mind that mental health and quality of life are conditions that characterize not only individuals but also collectivities, from families to work teams to societies. As noted earlier, the ability of a society to function as a democracy is thought in many ways to be dependent on the robustness of its citizens' mental health. Similarly, we might argue that the quality of life in a society depends on the robustness of its citizens' mental health.

Work and Mental Health

From the juxtaposition of the operational definitions just given, it is easy to see that some manifestations of work contribute more to mental health than others. As an extreme example, work that is carried out according to one's own whim on one's own behalf is likely to generate a greater sense of well-being than work that is imposed on an individual entirely according to another person's agenda and philosophy. Even in this extreme contrast, however, it is important not to assume the universality of the value placed on complete autonomy. People vary a great deal in their need for autonomy, and it is obvious that some are content to be directed, whereas others bridle at the suggestion. Because every person has his or her own threshold of desire for autonomy, it follows that mentally healthy work involves some match between the needs of individuals in this regard and the characteristics of the work they do. In addition, however, people need to feel that what they do is valued by others or, at least, by significant others. It is a rare individual who can sustain herself or himself indefinitely simply by drawing on his or her own sense of work's value.

Employment and Mental Health

Many of the studies that have been carried out on the relationship between work and mental health have, in fact, been narrower investigations of *employment* and mental health. As observed earlier, this amounts to a rather skewed approach to the subject even though the research has implications for work and mental health in general. By focusing on employment, the research has dwelt on one particular relational context in which work is carried out. Employment relationships are, by definition, situations in which one party, the employer, has the right (whether exercised or not) to control the behavior of another, the employee, at least for certain purposes. These purposes are supposed to revolve around performance of the job for which the employee was hired. Many instances can be cited, however, of situations in which employers seek to influence much more than this under the flag of management rights (Shain, 1992).

Because employment is a relationship defined by reference to control, it is immediately apparent that opportunities for the pursuit of mental health in this context have some basic limitations (Lennerlof, 1988). Abundant research over the past 25 years shows, in various ways, that lack of control or influence over the means, manner, and method of work has a profound influence on both the mental and physical health of employees (Karasek & Theorell, 1990). It appears from this literature that a sense of influence or efficacy consistent with individual needs is part of being well, whereas a deficiency in this regard—if severe enough—can place people at risk for all manner of mental and physical distress (e.g., see Kelloway & Barling, 1991; O'Leary, 1985).

Correspondingly, it has been observed that efficacy can be enhanced by workplace innovations aimed at increasing the participation of employees in the organization and design of key aspects of their work (Johnson & Johansson, 1991). Health and safety management, the introduction of new technology, reorganizations, downsizing, and plant relocations are among some of the leading candidates for such involvement (e.g., see Gardell, 1982). Productivity and quality control, problem solving, and design of workplace environments are others (Elden, 1986; Kolodny & Stjernberg, 1986). But efficacy, and thus well-being, can be defeated by ways of organizing and designing work that ignore employee needs for participation, impose superfluous stress, and generally ride roughshod over individual autonomy.

Therefore, the organization and design of work constitute a health issue. In consequence, it is also an efficiency and effectiveness issue because organizations do better when their employees feel better. And beyond that, even political democracies do better when peopled by voters who know how to think and whose ability to participate has not been sabotaged by chronic exposure to conditions of impotence (Emery, 1989; Pateman, 1970). The last point is of enormous social and political significance. If people learn to be helpless as a result of subservience-oriented socialization practices that are all too common in our major educational and workplace environments, we can expect little from them when it comes time to make decisions affecting all of us in the political arena. Therefore, if we want a robust and healthy democracy, we must encourage the development of workplace relations that foster the democratic competence of employees. In this sense, the way in which work is organized and designed is intimately connected with the political health of the nation.

Influences on Wellness in the Workplace

It is worth taking a closer look at how this process works. How do certain forms of the organization and design of work bring about these pernicious results? For this purpose, we may refer both to the general literature cited earlier and to recent empirical studies. One of these studies, *Influences on Wellness in the Workplace: A Multivariate Approach,* was conducted as a key part of the Corporate Health Model Development Project, a collaborative venture of Health and Welfare Canada and the Addiction Research Foundation of Ontario. This project was developed by the partners in response to the fact that workplace interventions aimed at improving the health of employees are hardly ever based on a clear understanding of what health is or what influences it (Shehadeh & Shain, 1990).

In developing a survey instrument that would assess employee health-related needs and risks, the investigators determined that the inquiry should be couched within a broad theoretical framework that would allow hypothesis testing about the influence of environmental, personal, and background variables on *wellness*. Wellness, in this study, refers to people's subjective evaluation of their overall health status. As such, it is considered to be a holistic reflection of how people weigh and interpret a wide variety of physical, mental, and spiritual signals from within their own experiential worlds. So, when people speak of how well they are, they are speaking essentially about the quality of their lives from a holistic health perspective (Zautra & Hempel, 1984).

A theoretical model of how several classes of variables influence wellness was accordingly developed, refined, and tested through the powerful multivariate statistical technique of covariance structure modeling (CSM) (Bentler, 1985; Jöreskog & Sörbom, 1983; Muthen, 1987). This theoretical model was tested in relation to three samples of employees: one male group in one site and a male group and a female group in another site. Our goal was to replicate the model developed in Site 1 on samples from Site 2. The influences considered in the study fell into four major categories: personal health practices and conditions (e.g., exercise, smoking, drinking, sleeping habits, and weight), perceived stressors at home and at work, personal resources (self-efficacy, or sense of influence in relation to work and health, and social support), and selected demographic and socioeconomic factors. The contribution of this study lies in its attempt to model all these influences simultaneously and then to replicate the results across samples. CSM has the capacity to demonstrate the degree to which a large number of individually hypothesized relationships are *simultaneously* as opposed to *independently* valid. It also has the ability to indicate the extent to which an entire set of hypotheses is valid, as opposed to the extent each hypothesis may be true independently of all the others (Fox, 1984). Thus each relationship depicted in the final statistical model shown in Figure 23.1 is found to hold true even when controlling for the influence of all the other variables in the equation.

Across all three samples, for females as well as for males, the results consistently demonstrate powerful lines of influence in which workplace pressures exacerbated by home stress contribute to the defeat of efficacy and, in turn, to the undermining of wellness. Social support is shown to mediate these negative effects to some extent. Certain health practices, in particular smoking, use of alcohol, and sleep, are interrelated and have significant effects on wellness.

In this model of influences, heavy alcohol use and smoking are seen to be correlated. Heavy alcohol use is implicated in sleep disorders. Job stress directly influences the probability of a person being a heavy drinker; home stress exacerbates job stress and increases the likelihood of heavy drinking. Home stress also raises the odds that people will sleep badly or not enough. The net effect of job stress, home stress, not getting enough rest, heavy drinking, and smoking is to weaken the extent to which people feel they have control over their work lives and over their health. This sense of weakened efficacy, together with the directly debilitating effect of heavy drinking and smoking, contributes to the perception of being under par or in less than optimum health (see Figure 23.1).

These results are generally consistent with the predictions of the biopsychosocial model of health and, in particular, with the work of Karasek and

Theorell (1990). In the biopsychosocial model, personal resources are seen mainly in a kind of brokerage or mediator role between individuals and their environments. In the quasi-causal model that emerged from this study, however, there is evidence that the personal resources of self-efficacy and social support are directly and indirectly influenced by the environment as well as being mediators or brokers of that environment. In other words, the personal resources that we bring to work with us can actually be eroded or reinforced by what happens to us once we get to work (for further discussion, see House, Strecher, Metzner, & Robbins, 1986; Israel, House, Schurman, Heaney, & Mero, 1989; Marcelissen, Winnubst, Buunk, & de Wolff, 1988).

This is not a static model of wellness. Personal resources can be enhanced; job pressures can be reduced; home stress can be managed; health practices can be improved. A major implication of this study, however, is that concerted efforts that deal simultaneously with environmental and personal influences on wellness are more likely to succeed than interventions aimed at either domain separately or alone. And in both cases, the empowerment of individuals—be it with regard to work or personal life—recommends itself as a central strategy for enhancing wellness. Otherwise stated, a primary strategy for promoting physical well-being and enhancing the quality of life is the development of measures that will augment mental health.

The crucial link between work and wellness in the research just described is stress: stress in the workplace that fuels and is fueled by stress at home (e.g., see Cohen, Tyrell, & Smith, 1991; Green & Johnson, 1990; Klitzman, House, Israel, & Mero, 1990). Stress can be both a direct and an indirect source of damage to efficacy and health and thus to organizational and social efficiency and effectiveness. An example of the direct effect of stress on mental health is to be found in managerial practices that are highly and unnecessarily directive, where control is exercised over even the minutiae of performance and where the objects of such surveillance are made to feel stupid or insignificant. A less direct but equally destructive effect occurs when employees are subject to unrealistic expectations, conflicting demands, role ambiguity, unrelieved and uncalled-for time pressure, work overload, discrimination in one or more of its many forms, and harassment. Indeed, the more stressors employees are exposed to, the more likely they are to experience a sense of assault on their ability to cope, an effect they may seek to counteract through the use of alcohol, tobacco, or other chemicals. Unfortunately, the use of these substances tends to become part of the problem rather than part of the solution. As we can see from Figure 23.1, for example, the heavy use of alcohol, particularly when combined with smoking, has not only directly negative effects on self-reported health but also indirectly negative effects through disruption of sleeping patterns, which leads, in turn, to a sense of being out of control or inefficacious.

In so far as stress leads to a sense of being out of control, it can do this either on an acute basis where its effects are limited to certain situations, times, and places or on a chronic basis where its effects are generalized and contribute to what has been aptly termed a state of learned helplessness (Lennerlof, 1988). This state can be accompanied by feelings of anxiety and depression that are debilitating enough in themselves but that are also believed to contribute, through a complex psychoneuroimmunological process, to disease conditions ranging from the common cold to cancer. In effect, empirical evidence supports the claim that sustained or cumulative stress can have a significantly negative effect on health in the absence of conditions that might be expected to mediate this outcome (Cohen et al., 1991; Jemmott & Locke, 1984; Kiecolt-Glaser & Glaser, 1986; Wiedenfeld et al., 1990).

One of these mediating conditions is the availability of social support to the individual employee. Social support helps to augment the sense of efficacy that is so important to health and well-being (Loscocco & Spitze, 1990). But there is evidence, too, that suggests that people have to enjoy at least a moderate level of health to engender social support (Marcelissen et al., 1988). So there appears to be a circularity to the relationship between social support, efficacy, and wellness. The process of the relationship appears to be one in which having people to call on in times of trouble contributes to feeling loved or cared for; this feeling is somehow empowering, leading to a sense of well-being and bonhomie that serves in turn to attract more social support, thus perpetuating the cycle (see Figure 23.1).

The Law of Employment and Mental Health

So far, we have identified stress as a key link between work and wellness. At the center of the stress vortex, we find lack of influence over or lack of participation in the organization and design of work (see Spector, 1986, for a review). Although lack of influence and participation share pride of place with other psychotoxic job factors, they are clearly major contributors to unwellness in the holistic sense described earlier. In this context, we have equated unwellness with impoverishment of quality of life. How, we might ask, is this state of affairs perpetuated in the workplace? Why do we tolerate institutional disempowerment of this order if its personal and social consequences are so grave? To address these questions, we must look to an engine of workplace organization so deeply buried that its workings are frequently inaudible to the naked ear yet so powerful that it influences our very

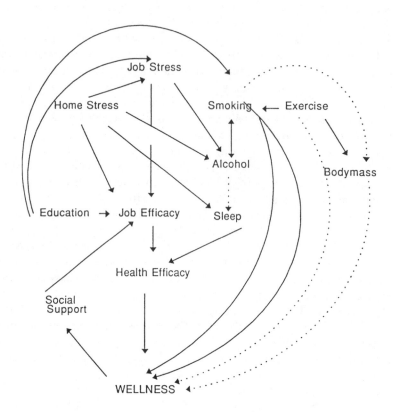

Figure 23.1. Major Influences on Wellness in Three Employee Groups

Adapted from Shehadeh and Shain (1990).

Legend: ..... = Significant in 2 of 3 samples

_____ = Significant in all 3 samples

NOTE: Type of analysis: covariance structure modeling.

consciousness of what it means to work and be employed in our society. This engine is the law of employment, or labor law. This law is such a strong influence on the governance of work and is so deeply implicated in lack of employee participation that we can justifiably identify it as a major culprit in the defeat of employees' mental and physical health (Shain, 1990, 1992). This critique of the law applies to all jurisdictions in which actual practice of labor relations revolves around the concept of employer as "master" and employee as "servant." Although some countries are attempting to lift themselves out of the master-servant paradigm (e.g., Norway, Sweden, and, to some extent, Germany) most, whether they are Common Law or Civil Law jurisdictions, still adhere to this model.

The law of employment harbors a very odd paradox with regard to its attitudes toward employee autonomy and participation. On the one hand, the language used by judges, arbitrators, and labor board members to describe the employment relationship is that of contract: That is, the language implies the idea of two (adult) parties who deal with each other as equals, bargaining freely and having complete information for an exchange of money and services. On the other hand, the actual rules of law as they are applied in courts, hearing rooms, and tribunals are shot through with the assumption that employer and employee are anything but equals. Indeed, in this context, they stand in relation to one another as parent to child or master to servant, and this situation reflects the permanently unequal status of the parties. Unfortunately, the law breathes the air of a time long past when the workplace was little more than the extension of the family and family members were little more than chattels of the husband and father. The dominant image of our labor law, that of master and servant (or controller and controlled), is reflected in the very definition of the employment relationship as one in which an employee ceases to be an employee if he or she exercises anything resembling autonomy with regard to the organization and design of his or her own work. This definition colors the attitude of the courts, tribunals, and arbitrators as they seek to apply rules pertaining to the governance of the employment relationship. Examples abound in rules concerning insubordination, how reorganizations are carried out, and how health and safety matters are decided. In all these areas, we find that employees (whether unionized or not) have very little say in the ordering of their own lives in the workplace. If they disagree with their employer about the best way of getting the job done, they court discipline or dismissal. If employers want to change the nature and content of employees' jobs, there is little that employees can do about it unless the change is fundamental, and even then, it can be legitimized under rules that allow employers to unilaterally reorganize the workplace if business reasons dictate it. With regard to health and safety rules, employees have a little more say under legislation that at least confirms their right to be involved (up to a point) in determining working conditions that put life and limb in jeopardy. But the boundaries of these rights are heavily patrolled by judges, arbitrators, and labor board members, who, with few exceptions, see entitlements in the area of health and safety as a major threat to the citadel of management prerogatives.

Some might argue that collective bargaining has made a difference to this state of affairs. Surely, the observations just made can only refer to labor relations in nonunion environments? Sadly, this is not the case to any great extent. In some ways, the explicitly adversarial nature of collective bargaining brings into even sharper focus the limits of employee influence because there are even more dramatic opportunities for public and theatrical demonstrations of management rights. It is true that some unions wield considerable economic power in the form of strike action but it is rarely exercised successfully to bring about meaningful changes in the extent to which employees can influence the organization and design of their own work. The fundamental reason for this is that the consciousness of master-servant relations that pervades the common law, applied by judges, has infused itself into the thought process of arbitrators and labor boards who apply collective bargaining law. The problem, again, is that the bargaining is in many ways still preregulated. The collective bargaining rules govern the way in which employees are defined, who is eligible to receive the benefits and protections of unionization, what can and cannot be negotiated during the course of contract discussions, and what can and cannot be disputed in the course of the employment relationship. All these rules bear the heavy imprint of common law consciousness, of the idea that employees are people who by definition do not participate meaningfully in the organization and design of their own work. This said, certain exceptions to the rather bleak picture just portrayed can be found.

So far, the contribution of collective bargaining to the cause of participation has lain mostly in the somewhat underused capacity of arbitrators to interpret collective agreements in ways that respect the interest of employees in being involved in the organization and design of their own work. Arbitral jurisprudence in this regard has tended to revolve around an emerging doctrine of reasonableness in contract administration. The central feature of this, for present purposes, is the principle that the exercise of management rights must be conditional on at least some recognition and acknowledgment of employee interests, even if these interests are not protected by specific language in the collective agreement. Most recently, it would appear that another foothold has been gained on the wall of management rights through endorsement by the courts of an arbitral doctrine that may be interpreted as requiring consultation of employees in changes to policies or rules affecting, at a minimum, their health and safety. It is possible, if not probable, that the effect of such doctrine is to reinforce the entitlement of employees to challenge employer policies and rules that are thought to be unreasonable, precisely because they fail to reflect employee input and advice. If this is correct, it will go a long way toward underpinning the statutory right to participate that is found in the context of health and safety law. For example, it will allow joint health and safety committees to challenge management policies or rules that could lead to injury or disease, thus supplementing the right of individuals to refuse work that is dangerous.

Important though those developments are, they stop short of acknowledging a right of employees to be involved in the original formulation of policies and rules. Currently, the entitlement to challenge management is a reactive one that allows employees to dispute the reasonableness of changes that their employers wish to make in the area of health and safety regulation. It is possible that this right to challenge will be interpreted more broadly in the future to encompass rules and policies beyond the realm of health and safety. If this turns out to be the case, an effective participative vehicle will have been introduced into collective bargaining environments in cases where, formerly, employee challenges to management policies and rules would have attracted discipline for insubordination.

Toward Employment That
Promotes Mental Health

The argument so far has been that employment relations have a tendency to be *psychotoxic* (a term coined by Shain, 1990/1991), or damaging to employees' mental health, and that the law tends to keep them this way (see Shain, 1993). The dynamic of psychotoxicity has been portrayed as lack of employee influence or control over the means, manner, and method of work.

What can be done about this? Can work in the context of employment be made more "psychosalubrious"? How can we make employment contribute more and detract less from quality of life? The answer depends in large part on the acknowledgment by management (and indeed by unions) that the organization of work is a health issue. Central to this issue and to this acknowledgment is the recognition that employee participation must be at the heart of any proposed initiative to make the workplace healthier. This clearly points the way to a political agenda. For further discussion of this key issue, see Emery (1989), Halpern (1992), Johnson and Johansson (1991), Karasek (1989), Pelletier (1992), and Sass (1989).

Participation, however, is a term that can be and often is used to describe forms of involvement that fall far short of what is needed to serve the mental health needs of employees. In fact, the concept of participation is amenable to exploitation by those who see it as an opportunity to get more out of employees for the same amount of money or less (Vogt & Hunt, 1988). Justifiably, labor organizations have rejected such manipulations out of hand. But in its authentic form, participation really means that managerial authority is exercised subject to the input and influence of employees. In short, it implies a way of doing business that is careful of employees' autonomy and respectful of the need for this autonomy to be expressed through informed choices about the organization and design of work. Thus participation implies a system of labor relations that is characterized by a high degree of cooperation between employers and employees while leaving intact the legitimacy of management rights in the direction of organizations.

A fully developed vision of the healthy workplace therefore involves a concept of the *just workplace* in which managerial authority is legitimized by the ongoing consent of employees to the relations of production as ensured by continuous influence over the organization and design of work.

There are many obstacles in the way of achieving a healthy workplace that would be typified by such cooperative relations. But in the end, it is a matter of will: the will to make participation a priority. We know full well that it can work. One of the best examples known to the writer comes from the logging industry in British Columbia, Canada, where the genuine participation of workers in the management of safety led to dramatic improvements in the accident record and in employee spirit and morale (Painter & Smith, 1986). The protection of physical welfare became, through participation, a means by which the mental health of employees was also served and served well.

Our time for acknowledging and acting on the evidence that confirms the contribution of participation to the mental and physical health of employees may be fast running out as we contemplate the fierce competition to which some economies experience from countries where cooperation is fast becoming the norm in relations of production. In the end, we must look for those conditions of work that contribute to quality of services and products as well as to quality of life. There is increasingly compelling research evidence that there is a strong link between these sets of conditions (Karasek & Theorell, 1990; Rosenberg & Rosenstein, 1980). We should not be surprised to find, then, that workplaces that are most attentive to the mental health of their employees are also the most successful in terms of quality of products and services.

Toward Employment That
Promotes Quality of Life

The premise of this chapter has been that different forms of work organization affect mental health, and thus quality of life, in different ways. The specific relationship of employment was chosen to illustrate a form of work organization that has a particularly corrosive effect on mental health and quality of life when regulated in ways that deprive employees of the right to participate meaningfully in the governance of their own labor. How can one realize the important possibilities of life when the core resource required to exploit such possibilities—namely, a sense of confidence, competence, and self-efficacy—is corroded by relations of employment? Such corrosion of a central pier supporting mental health virtually guarantees the structural collapse of any life plan built on it, whether this plan relates to work, family, leisure, or involvement in the polity of community and society.

The point here is not so much that work becomes meaningless and unfulfilling as a result of psychotoxic labor relations but rather, that life itself can become meaningless and unfulfilling as a result of the kind of work we do. Consequently, the reform of labor relations has a direct bearing on quality of life not only, or even principally, because it improves the experience and satisfaction of work but because it frees the mind and spirit to contemplate and pursue the vast range of possibilities that lie outside the workplace.

24

Leisure, Living, and Quality of Life

Aubrey H. Fine

A remarkable accomplishment occurred in 1989. Mark Wellman, a park ranger, captured national attention by climbing a sheer rock cliff in Yosemite National Park. What made this accomplishment particularly challenging, and hence interesting, was the fact that Mark Wellman was paraplegic.

The piece illustrated how all people can capture dreams. Twenty-five years ago, this story probably would have not been reported. On the contrary, people would probably have questioned why it was so important for such an event to occur and might have viewed the story in a paternalistic manner. Today, stories of remarkable accomplishments, of which this is admittedly an extreme, are becoming more commonplace and are being reported as worthwhile endeavors.

Numerous worldwide legislative initiatives are helping to make more people cognizant of the rights and needs of people with disabilities. For example, in the United States, on July 26, 1990, the 101st Congress passed Public Law 101-336, which is known as the *Americans with Disabilities Act of 1990.* The purpose of the act is to provide a clear and inclusive national mandate to help end discriminatory acts against people with disabilities. Furthermore, the act promotes and encourages people with disabilities to be integrated into the economic and social mainstream of life. This and other laws function as supports to providing opportunities for, and promoting a clearer understanding of, the rights of people with disabilities. As a consequence of such legislation as well as proactive advocacy in general, community members are becoming more aware of the fact that people with disabilities have the same needs and desires as all members of the community at large. Such awareness extends to all aspects of life, including social and leisure pursuits.

Tremendous efforts within the field of disabilities in recent years have led to people with disabilities securing better educational, vocational, and accommodation opportunities. Still, the importance of leisure and social activities has not been adequately recognized. This is all the more important given that leisure involvement appears to be a fundamental element to life satisfaction (Fine, 1991).

What Is Leisure?

The English word *leisure* derives from the Latin word *licere,* which means "to be permitted" (Rybczynski, 1991). The French refined the term and developed the word *loisir,* which means "free time." From this evolved the closely related English word, *license.* Thus the word leisure literally means "exception" or "permission" as applied to an opportunity. According to Rybczynski (1991), leisure referred more specifically to the opportunity to do nothing, where doing nothing was not an emptiness but, rather, an occasion for self-reflection. Today, leisure is often thought of as occupying oneself in one's free time.

But leisure is much more than occupying oneself in free time. Although a concise definition of leisure is difficult to formulate, one way of describing it is to do so in terms of the benefits ascribed to it. First, many general human needs are met through leisure. Kabanoff (1982) identified 11 such needs: autonomy, relaxation, family activity, interaction with others, stimulation, skill development and use, challenge or competition, leadership or social power, and health. Leisure may be especially instrumental in satisfying needs associated with good emotional health. Iso-Ahola (1980) pointed out that there is a significant body of research that suggests that leisure satisfaction is a principal source of perceived happiness, life satisfaction, and quality of life. Tinsley and Johnson (1984) identified seven psychological benefits of leisure: intellectual stimulation, catharsis, hedonistic companionship, secure solitude, moderate security, and expressive aestheticism. In addition, leisure can help people learn to relax and to cope with many stressors in life (Fine & Fine, 1988).

Second, meaningful leisure can be tremendously helpful in reducing feelings of helplessness (Iso-Ahola, 1980). Iso-Ahola (1980) contended that the most important dimension within the leisure experience is that of perceived freedom. A perception of freedom makes it possible to exercise individual choice within productive leisure experiences. This leads to the view that leisure offers one of the best opportunities for people to experience a sense of self-determination because it offers a chance for an individual to be in control (Austin & Crawford, 1991). Thus it can contribute to a person's sense of self-efficacy as well as empowerment.

Third, leisure experiences are very likely to become critical dimensions of an individual's personal lifestyle. For example, in Mark Wellman's case, the cliff climber who was paraplegic, leisure pursuits were a strong element of his being—an expression of who he is. This implies that a person's self-identity is enhanced (or, for that matter, diminished) by the quality of activities he or she engages in.

Last, leisure participation offers people occasions to escape from everyday personal and interpersonal environments, to set aside issues and difficulties, and to engage in activities that are enjoyable and personally satisfying (Iso-Ahola, 1984; Kabanoff, 1982; Tinsley & Johnson, 1984). At the same time, they are afforded opportunities to demonstrate mastery and competence over activities. In the past, these benefits of leisure went largely unrecognized (Fine & Fine, 1988). However, this position appears to be changing. For example, the American Psychiatric Association, a few years ago, developed a task force to study the effect of the leisure phenomenon.

Fine (1988) addressed the relationship between intrinsic motivation and satisfying leisure options. It appears that when people want to be involved in leisure activities, they feel that they are in control of the outcomes and, as a result, they are more willing to become invested. As their feelings of competence in the activities increase and as they become more internally driven, they become more willing to take risks within that leisure context. In addition, people who want to be involved in leisure activities are more likely to be involved over time. This, along with the work of Smith and Theberge (1987), suggests that perceived freedom and intrinsic motivation are the central defining properties of leisure.

It is important to highlight, though, that some of the greatest joys in life are not intrinsically motivated or planned but are discovered through serendipity. The concept of *serendipity* involves the discovery of desirable outcomes that were not sought out. The term itself originated from an ancient

Persian fairy tale about the three princes of the Isle of Serendip (Ceylon) who repeatedly traveled to the mainland to complete specific tasks. During their various excursions, they never completed their entire objective but they always had valuable discoveries or experiences (Dixon, 1988). Fine (1988) suggested that many active leisure preferences may be discovered in this manner. For example, encountering a crowded amusement area and experiencing some difficulty in accessing an activity could lead an individual to alter a plan and discover a new entertainment option or another source of recreation (e.g., a new restaurant, a movie theater) that would have been ignored due to previous planning.

However leisure comes into being, leisure as a concept is embedded within the cultural context where it occurs. This may mean that whether an activity is considered to be leisure or not depends on the subjective meaning attached to it.

All this suggests that engaging in satisfying leisure activities can contribute to the well-being of an individual and assist in the process of self-actualization. Leisure activities help people toward feelings of mastery, self-efficacy, and sheer pleasure and joy. The purpose of this chapter is to present a view on how leisure is a vital contributor to quality of life. Furthermore, several of the key concepts that need to be addressed in formulating a plan for a quality leisure lifestyle will be provided.

Leisure and Quality of Life

VIEWS OF QUALITY OF LIFE

There are numerous views of quality of life that can be used conceptually to describe the role of leisure in enhancing quality of life. For example, Malbraith (1982) described quality of life as an outcome that results from personal values and from lifestyles that attempt to fulfill those values. These lifestyles represent the interaction between a person's desires and the environmental demands placed on that person. Taylor and Bogdan (1990) maintained that quality of life is a matter of subjective experience. That is, the concept has no meaning apart from what a person feels and experiences. As a corollary to this proposition, these authors claimed that people may experience the same circumstances differently: "What enhances one person's quality may detract from another's" (pp. 34-35).

Halpern (1993) pointed out that there are a number of dichotomies that exist within quality of life conceptualizations, such as subjective versus objective perspectives, personal choice versus social expectations, and personal needs versus social expectations, among others. Although these dichotomies result in quality of life being addressed in different manners, each can be used to advance the role of leisure within quality of life. For example, the dichotomy that highlights the issue of personal choice versus social expectation suggests that, although leisure experiences should be considered an entitlement deserved by all people, the actual choices for activity involvement need to be personal.

THE IMPORTANCE OF
LEISURE IN QUALITY IN LIFE

However quality of life is conceptualized, Edgar (1987) claimed that everyone is entitled to quality of many areas of life, such as safety, pleasantness, friends and companions, self-esteem, fun, accomplishments or productivity, and excitement. The role of leisure in enhancing quality of life across the various areas of life stems from the fact that it is not a distinct category or social behavior but, rather, occurs within other activities (Kando, 1980). The role of leisure in enhancing quality of life in general has become increasingly better known during the past 20 years. Early studies by Brooks and Elliot (1971) and by Flanagan (1978) implied that leisure participation contributes to perceived quality of life and psychological well-being. For example, Flanagan (1978) found that active involvement in recreation was one of the six areas showing strong correlation with overall quality of life.

More recently, Gold (1989) broadened the role of leisure in quality of life by emphasizing that leisure is much more than recreation programming and involvement. Leisure, in this view, has to do with freedom, choices, and growth. In short, leisure is about all of life. Ferrel (1989) supported this broader view of leisure's role in the quality of life in her poignant article on community recreation in which she stated that recreation "enables us to function differently in a world that demands conformity" (p. 6).

This view of leisure's role can provide strong support for people with disabilities becoming integrated into the communities where they live in a quality way. In the past, recreational opportunities and leisure experiences have been given low priority in the education and preparation of people with disabilities (Dattilo & Schleien, 1994; Fine, 1991). Today, however, the community as a whole seems to appreciate that there has to be quality in life if people are to lead satisfying and enriched existences (Fine, 1994) and that recreation and leisure activities are critical elements for generating joy and satisfaction. For example, Marinoble and Hegenauer (1988) reported the growing need to examine the key variables in transition planning for young people with disabilities. Students judged the importance of the training they received in school and identified elements that were most helpful to them in securing quality living. They rated social skills and independent living training along with the use of leisure time as far more valuable to them than traditional academic training.

For people with severe disabilities, the role of leisure may be just as crucial. Interviews conducted with families by Fine (1992) indicated that many individuals believed that loneliness, isolation, and boredom were three variables that many adults with severe disabilities face when living independently. Ferrel (1989) noted that a person's home may be void of social opportunities. She reported that many persons with disabilities are, unfortunately, taught to follow very rigid domestic routines so they can learn to live independently. She questioned whether a majority of professionals might be more concerned with task mastery than human relationships. Could some of the voids in community living be avoided if efforts early in life attempted to train and develop more self-initiated leisure choices?

IMPORTANCE OF SUCCESSFUL
LIFELONG LEISURE IN QUALITY OF LIFE

The question of whether there really can be quality in life without expression of leisure was explored by Fine (1994). It was suggested that life cannot be celebrated in its entirety without the contribution of productive avocational activities. Furthermore, healthy lifestyles that are stable and foster well-being are achieved through involvement in the major life settings (e.g., home, community, and work), but leisure involvement needs to be superimposed on these other life settings. People may appear to have a variety of opportunities in home and work life, but if they cannot access enjoyable activities within the home or the community when the more practical life activities end (e.g., work, activities of daily life), the home merely becomes an asylum and life is considerably empty. It is the contention here that satisfactory and appreciated lifelong leisure that becomes part of healthy lifestyles can enhance the quality of one's life as it is celebrated in both the community and the home.

The methods by which people secure quality of life in many ways assist in attaining higher levels of community adjustment and independent living. Halpern (1993) pointed out that adults have many options but that developing and maintaining personal and social networks are critical. Such networks relate to a person's ability to maintain positive involvement with friends and naturally fit into how people use their free time to pursue leisure interests and activities. Fortunately, professionals from many disciplines are now attempting to support people with disabilities in developing such networks to enable them to be more active participants in their rehabilitation, not just in the planning process but also in putting together the supports that they need both to get along and to get involved.

Securing Successful Lifelong Leisure

The overall goal in securing successful lifelong leisure is to improve the quality of people's lives by enabling them to have the freedom to make choices that improve their lifestyles in healthy ways. Four guidelines for planning and ensuring successful lifelong leisure, building on those previously suggested by the author (Fine, 1994), are provided in the subsections that follow.

LEISURE WITH A PLAN

Too little emphasis has been given to the importance of lifelong leisure planning. Professionals and family members need to recognize that, to express leisure as an adult, the value of daily leisure experiences within one's whole life must begin in childhood and developed as a life skill. If we anticipate that most adults will be able to function independently, emphasis on assisting children to prepare for lifelong independent leisure functioning is essential. Fine (1994) suggested comparing leisure planning to eating a balanced and nutritious diet: Parents, presumably, would feel disturbed to learn that their children were not eating a sufficiently nutritious diet and should feel just as disturbed to learn that leisure experiences were not being incorporated into their children's lifestyles. The inference here was that the ability and desire to engage in satisfying leisure activities are critical for all individuals—equally for people with and without disabilities. Preparing for a life with quality, then, must include building a lifestyle that includes an optimal portion of leisure participation.

SELF-INITIATED LEISURE CHOICES

Productive leisure that is practiced naturally, working to enhance healthy lifestyles for specific individuals, involves leisure behaviors that are self-initiated. A problem that is frequently discussed, regarding both children and adults, is that they often have the time but do not appear to have the drive to initiate the opportunities. In actual fact, they may simply not have developed sufficient skills in self-selection to initiate opportunities. As a result, what has developed for many people is that they become involved in activities for which the outcomes are structured by others. Although involvement may be enjoyable, they selected neither the activity nor the outcome and there is usually little attention given to developing skills to support self-selection of future leisure activities.

This implies that professionals should be not only providing recreational programs but also spending the necessary time to teach and demonstrate where and how individuals can apply these and other activities independently (Fine, 1994; Fine & Fine, 1988). This can be accomplished by emphasizing the enjoyment inherent within activity involvement, by enhancing perceived competence within the framework of a leisure lifestyle, and by focusing on teaching people how to use leisure in their lives. The goal of leisure instruction, then, is to educate and train people to apply their leisure skills and knowledge and to appreciate its benefits (Iso-Ahola, 1980). The broader goal is to expose the individual to a whole reservoir of different activities that are adaptable and pertinent to different situations and environments.

Achieving this goal leads to what Gerson, Ibrahim, deVries, Eisen, and Lollar (1991) have termed the *leisure educated adult,* a phrase used to describe a person who has a well-balanced leisure lifestyle. These authors suggested that a leisure-educated adult needs to have diversified interests and should be able to participate in leisure activities both individually and with others, such as family and friends. They go on to explain that key to developing a healthy leisure lifestyle is acquiring a frame of mind that recognizes leisure as distinctly different from just free time. This frame of mind develops over time and is affected by many factors, such as living environment, age, interests, physical ability, social maturity, and intellectual capacity. Becoming a leisure-educated adult, then, is an ongoing process that progressively enriches healthy lifestyles by including opportunities to self-initiate and apply a wide variety of leisure experiences.

OPPORTUNITIES FOR INTEGRATION

The ultimate goal of leisure service delivery for people with disabilities is total inclusion of people with disabilities in community-based leisure experiences in an ongoing way. Nevertheless, despite recent advances that have seen the leisure-recreation field support integrative experiences for people with disabilities (Fine, 1994), there still exists a tremendous gap between this goal and actual practice. Some people, especially those with more severe disabilities, have been involved in activities with some degree of integration, but on the whole, attempts at integration have not met with a high degree of success.

For too long, professionals have debated how to put leisure integration into effect. The literature contains numerous arguments in favor of integrated leisure experiences (e.g., Dattilo, 1991; Howe-Murphy & Charboneau, 1987; Hutchinson & Lord, 1979; Knapczyk & Yoppi, 1975). It does not seem necessary in this chapter to add any more to those arguments but, rather, to give some ideas on how professionals can make the process of integration more natural and pleasant, and hence more successful, for all those involved.

It is vital that practitioners promote, within the larger community, a vital, positive view toward integration so that those who provide leisure opportunities will have a better understanding of its importance. One problem that arises from attempts to integrate is that many laypersons are skeptical about the potential success of integrated leisure activities, and, to the extent that such skepticism arises from discomfort with the unknown, it is essential to decrease insensitivity and bias toward people with disabilities by promoting awareness in the community as a whole.

It appears that tremendous energies may need to be expended to ensure that this type of community awareness occurs. Biklen (1985) claimed that we are currently at a crossroads with regard to integration, with our ability to promote integration depending on our commitment to it. If we can act on a strong commitment in a proactive way, we should be able to assist the general population to become more aware of and comfortable with the integration needs of people with disabilities, but if this does not occur, it is very possible that full integration will never become a reality (Fine, 1987).

There have been many projects that have been established to generate more community enthusiasm in sponsoring integrated activities. One example is provided here, a communitywide project that emphasized the value and importance of integration and strategies in facilitating transition (Fine, 1988). The project established a working network of recreational professionals, community and social service leaders, educators, and parents who interacted to formulate a plan to ensure the expansion of leisure options. Although in theory, the notion of forming community networks makes tremendous sense, the project initially received some resistance from many community agencies. They were not comfortable with the suggested expansion of services and believed that the needs of people with disabilities could be best served through traditional recreational therapy. After some time and information sharing, most of those in the network gained a new perspective on the importance of community leisure options for people with disabilities. They also seemed to develop a better understanding of how they could help all people within their communities to acquire the richest and most diverse leisure options.

This form of networking and collaboration is now being carried out in various parts of the world as a "best practice" in encouraging cooperation between various service providers. Traditional leisure programs are now taking advantage of a great many additional community resources to optimize leisure opportunities, making integration into a wide variety of community leisure options more of a reality. In doing so, community people (e.g., educators, social workers, parents, and laypersons) acquire knowledge and skills in teaching leisure participants to apply leisure lifestyles successfully, thus creating a community network through which responsibility for such teaching can be distributed. This in turn should broaden the scope of services and make them more efficient.

Implementing Circles of Support

Implementing circles of support is one method for encouraging quality integrative experiences that support successful lifelong leisure. For successful leisure to occur smoothly and in an optimal way, natural supports in the community need to be in place. Sometimes, especially for people with disabilities, these need to be developed.

The concept *circle of support* itself includes support people and services, identifying the purpose and functions of the services, and specifying the intensities of supports necessary for the outcome to occur. One explanation of this concept was provided by the American Association on Mental Retardation (1992). It defined several subconcepts, including *support resources,* the individuals who could be used to assist the person in accessing the desired community activities (e.g., family, friends, nonpaid support individuals, and generic and specialized services); *support function,* the area to which the support resources will be applied (e.g., befriending, in-home living assistance, and behavioral assistance); and *intensity of supports,* the degree of support needed by individuals (e.g., intermittent, limited, extensive, and pervasive) to access the desired opportunities and lifestyles or opportunity.

Developing circles of support appears to make remarkable sense when helping persons with disabilities to apply their leisure lifestyles (Fine, 1994). At times, just having a friend or a family member assist a person to get to an activity may be all that is needed. In other cases, more extensive supports may be required (e.g., leisure coaches). Whatever form they take, however, circles of support need to be viewed as dynamic, changing things that take on different forms and assume different values at different stages of life. This process requires ongoing commitment and energy.

Pursuing Lifelong Friendships

Pursuing lifelong friendships is key to establishing opportunities for integration and for true integration to become a reality. Practitioners must continue to give attention to improving the likelihood that people, and especially those with disabilities, have long-lasting and realistic friendships. Some people with disabilities have very limited social networks and very few friends, and the resulting loneliness is thought to contribute to overall health, mood, and behavior problems (Amado, 1993).

One of the great challenges for adults with disabilities is dealing with the emergence of isolation and loneliness. Although living independently has merit, a life spent alone is a dreadful human tragedy. Simply locating people with disabilities in community settings does not necessarily lead to positive changes in overall quality of life (Crapps, Langone, & Swaim, 1985). What is strongly needed for high quality, it appears, is that people have and use choice for active involvement in leisure opportunities.

A problem in adulthood for people with disabilities is that many of the social supports that were available in childhood decline. As a result, the opportunities and experiences for integrative leisure experiences that were celebrated in childhood are more limited. This decline is unfortunate and may not have to occur. Processes that contribute to the loneliness of people with disabilities must be identified and altered for the sake of people's well-being, longevity, mental health, and positive social and emotional growth (Amado, 1993). Amado (1993) claimed that working on friendship must be a priority with people with disabilities and suggested that supporting friendships and building on a sense of involvement can realign and enhance the lives of many individuals. This implies that having friends in one's life should be considered not as a luxury but, rather, a necessity for quality of life.

The professional community must give credence to this position to ensure lifelong quality living. Too often, the friendships of childhood are merely associations. Not enough has been done to help children learn social skills that lead to developing and sustaining true friendships. As children age, there are new barriers that develop, and ways need to be found to diminish the effects of these barriers.

Social competence implicitly supports involvement in integrative leisure experiences. By cultivating more and better prosocial skills and, as a consequence, by fitting in better, people with disabilities should be more comfortable with and competent at leisure activities. A number of conceptualizations and methods for helping individuals to develop social competence have been suggested in the literature (e.g., Novak-Amado, 1993).

LEISURE WITHIN THE HOME

Too much attention is always given to formal leisure participation outside the home. The reality is that most people learn to entertain themselves within the confinement of their own homes. The home is the first school and recreation center; the parent is the first teacher and recreation leader. The family provides the foundation of learning, including guidance in play and recreation, which in turn provides opportunities for growth. A home that provides options for wholesome leisure is developing skills that children will use in their adult years. When children recognize the wealth of options that can be selected and begin to participate naturally, they prepare themselves for the future.

Families that have a member with a disability need to be encouraged to try to remove any obstacles that might prevent the success of family leisure activities. Success may be slow, especially at first. Efforts will have to be made to involve the child (or adolescent or adult) in diverse opportunities for leisure that can be engaged in at home. After exposure, it is more realistic to expect that the individual will gradually become more self-motivated to make leisure choices. Adults with disabilities who, as children, had a strong positive foundation of leisure within the home, are more likely to continue this process as they age.

In many cases, families cannot initiate successful leisure activities within the home on their own. Recreation within the home may differ depending on the age of the individual as well as the individual's abilities and preferences. It is imperative that attention be given at an early age to encourage families to learn about how they can help their child develop a routine at home that incorporates positive practices of leisure. In the early years of a child's life, professionals can share with families the position that to obtain optimal life satisfaction, families must emphasize productive use of free time. If the view is accepted that developing an effective leisure lifestyle is a fundamental ingredient contributing to the quality of life, parents and other support individuals may become motivated to expend energy on promoting leisure activities. Their efforts should be used to ensure that a home environment is established that offers diverse choices of activities in which to participate, both with others and by oneself, and encourages children to participate in them actively. In doing this, we may be helping to prepare the child for independent life as an adult (Fine, 1994). Practitioners need to emphasize this position with families so that they become more aware of their role in assisting maturation in applied leisure functioning.

Conclusion: Future Directions

Aristotle claimed that friendship is a thing most necessary to life because without friends, no one would choose to live, though possessed of all other advantages. A human life is shallow without the friendships that can be shared and the joyful experiences that make it meaningful. A well-rounded lifestyle that includes active leisure participation will issue tremendous joy to daily living because one has something to look forward to.

It is imperative that attention be given by researchers in the future to investigating how perceived competence and freedom in leisure contribute to overall quality in life. Furthermore, researchers should make a serious effort to study the value and benefits of establishing circles of support and their overall contribution to optimal leisure lifestyles. The primary research trends of the 1980s in the field of leisure-recreation (addressing leisure and people with disabilities) focused strongly on therapeutic by-products of leisure-recreation participation. Nevertheless, there has been a tremendous shift in viewing the value of leisure experiences. A major element in this shift has been the global acceptance of the importance of securing rich and quality lifestyles for all people.

As cited in Safire and Safire (1989), Thoreau noted that it is

> something to be able to paint a particular picture, or to carve a statue and so to make a few objects beautiful; but it is more glorious to carve and paint the very atmosphere and medium through which we look, which morally we can do. To affect the quality of day, that is the highest of arts. (p. 312)

Pleasure with one's lifestyle and leisure experiences can promote within an individual a tremendous source of joy and life fulfillment. Involvement with positive leisure experiences may not be the only panacea for exceptional living but its contribution may represent a strong source for its quality.

PART

V

FUTURE DIRECTIONS

25

Conceptualization, Research, and Application

Future Directions

Rebecca Renwick
Ivan Brown
Irving Rootman
Mark Nagler

Part of the value of a volume such as this one is that it allows readers to choose from among the offerings, to draw their own conclusions, and, we hope, to be stimulated and inspired by new ideas. Still, a number of important and recurring themes emerge from the collective work presented in this volume and these bear specific mention here. Some of these themes will be valuable in guiding our future conceptualizations and applications of quality of life in the context of health promotion and rehabilitation. Several of these themes, which refer to both the content of such frameworks and the methodology for developing them, are discussed in the next section and summarized in Table 25.1. Our intention in setting them out in this manner is to present them as a set of recommendations for conceptual development. Other themes that are more relevant to a range of issues pertaining to future

TABLE 25.1 Guidelines for Development of Conceptual Frameworks of Quality of
Life in Health Promotion and Rehabilitation

Content of Conceptual Frameworks

Consider

Complexity of person-environment interactions, including interplay of environmental factors

Important aspects of environment (e.g., opportunities for enhancing quality of life,
environmental supports for and barriers to a good quality of life)

Empowerment of individuals: Control over own life (choices and decision making)

Generic approaches applicable to both general and specific populations

Personal meanings attached to quality of life (e.g., importance attached to and satisfaction
with its various dimensions or domains)

Broad range of life domains, which are common to people with and without disabilities, as a
context for a understanding of people's quality of life

Relationship between health and quality of life

Methodology for Developing Conceptual Frameworks

Consider

Inclusion and participation in the development process of persons whose lives and quality of
life are likely to be influenced by applications of the conceptual framework (e.g., research,
policy, program development)

Use of qualitative data from real people as a foundation for conceptual framework

Making explicit the assumptions underlying the framework and using these to guide
development of the framework

research, service practice, and policy development are discussed in subsequent sections.

Conceptual Development

CONCEPTUAL CONTENT

Several themes recurring throughout the volume are associated with the
appropriate or desirable content of conceptual frameworks (see Table 25.1).
The importance of attention to ongoing, complex interactions between persons and environments was highlighted by several authors (e.g., R. Brown;
Day & Jankey; Renwick & Brown). As Renwick and Friefeld noted, however, many approaches to quality of life strongly emphasize the personal
aspects of such interactions. Perhaps as a way of redressing this imbalance,

several contributors have refocused our attention on the environmental aspects of these interactions. The chapters by Bach and Rioux (on social well-being), O'Keefe (which addresses the issues of invisible environmental barriers for persons with disabilities), Raphael (on adolescents), and Rioux (on social inequality) exemplify this focus. Other authors underscored the need to include the interplay of environmental factors in various areas of life, such as work and home, that can affect perceptions about quality of life and our understanding of this construct (e.g., McPhail; Shain). The presence of supports for individuals and opportunities for enhancing one's quality of life were discussed as specific environmental elements of quality of life (Fine; McPhail; Nagler; Ouellette-Kuntz & McCreary; Raphael on adolescents; Renwick & Brown).

Three broad, related concepts—power relations; empowerment; and personal control over one's life, including one's health—were considered from several different perspectives (e.g., Bach & Rioux; R. Brown; Labonté; Renwick & Brown) and appear to be germane to models of quality of life that would be useful for both fields. Two narrower, more specific concepts related to the issue of power—namely, personal choices and decision making—were raised by several authors (e.g., I. Brown; Fine; Renwick & Brown). These narrower concepts are relevant to the manifestations of power within the person and the balance of power within relationships. Such notions (both narrow and broad) are particularly salient when we want to understand the quality of life experienced by those persons or groups who are often considered different (e.g., persons with disabilities) or marginal (e.g., individuals who are homeless) by their societies. Given the economic constraints and the emphasis on person-centered health and social services noted in the opening chapter, these issues also have wider relevance to the general population.

The usefulness of generic models that can be applied to the general population or more specific ones (e.g., persons with disabilities) was a common theme and highlights the principle that the basic components of quality of life are the same for all people (e.g., Day & Jankey; Felce & Perry). Other key ideas that emerged include the acknowledgment of personal meanings individuals attach to quality of life and individual variations in perceived quality of life (I. Brown; Renwick & Brown). Some contributors noted that models of quality of life could incorporate these concepts through attention to the relative importance individuals attach to, and satisfaction they experience in, various life areas (e.g., Day & Jankey; Renwick & Brown).

Development of conceptual approaches to quality of life that are broader than some of the health-related ones generally used in both fields was encouraged by several contributors (e.g., Bach & Rioux; Day & Jankey; Felce & Perry; Renwick & Friefeld; Schalock). This is not to suggest that health promotion or rehabilitation must necessarily deal with all dimensions or domains of quality of life within such broader frameworks, as Raeburn and Rootman noted in their chapter. Such frameworks, however, provide the necessary context for a meaningful, holistic understanding of how people, singly and in groups (Green & Kreuter, 1991), experience quality in their lives.

The material in several chapters pointed to the need to conceptualize the relationship between health and quality of life in a clear way (e.g., Parmenter; Raeburn & Rootman; Raphael on older adults; Renwick & Friedland). For instance, health may be conceptualized as a component, an outcome, or a determinant of quality of life (see Epp, 1986; Raphael, Brown, Renwick, & Rootman, 1994b). Alternatively, as Raeburn and Rootman (this volume) proposed, health and quality of life may reciprocally influence one another. It is readily apparent that this is a complex and intriguing issue. Future conceptualizations of quality of life with the potential to guide instrument development and research might contribute significantly to our knowledge about quality of life by addressing its relationship to health.

There is a dearth of well-developed conceptualizations of quality of life. The models presented in Part II of this book offer some fruitful approaches and may be the foundations and catalysts (or both) for development of new approaches in both fields. These models and new ones (to be developed) could guide research, service practice, and policy development in both fields and thus could draw the two fields even closer together.

Because both health promotion and rehabilitation have a strong emphasis on research, service practice, and policy development, it is essential that conceptualizations of quality of life be readily applicable to these endeavors (see chapters by I. Brown; Raphael on older adults; Renwick & Brown; Schalock). Models incorporating the themes outlined in this section are likely to be valuable for guiding research (including instrument development), practice, and policy development in health promotion and rehabilitation.

METHODOLOGICAL CONSIDERATIONS

Three major themes emerged that are particularly informative with regard to the methods for developing conceptual approaches to quality of life in the two fields (see Table 25.1). One theme was the inclusion of persons whose quality of life is being conceptualized. Inclusion was discussed in detail by some authors (see the chapters by Labonté; Rioux) and emerged as a recommendation from the research or analysis of other contributors (e.g., Mason; McPhail; Renwick & Brown). This theme of inclusion is related to balances of power between the persons doing the conceptual work and the persons whose lives might be influenced by application of the framework developed (see the Labonté chapter). This issue becomes especially important when the persons whose lives will be influenced are commonly perceived as different, of lower status, unequal, or marginal (see the chapters by I. Brown; Mason; Rioux). Inclusionary, participatory approaches to developing conceptual frameworks can help to balance some of these power issues and result in models that accurately reflect the voices of the persons whose lives may be affected by the use of the frameworks. Similar approaches certainly have been employed in other endeavors in health promotion (McQueen, 1994). These kinds of approaches have also begun to be used in the context of rehabilitation to develop (Goode, 1990b) and test the relevance of quality of life frameworks (Rudman, Renwick, Raphael, & Brown, 1995).

A second, related theme pertains to the use of qualitative data as a foundation for constructing conceptual frameworks for quality of life. This information may be obtained in the context of personal interviews or written materials concerning what people think makes life good or not so good for them and others they care about. Such information may also be shared by groups of individuals in the context of carefully designed focus groups or larger community meetings that encourage active involvement by all participants. For instance, the Day and Jankey chapter reported the use of a phenomenological, grounded theory approach for developing the content of a conceptual framework of quality of life. The chapter by Renwick and Brown referred to the combined use of personal interviews and focus groups as a basis for developing conceptual content as well for testing how well the new content fit with the perceptions of quality of life held by people with and without disabilities.

The third theme that has implications for the methods used to develop conceptual frameworks of quality of life concerns the assumptions on which such frameworks are based. Although Raphael's chapter on the 11 debates concerning approaches to quality of life focused on the measurement of the construct, the debates he presented constitute a framework that is also useful for examining and making explicit the assumptions underpinning the development of conceptual models. If this set of assumptions is identified early in the process, it can be useful for guiding the methods used for developing the conceptual framework (e.g., participatory versus nonparticipatory approach, qualitative versus quantitative methods of model development).

Research, Practice, and Policy

Some key gaps in our current knowledge about quality of life as it relates to health promotion and rehabilitation need further attention. The contributors to this volume have identified and begun to address many of these issues. The gaps in our knowledge about quality of life are sufficiently substantial, however, so that considerable future work is still needed. Several major gaps in the areas of research, practice, and policy are outlined in the discussion that follows and summarized in Table 25.2.

Relationships Between Quality of Life, Health, Health Status, and Functional Status. A great deal of rehabilitation research on quality of life has focused on functional and health status, yet not much is known about the relationships between quality of life, health, health status, and functional status. Several authors in this volume highlighted the nature and significance of some of these interrelationships (e.g., Parmenter; Raphael on older adults; Renwick & Friedland; Renwick & Friefeld). The Raeburn and Rootman chapter examined several of these relationships in the context of health promotion and opens what promises to be a continuing and lively debate on the topic. Many aspects of the relationships among these concepts remain to be explored, however.

Relationships Between Quality of Life, Life Satisfaction, Well-Being, Happiness, Morale, and Others. Several contributors have highlighted some of these concepts and the importance of understanding their interrelationships (e.g., Bach & Rioux; Brown, Renwick, & Nagler; Renwick & Friedland). These relationships need to be more fully explored, however, through future research based on careful conceptual work in order to illuminate some of the complexities of quality of life.

Quality-Promoting Features of Environments. Although several authors in this book (e.g., McPhail; O'Keefe; Renwick & Friefeld; Rioux; Shain) have underscored the need to better understand the contribution of particular environmental features to quality of life, relatively little work has been done in the context of health promotion and rehabilitation research. Because environmental factors are receiving increasing attention in both fields, this area of quality of life research offers many opportunities for collaborative projects between the two fields.

A Multimethod Approach to Research. Quality of life of individuals and groups in the context of health promotion and rehabilitation needs to be

TABLE 25.2 Quality of Life in Health Promotion and Rehabilitation:
Future Areas for Development

Research
  Relationships between quality of life, health, health status, and functional status
  Relationships between quality of life and similar constructs (e.g., well-being, life satisfaction)
  Environmental factors that foster quality of life
  Multimethod research approaches
  Instrument development and validation

Service Practice
  Assessment instrument development and validation
  Interventions focused on quality of life
  Program evaluation based on quality of life outcomes
  Quality assurance guided by quality of life conceptual frameworks

Policy
  Development of quality of life frameworks to integrate social and health policy issues
  Application of quality of life frameworks to policy development and analysis

studied using a variety of methods. Several chapter authors made suggestions that are useful in this regard (e.g., Raphael on measurement; Renwick & Brown; Renwick & Friedland). For example, qualitative and quantitative methods, as well as combinations of the two, are fruitful approaches for illuminating the complexities of quality of life. As Raphael pointed out, quality of life entails an understanding of some of the most personal and fundamental aspects of people's lives. Thus, qualitative information is a valuable means of understanding it. When decisions about people's lives are based on quality of life information, having subjective, qualitative data becomes even more important. Although financial factors generally make cross-sectional studies more feasible, there is a need for longitudinal research on quality of life. Such longitudinal research is necessary if we are to gain an understanding of some of the dynamic aspects of quality of life and patterns of change over time.

Instruments to Assess Quality of Life. There has been growing attention to quality of life in both health promotion and rehabilitation. Nevertheless, little has been done with regard to developing and validating instruments to assess quality of life based on clear, well-developed conceptual frameworks for quality of life. Such instruments could contribute to both research and practice (e.g., assessment and program evaluation) focused on quality of life. The most commonly used measures of quality of life in both fields were designed to tap various aspects of health or function. Not surprisingly, most of these approaches are operational in nature and not explicitly linked to any conceptual framework for quality of life. Several contributors to the current volume have begun to address this issue. For example, Raphael's chapter on measurement sets out 11 key points that can serve as a context for developing quality of life instrumentation. The chapters by Ouellette-Kuntz and McCreary and by Raphael (on older adults) discussed some recently developed quality of life instrumentation. Other authors (Raphael on adolescents; Renwick & Brown; Schalock) referred to instrumentation that they have developed on the basis of quality of life conceptual frameworks. Several quality of life frameworks in which such instrumentation could be grounded were presented in Part II of the book. Much work remains to be done, however, on the development of both quantitative and qualitative (e.g., interview formats) measurement tools.

Quality-of-Life-Focused Interventions. Specific interventions and methods of implementing them, based on clear conceptualizations of quality of life and focused on quality of life, need to be developed. Quality of life interventions can be developed for individuals, groups, or populations. Both the process and outcome aspects of such interventions would need to be evaluated in terms of quality of life measures. Approaches to quality assurance of program and service delivery can also be developed around a quality of life framework. Schalock has set out one such approach in this volume. Several contributors discussed issues relevant to quality of life interventions and their evaluation (e.g., R. Brown; Renwick & Friedland; Schalock).

Policy Analysis and Development. Policy and legislation can also be developed around quality of life as an organizing framework for integrating health and social issues. For example, this approach is relevant in the area of work and labor relations (see Shain's chapter) and with respect to access to, and participation in, leisure activities (see Fine's chapter). It is also germane to policies affecting persons with disabilities as well as the services and resources they use (e.g., policies concerning deinstitutionalization, habilitation programs, and accessible public transportation). Analysis and refinement of policy can also be guided by quality of life principles and conceptual frameworks, as proposed by several contributing authors (e.g., Felce & Perry; Ouellette-Kuntz & McCreary; Parmenter). The processes of policy development, analysis, and refinement should be influenced by those receiving the programs or services affected by the particular policy (see the chapters by Bach & Rioux; Mason; O'Keefe). Much future work is still needed with respect to health and social policy formulation structured around quality of life issues.

This book begins to explore and offers valuable insights into the foregoing issues. Although much remains to be accomplished, this volume represents a promising foundation on which to build future work.

Strengthening Bonds Between
Health Promotion and Rehabilitation

The higher order goals, underlying principles, and foci of interest of health promotion and rehabilitation have much in common. Quality of life promises to be a significant and useful construct to facilitate exploration of that common ground. Future collaborative work in the areas of conceptualization, research, joint practice-related projects (e.g., quality of life assessment and intervention), and policy formulation can serve to draw the two fields closer together to enrich and cross-fertilize one another. This volume represents one type of collaborative project between the two fields. Examples of conceptual development and research jointly undertaken by researchers in the two fields are illustrated in the work described in the chapters by Renwick and Brown, and Raphael (on older adults).

Health promotion is a growing field open to many different disciplines and constituencies, and new players will continue to become involved in this field. Rehabilitation is a discipline that has begun to be involved in health promotion and probably will do so more and more in the future. Both fields have a great deal to contribute and to gain from closer ties with one another (e.g., see the chapters by Brown, Renwick, & Nagler; Raphael on adolescents and on older adults; Renwick & Friefeld).

Both fields are concerned with promoting healthy and health-fostering environments. Health promotion has led the way on these issues and thus can enrich rehabilitation in this respect. On the other hand, rehabilitation can help to make health promotion relevant to people in their everyday lives and activities, especially for individuals with disabilities. For example, some rehabilitation researchers and professionals are experts in developing and adapting technology and environments to suit the needs of persons with disabilities. Thus, they do (and could increasingly) participate in health promotion strategies for persons with disabilities.

Some disciplines within rehabilitation have a tradition of using a person-centered or client-centered approach, and they continue to refine this approach (e.g., Townsend, 1993). Person-centered approaches are central to the thinking of many of the authors in Part IV of this volume on applications of quality of life concepts (e.g., I. Brown; R. Brown; McPhail). People-centered health promotion is an emerging approach that is critical to the field (Raeburn & Rootman, 1995). Thus, rehabilitation has strong potential as a collaborator in the process of making health promotion people-centered in that it has collective expertise in client centeredness at the individual level of analysis and application. On the other hand, rehabilitation stands to benefit from health promotion's knowledge base in the area of people-centered approaches with neighborhoods and communities.

Rehabilitation can also benefit from theoretical and methodological developments within health promotion (McComas & Carswell, 1994; Stuifbergen & Becker, 1994; Teague, Cipriano, & McGhee, 1990) as well as from its increasingly effective international network of researchers, practitioners, and organizations. Leadership in health promotion is likely to continue to become increasingly diffused. This will mean that rehabilitation as a field, as well as its researchers and professionals, will have more opportunities to influence the direction of health promotion and become more visible in its organization.

Local communities are likely to become more important in health promotion (Pederson, O'Neill, & Rootman, 1994). An example of this is the Healthy Cities movement that is rapidly spreading around the world (e.g., Hancock, 1994). This represents another opportunity for rehabilitation researchers and professionals worldwide to collaborate in developing approaches and policies that will have a significant effect on people's health and, ultimately, on their quality of life.

More integrated and comprehensive approaches that have been predicted for health promotion (Pederson et al., 1994) would also offer opportunities for rehabilitation researchers and professionals. Given the growing attention to the effects of a spectrum of environmental factors on health (and, ultimately, on quality of life), their perspectives and skills could inform the development and implementation of such comprehensive approaches to health promotion. In particular, based on the collective contributions to this volume, both fields are likely to focus increasing attention on research, assessment, intervention, program evaluation, and policy that are organized around the construct of quality of life (see Sartorius, 1992).

Quality of life measurement will become increasingly important. Measurement of this construct needs to be developed within health promotion (e.g., better grounded in theory, broader, and focused more on the environment), and the field may learn from the experiences of rehabilitation researchers in attempting to measure this multifaceted and complex construct. Despite the shortcomings of rehabilitation approaches to quality of life measurement (see the Renwick & Friefeld chapter), there is a body of literature on this that could inform developments in health promotion.

Work in the area of quality of life is central to the shared, elemental goal of the two fields—namely, enhancing the quality in people's lives. Quality of life constitutes a unifying framework that coherently draws together common concepts, principles, and issues. As such, it represents the common ground that the two fields share. In partnership, health promotion and rehabilitation can address quality of life issues in a wide spectrum of life domains. Quality of life is the area that has the greatest potential for facilitating the kinds of cross-fertilization and collaboration between the two fields that have been discussed here as well as for advancing both fields. This chapter underscores the complex challenges that lie ahead in conceptual development, research, service practice, and policy formulation related to quality of life. The partnership between the two fields will better equip us for the challenges ahead and add depth and richness to our understanding of quality of life.

References

Abbott, D., & Meredith, W. (1986). Strength of parents with retarded children. *Family Relations, 35,* 371-375.

Abella, R. S. (1985). *Equality in employment* (A Report of the Commission on Equality in Employment). Ottawa, Ontario: Minister of Supply and Services.

Ackoff, R. L. (1976). Does quality of life have to be quantified? *Operational Research Quarterly, 27*(2i), 289-303.

Adam, H., & Gudalefsky, A. B. (1986, August). *Sexuality and mental retardation.* Paper presented at the meeting of the World Congress of the International League of Societies for Persons With Mental Handicaps, Rio de Janeiro, Brazil.

Adler, R. (1986). Physical maltreatment of children. *Australian and New Zealand Journal of Psychiatry, 20,* 404-412.

Adorno, T. (1976). Sociology and empirical research. In P. Connerton (Ed.), *Critical sociology* (pp. 237-257). Markham, Ontario, Canada: Penguin.

Albin, J. M. (1992). *Quality improvement in employment and other human services: Managing for quality through change.* Baltimore: Brookes.

Albo, G., Langille, D., & Panitch, L. (1993). *A different kind of state? Popular power and democratic administration.* Toronto: Oxford University Press.

All, A. C., & Fried, J. H. (1994). Psychosocial issues surrounding HIV infection that affect rehabilitation. *Journal of Rehabilitation, 60,* 8-12.

Allen, D. (1989). The effects of deinstitutionalization on people with mental handicaps: A review. *Mental Handicap Research, 2,* 18-37.

Allison, K. (1992). Academic stream and tobacco, alcohol, and cannabis use among Ontario high school students. *International Journal of the Addictions, 27,* 561-570.

Alonzo, A. A. (1985). Health as situational adaption: A social psychological perspective. *Social Science and Medicine, 21,* 1341-1344.

Amado, R. (1993). Loneliness: Effects and implications. In A. Novak-Amado (Ed.), *Friendships and community connections between people with and without developmental disabilities* (pp. 67-84). Baltimore: Brookes.

American Association on Mental Retardation. (1992). *Mental retardation: Definition, classification, and systems of support* (9th ed.). Washington, DC: Author.

American Psychiatric Association. (1987). *Diagnostic and statistical manual of mental disorders* (3rd ed. rev.). Washington, DC: Author.

American Society for Quality Control. (1992). *Malcolm Baldrige 1993 award criteria.* Milwaukee, WI: ASQC Quality Press.

Americans With Disabilities Act of 1990, 42 U.S.C.A. §12101 *et seq.* (West 1993).

Ames, T. R. H., & Boyle, P. S. (1980). The rehabilitation counselor's role in the sexual adjustment of the handicapped client: The need for trained professionals. *Journal of Applied Rehabilitation Counselling, 11*(4), 173-178.

Ammerman, R. T., Van Hasselt, V., Hersen, M., McGonigle, J. J., & Lubetsky, M. J. (1989). Abuse and neglect in psychiatrically hospitalized multihandicapped children. *Child Abuse and Neglect, 13,* 335-343.

Andersson, Y. (1994). Single-disability organizations: The best experts of their cause. *World Federation of the Deaf News,* p. 2.

Andrews v. Law Society of British Columbia (1989) 1 S.C.R. 143, 56 D.L.R. (4th) 1.

Andrews, F. M. (Ed.). (1986). *Research on the quality of life.* Ann Arbor: University of Michigan, Institute for Social Research.

Andrews, F. M., & Withey, S. B. (1976). *Social indicators of well-being: Americans' perceptions of life quality.* New York: Plenum.

Antonovsky, A. (1987). *Unraveling the mystery of health: How people manage stress and stay well.* San Francisco: Jossey-Bass.

Argyris, C., Putnam, R., & Smith, D. (1987). *Action science.* San Francisco: Jossey-Bass.

Aristotle. (1980). The varieties of justice. In J. Sterba (Ed.), *Justice: Alternative political perspectives* (pp. 14-25). Belmont, CA: Wadsworth.

Arnold, S. (1991). Measurement of quality of life in the frail elderly. In J. Birren, J. Lubben, J. Rowe, & D. Deutchman (Eds.), *The concept and measurement of quality of life in the frail elderly* (pp. 50-74). New York: Academic Press.

Austin, D., & Crawford, M. (1991). *Therapeutic recreation.* Englewood Cliffs, NJ: Prentice Hall.

Bach, M. (1994). Quality of life: Questioning the vantage points for research. In M. H. Rioux & M. Bach (Eds.), *Disability is not measles: New research paradigms in disability* (pp. 127-152). North York, Ontario, Canada: Roeher Institute.

Backman, L., Mamtyla, T., & Herlitz, A. (1990). The optimization of episodic remembering in old age. In P. Baltes & M. Baltes (Eds.), *Successful aging: Perspectives from the social sciences* (pp. 118-163). New York: Cambridge University Press.

Badgley, R. F. (1984). *Sexual offenses against children* (Vols. 1 & 2). Ottawa, Ontario: Canadian Government Printing Centre.

Baer, J. (in press). Quality of life and brain injury: Searching for solutions. In R. I. Brown (Ed.), *Issues in quality of life.* Toronto, Ontario, Canada: Captus.

Bakan, D. (1964). *The duality of human existence: Isolation and communion in Western man.* Boston: Beacon.

Baker, C. E. (1983). Outcome quality or equality of respect: The substantive content of equal protection. *University of Pennsylvania Law Review, 131,* 933.

Baker, F., & Intagliata, J. (1982). Quality of life in the evaluation of community support systems. *Evaluation and Program Planning, 5*, 69-79.

Baltes, M., & Baltes, P. (1986). *The psychology of control and aging.* Hillsdale, NJ: Lawrence Erlbaum.

Baltes, M., & Reisenzein, R. (1986). The social world in long-term care institutions: Psychological control towards dependency. In M. Baltes & P. Baltes (Eds.), *The psychology of control and aging* (pp. 315-344). Hillsdale, NJ: Lawrence Erlbaum.

Baltes, M., & Wahl, H. (1987). Dependency and aging. In L. L. Carstensen & B. A. Edelstein (Eds.), *Handbook of clinical gerontology* (pp. 204-221). New York: Pergamon.

Baltes, P. (1968). Longitudinal and cross-sectional sequences in the study of age and generation effects. *Human Development, 11*(3), 145-171.

Baltes, P. (1973). Prototypical paradigms and questions in life-span research on development and aging. *The Gerontologist, 13,* 458-467.

Baltes, P. (1987). Theoretical propositions of life-span developmental psychology: On the dynamics between growth and decline. *Developmental Psychology, 23,* 611-626.

Baltes, P., & Baltes, M. (1990a). Psychological perspectives on successful aging: The model of selective optimization with compensation. In P. Baltes & M. Baltes (Eds.), *Successful aging: Perspectives from the social sciences* (pp. 1-34). New York: Cambridge University Press.

Baltes, P., & Baltes, M. (1990b). *Successful aging: Perspectives from the social sciences.* New York: Cambridge University Press.

Baltes, P., Reese, W., & Lipsett, L. (1980). Life-span developmental psychology. In M. Rosenzweig & L. Porter (Eds.), *Annual review of psychology* (pp. 65-110). Palo Alto, CA: Annual Reviews.

Baltes, P., Reese, W., & Nesselroad, J. (1977). *Life-span developmental psychology: Research methods.* Monterey, CA: Brooks/Cole.

Baltes, P., & Schaie, W. (1976). On the plasticity of intelligence in adulthood and old age: Where Horn and Donaldson fail. *American Psychologist, 31,* 720-725.

Barnhart, J. (1994). Deaf and deafened have different needs. *Silent News, 26*(10), 6.

Bartlett, J. (Ed.). (1980). *Familiar quotations.* Boston: Little, Brown.

Barton, L. (1993). The struggle for citizenship: The case of disabled people. *Disability, Handicap & Society, 8,* 235-248.

Barton, L., Ballard, K., & Folcher, G. (1991). *Disability and the necessity for a socio-political perspective (Monograph 51).* Durham: University of New Hampshire.

Bauer, H. (1983). Preparation of the sexually abused child for court testimony. *Bulletin of the American Academy of Psychiatry and the Law, 11*(3), 287-289.

Bayefsky, A., & Eberts, M. (Eds.). (1985). *Equality rights and the Canadian charter of rights and freedoms.* Agincourt, Ontario, Canada: Carswell.

Bayer, M. B., Brown, R. I., & Brown, P. M. (1988). Costs and benefits of alternative rehabilitation models. *Australian & New Zealand Journal of Developmental Disabilities, 14,* 277-281.

Beauchamp, T. L., & Childress, J. F. (1983). *Principles of biomedical ethics* (2nd ed.). New York: Oxford University Press.

Becker, E. (1971). *The birth and death of meaning* (2nd ed.). New York: Free Press.

Bellamy, G., Clark, G. M., Hamre-Nietupski, S., & Williams, W. (1977). Implementation of selected sex education and social skills to severely handicapped students. *Education and Training of the Mentally Retarded, 12*(4), 364-372.

Bellamy, G. T., Newton, J. S., LeBaron, N. M., & Horner, R. H. (1990). Quality of lifestyle outcomes: A challenge for residential programs. In R. L. Schalock (Ed.), *Quality of life: Perspectives and issues* (pp. 127-137). Washington, DC: American Association on Mental Retardation.

Benhabib, S. (1986). *Critique, norm, and utopia: A study of the critical foundations of society.* New York: Columbia University Press.

Bentler, P. M. (1985). *Theory and implementation of EQS: A structural equations program.* Los Angeles: BMDP Statistical Software.

Beresford, P., & Campbell, J. (1994). Disabled people, service users, user involvement, and representation. *Disability & Society, 9,* 315-325.

Bergner, M. (1989). Quality of life, health status, and clinical research. *Medical Care, 27*[Suppl.], 148-156.

Bergner, M., Bobbitt, R. A., Carter, W. B., & Gilson, B. S. (1981). The Sickness Impact Profile: Development and final revision of a health status measure. *Medical Care, 19,* 787-806.

Berkman, L. F., & Breslow, L. (1983). *Health and ways of living: The Alameda County study.* New York: Oxford University Press.

Berkman, L. F., & Smye, S. L. (1979). Social networks, host resistance, and mortality: A nine-year follow-up study of Alameda County residents. *American Journal of Epidemiology, 109,* 186-204.

Bernstein, E., Wallerstein, N., Braithwaite, R., Gutierrez, L., Labonté, R., & Zimmerman, M. (1994). Empowerment forum: A dialogue between guest editorial board members. *Health Education Quarterly, 21,* 281-294.

Bervovici, S. (1983). *Barriers to normalization: The restrictive management of retarded persons.* Baltimore: University Park Press.

Bess, F., & McConnell, F. (1981). *Audiology, education and the hearing impaired child.* St. Louis: C. V. Mosby.

Beukelman, D. R., & Mirenda, P. (1992). *Augmentative and alternative communication.* Baltimore: Brookes.

Bigelow, D. A., McFarland, B. H., & Olson, M. (1991). Quality of life of community mental health program clients: Validating a measure. *Community Mental Health Journal, 27,* 43-55.

Biklen, D. (1985). Integration in school and society. In D. Biklen (Ed.), *Achieving the complete school* (pp. 174-186). New York: Teachers College Press.

Birren, J., Lubben, J., Rowe, J., & Deutchman, D. (1991). *The concept and measurement of quality of life in the frail elderly.* New York: Academic Press.

Blackman, D. K., Howe, M., & Pinkston, E. (1976). Increasing participation in social interaction of the institutionalised elderly. *The Gerontologist, 16,* 69-76.

Blatt, B. (1980). The pariah industry: A diary from purgatory and other places. In G. Gerber, C. J. Ross, & E. Zigler (Eds.), *Child abuse: An agenda for action* (pp. 185-203). New York: Oxford University Press.

Block, F. (1990). *Postindustrial possibilities: A critique of economic discourse.* Berkeley, CA: University of California Press.

Bo, I. (1990). Social networks as resources: Relationships between background variables and social behavior. In K. Hurrelman & F. Losel (Eds.), *Health hazards in adolescence* (pp. 433-458). New York: Walter de Gruyter.

Borthwick-Duffy, S. (1990). Quality of life of persons with severe or profound mental retardation. In R. L. Schalock (Ed.), *Quality of life: Perspectives and issues* (pp. 177-189). Washington, DC: American Association on Mental Retardation.

Borthwick-Duffy, S. (1992). Quality of life and quality of care in mental retardation. In L. Rowitz (Ed.), *Mental retardation in the year 2000* (pp. 52-66). Berlin, Germany: Springer-Verlag.

Boucher, P. (1992). Reclaiming the power of community. In J. Plant & C. Plant (Eds.), *Putting power in its place: Create community control!* (pp. 47-48). Philadelphia: New Society.

Bourgeois, M. (1975). Sexualite et l'institution psychiatrique [Sexuality and the psychiatric institution]. *Evolution Psychiatrique, 40*(3), 551-573.

Bowles, S., & Gintis, H. (1986). *Democracy and capitalism: Property, community, and the contradictions of modern social thought.* New York: Basic Books.

Bowling, A. (1991). *Measuring health: A review of quality of life measurement scales.* Philadelphia: Open University Press.

Boyle, G., Rioux, M., Ticoll, M., & Feiske, A. W. (1988). Women and disabilities: A national forum. *Entourage, 3*(4), 9-13.

Bradburn, N. M. (1969). *The structure of psychological well-being.* Chicago: Aldine.

Bradley, V. J., Ashbaugh, J. W., & Blaney, B. (Eds.). (1993). *Creating individual supports for people with developmental disabilities: A mandate for change at many levels.* Baltimore: Brookes.

Bradley, V. J., & Bersani, H. A. (Eds.). (1990). *Quality assurance for individuals with developmental disabilities: It's everybody's business.* Baltimore: Brookes.

Brahams, D. (1991). Rationing health care: Ethical and legal considerations and QALYs [Editorial]. *Medico-Legal Journal, 59,* 3-6.

Bramston, P. (1994). *Lifestress test manual.* Toowooba, Queensland: University of Southern Queensland Psychology Department.

Brandt, A. S. (1979/1980). Relationship of locus of control, environmental constraint, length of time in the institution and twenty-one other variables to morale and life-satisfaction in the institutionalized elderly (Doctoral dissertation, Texas Women's University, 1979). *Dissertation Abstracts International, 40,* 5802B.

Brandtstadter, J., & Baltes-Gotz, B. (1990). Personal control over development and quality of life perspectives in adulthood. In P. Baltes & M. Baltes (Eds.), *Successful aging: Perspectives from the social sciences* (pp. 197-224). New York: Cambridge University Press.

Braybrooke, D. (1987). *Meeting needs.* Princeton, NJ: Princeton University Press.

Braybrooke, D. (1991). *Meeting needs: Towards a new needs-based ethics.* Paper presented at the meeting of the Montclair Conference for the Department of Philosophy, Dalhousie University, Halifax, Nova Scotia, Canada.

Bredo, E., & Feinberg, W. (1982). Introduction: Competing modes of social and educational research. In E. Bredo & W. Feinberg (Eds.), *Knowledge and values in social and educational research* (pp. 3-11). Philadelphia: Temple University Press.

Brodsky, G., & Day, S. (1989). *Canadian charter equality rights for women: One step forward or two steps back.* Ottawa, Ontario: Canadian Advisory Council on the Status of Women.

Brooks, J., & Elliot, D. (1971). Prediction of psychological adjustment at age thirty from leisure time activities and satisfactions in childhood. *Human Development, 14,* 51-61.

Brooks, N. A. (1984). Opportunities for health promotion: Including the chronically ill and disabled. *Social Science and Medicine, 19,* 405-409.

Brooks, W. D., & Heath, R. W. (1993). *Speech communication* (7th ed.). Madison, WI: Brown & Benchmark.

Brooks-Gunn, J., & Petersen, A. C. (1983). *Girls at puberty: Biological, psychological, and social perspectives.* New York: Plenum.

Brown, I. (1994). Promoting quality within service delivery systems. *Journal on Developmental Disabilities, 3*(2), i-iv.

Brown, I. (in press). Fools and foolishness as entertainment and power. In G. Woodill (Ed.), *The history of disabilities: International perspectives.* New York: Garland.

Brown, I., Raphael, D., & Renwick, R. (1993). *The quality of life profile.* Toronto: University of Toronto, Centre for Health Promotion.

Brown, I., Renwick, R., & Raphael, D. (1995). Frailty: Constructing a common meaning, definition, and conceptual framework. *International Journal of Rehabilitation Research, 18,* 93-102.

Brown, R. I. (1991). Changing concepts of disability in developed and developing communities. In D. Mitchell & R. I. Brown (Eds.), *Early intervention studies for young children with special needs* (pp. 1-15). London: Chapman & Hall.

Brown, R. I., & Bayer, M. B. (1992). *Rehabilitation Questionnaire and manual: A personal guide to the individual's quality of life.* Toronto: Captus.

Brown, R. I., Bayer, M. B., & Brown, P. M. (1992). *Empowerment and developmental handicaps: Choices and quality of life.* Toronto: Captus.

Brown, R. I., Bayer, M., & MacFarlane, C. (1988). Quality of life amongst handicapped adults. In R. I. Brown (Ed.), *Quality of life for handicapped people: A series in rehabilitation education* (pp. 107-123). London: Croom Helm.

Brown, R. I., Bayer, M. B., & MacFarlane, C. (Eds.). (1989). *Rehabilitation programmes: Performance and quality of life of adults with developmental handicaps.* Toronto: Lugus.

Brown, R. I., Brown, P. M., & Bayer, M. B. (1994). A quality of life model: New challenges arising from a six year study. In D. Goode (Ed.), *Quality of life for persons with disabilities: International perspectives and issues* (pp. 39-56). Cambridge, MA: Brookline.

Brown, R. I., & Timmons, V. (1994). Quality of life—Adults and adolescents with disabilities. *Exceptionality Education Canada, 4,* 1-11.

Bruce, L. (1994). *Identifying confusion among hard of hearing people.* Unpublished manuscript, University of Alberta, Edmonton.

Bryman, A. (1988). *Quantity and quality in social research.* Boston: Unwin Hyman.

Brynelson, D. (1990, May). *Historical perspective on infant development programs in Canada.* Paper presented at the Atlantic Conference on Early Intervention: Current Issues and Future Directions, Halifax, Nova Scotia, Canada.

Bunch, G. (1987). *The curriculum and the hearing impaired students: Theoretical and practical considerations.* Boston: Little, Brown.

Bunge, M. (1975). What is a quality of life indicator? *Social Indicator Research, 2,* 65-79.

Burchard, S. N., Hasazi, J. S., Gordon, L. R., & Yoe, J. (1991). An examination of lifestyles and adjustment in three community residential alternatives. *Research in Developmental Disabilities, 12,* 127-142.

Burgess, A. W., & Hartman, C. R. (Eds.). (1986). *Sexual exploitation of patients by health care professionals.* New York: Praeger.

Burt, M., & Cohen, B. (1989). *America's homeless: Numbers, characteristics, and programs that serve them* (Urban Institute report 89-3). Washington, DC: Urban Institute Press.

Calkins, C. F., Schalock, R. L., Griggs, P. A., Kiernan, W. E., & Gibson, C. A. (1990). Program planning. In C. F. Calkins & H. M. Walker (Eds.), *Social competence for workers with developmental disabilities: A guide to enhancing employment outcomes in integrated settings* (pp. 51-64). Baltimore: Brookes.

Cameron, P., Titus, D. G., Kostin, J., & Kostin, M. (1973). The life satisfaction of nonnormal persons. *Journal of Consulting and Clinical Psychology, 41,* 207-214.

Campbell, A. (1981). *The sense of well-being in America: Recent patterns and trends.* New York: McGraw-Hill.

Campbell, A., Converse, P. E., & Rodgers, W. L. (1976). *The quality of American life: Perceptions, evaluations, and satisfactions.* New York: Russell Sage.

Campbell, A., & Rodgers, W. L. (1972). *The human meaning of social change.* New York: Russell Sage.

Canadian Association of Independent Living Centres. (1994). *A time for change/The time for choices: A proposal for improving social security arrangements for Canadians with disabilities.* Ottawa, Ontario: Author.

Canadian Society for ICIDH. (1991). The handicap creation process [Special issue]. *ICIDH International Network, 4*(3).

Cantwell, D., & Baker, L. (1991). *Psychiatric and developmental disorder in children with a communication disorder.* Washington, DC: American Psychiatric Press.

Caparulo, F. (1987). *A comprehensive evaluation of a victim/offender of sexual abuse who is intellectually disabled.* Orange, CT: Center for Sexual Health and Education.

Carley, M. (1981). *Social measurement and social indicators.* London: George Allen & Unwin.

Carnegie Council. (1989). *Turning points: Preparing American youth for the 21st century.* New York: Author.

Carnegie Council. (1992). *Fateful choices: Healthy youth for the 21st century.* New York: Author.

Carpenter, S. (1991). The Canadian model of independent living centres: Trends and issues. *Rehabilitation Digest, 22*(2), 3-7.

Carver, R. (1989). *Deaf illiteracy: A genuine educational puzzle or an instrument of oppression? A critical review.* Toronto: Canadian Association of the Deaf.

Cella, D. F., & Tulsky, D. S. (1993). Quality of life in cancer: Definition, purpose, and method of measurement. *Cancer Investigation, 11,* 327-336.

Chakraborti, D. (1987). Sterilization and the mentally handicapped [Editorial]. *British Medical Journal [Clinical Research], 294*(6575), 794.

Chappell, A. L. (1992). Towards a sociological critique of the normalization principle. *Disability, Handicap and Society, 7,* 101-113.

Charness, N. (1985). *Aging and human performance.* New York: John Wiley.

Chesney, M. A. (1993). Health psychology in the 21st century: Acquired immunodeficiency syndrome as a harbinger of things to come. *Health Psychology, 12,* 259-268.

Cholewinski, R. (1990). *Human rights in Canada: Into the 1990s and beyond.* Ottawa, Ontario: Human Rights Research and Education Centre, University of Ottawa.

Chuang, H. T., Devins, G. M., Hunsley, J., & Gill, M. J. (1989). Psychosocial distress and well-being among gay and bi-sexual men with human immunodeficiency virus infection. *American Journal of Psychiatry, 146*(7), 876-880.

Cleary, P. D., Fowler, F. J., Jr., Weissmann, J., Massagli, M. P., Wilson, I., Seage, G. R., Gastonis, C., & Epstein, A. (1993). Health-related quality of life in acquired immune deficiency syndrome. *Medical Care, 31,* 569-580.

Clifford, D. L., & Sherman, P. (1983). Internal evaluation: Integrating program evaluation and management. In A. J. Love (Ed.), *Developing effective internal evaluation: New directions for program evaluation* (No. 20). San Francisco: Jossey-Bass.

Close, D. W., & Halpern, A. S. (1988). Transitions to supported living. In M. P. Janicki, M. W. Krauss, & M. M. Seltzer (Eds.), *Community residences for persons with developmental disabilities: Here to stay* (pp. 159-171). Baltimore: Brookes.

Coalition for Education Reform. (1994). *Could do better: What's wrong with public education in Ontario and how to fix it.* Toronto: Coalition for Education Reform.

Cobb, S. (1976). Social support as a moderator of life stress. *Psychosomatic Medicine, 38,* 300-314.

Cohen, S. (1985). *Visions of social control: Crime, punishment and classification.* Cambridge, MA: Polity.

Cohen, S., Mermelstein, R., Kamarck, T., & Hoberman, H. M. (1985). Measuring the functional components of social support. In I. G. Sarason & B. R. Sarason (Eds.), *Social support: Theory, research and application* (pp. 73-94). Boston: Martinus Nijhoff.

Cohen, S. R., & Mount, B. (1992). Quality of life in terminal illness: Defining and measuring subjective well-being in the dying. *Journal of Palliative Care, 8,* 40-45.

Cohen, S., & Scull, A. (Eds.). (1983). *Social control and the state.* Oxford, UK: Martin Robertson.

Cohen, S., & Smye, S. L. (1985). *Social support and health.* Orlando, FL: Academic Press.

Cohen, S., Tyrell, D. A. J., & Smith, A. P. (1991). Psychological stress and susceptibility to the common cold. *New England Journal of Medicine, 325,* 606-612.

Cohen, S., & Wills, T. A. (1985). Stress, social support and buffering hypothesis. *Psychological Bulletin, 98*(2), 310-357.

Cole, G. D. H. (1919). *Self-government in industry.* London: G. Bell.

Cole, S. S. (1986). Facing the challenges of sexual abuse in persons with disabilities. *Sexuality and Disability, 7*(3/4), 71-88.

Coleman, J. S. (1972). *Policy research in the social sciences.* Morristown, NJ: General Learning Press.

Collier, A. C. (1994). Early intervention in HIV infection: Where are we? *AIDS Research and Human Retroviruses, 10,* 893-899.

Comfort, M. B. (1978). Sexuality and the institutionalized patient. In A. Comfort (Ed.), *Sexual consequences of disability* (pp. 249-253). Philadelphia: George F. Stickley.

Conger, J. J. (1991). *Adolescence and youth: Psychological development in a changing world* (4th ed.). New York: HarperCollins.

Conroy, J. W., & Bradley, V. J. (1985). *The Pennhurst longitudinal study: A report of five years research and analysis.* Philadelphia: Temple University, Developmental Disabilities Center.

Corthell, D., & Oliverio, M. (Eds.). (1989). *Vocational rehabilitation services to persons with H.I.V. (AIDS)* (Sixteenth Institute on Rehabilitation Issues). Menomonie: University of Wisconsin-Stout, Stout Vocational Rehabilitation Institute, Research and Training Center.

Counting the cost of the good life. (1991, May 11). *Courier Mail* (Brisbane, Australia), p. 9.

Crapps, J. M., Langone, J., & Swaim, S. (1985). Quality and quantity of participation in community environments by mentally retarded adults. *Educating and Training in Mental Retardation, 20,* 123-129.

Crewe, N. M. (1980). Quality of life: The ultimate goal of rehabilitation. *Minnesota Medicine, 63,* 207-214.

Crutcher, D. (1990). Quality of life versus quality of life judgements: A parent's perspective. In R. Schalock (Ed.), *Quality of life: Perspectives and issues* (pp. 17-22). Washington, DC: American Association on Mental Retardation.

Csikszentmihalyi, M., & Larson, R. (1984). *Being adolescent: Conflict and growth in the teenage years.* New York: Basic Books.

Cummins, R. (1993). *The Comprehensive Quality of Life Scale: Intellectual disability* (4th ed.). Melbourne, Australia: Deakin University.

Cummins, R. A. (1992). *Comprehensive Quality of Life Scale: Intellectual disability.* Melbourne, Australia: Deakin University.

Cwikel, J., & Israel, B. (1987). Examining mechanisms of social support and social networks: A review of health-related intervention studies. *Public Health Reviews, 15*(3), 159-193.

Dattilo, J. (1991). Mental retardation. In D. R. Austin & M. E. Crawford (Eds.), *Therapeutic recreation: An introduction* (pp. 163-188). Englewood Cliffs, NJ: Prentice Hall.

Dattilo, J., & Schleien, S. (1994). Understanding leisure services for individuals with mental retardation. *Mental Retardation, 32,* 53-59.

Day, H. (1981). Rehabilitation for leisure: Attitudes and opportunities. *Final report to Ontario Ministry of Culture and Recreation.* Toronto: Ontario Ministry of Culture and Recreation.

Day, H. (1993). Quality of life: Counterpoint. *Canadian Journal of Rehabilitation, 6,* 135-142.

Day, H., Jankey, S., Alon, E., Clingbine, G., & Reznicek, P. (1993, October). *Quality of life: A qualitative study.* Paper presented at the meeting of the First North American Conference of Rehabilitation International, Atlanta, GA.

de Kock, U., Saxby, H., Thomas, M., & Felce, D. (1988). Community and family contact: An evaluation of small community homes for adults. *Mental Handicap Research, 1,* 127-140.

DeJong, G. (1979). *The movement for independent living: Origins, ideology, and implications for disability research.* East Lansing: Michigan State University, University Center for International Rehabilitation.

Deming, W. E. (1986). *Out of crisis.* Cambridge: Massachusetts Institute of Technology, Center for Advanced Engineering Study.

Dennis, R. E., Williams, W., Giangreco, M. F., & Cloninger, G. J. (1993). Quality of life as context for planning and evaluation of services for people with disabilities. *Exceptional Children, 59,* 499-512.

Desjardins, B. (1993). *Population ageing and the elderly: Current demographic analysis.* Ottawa, Ontario: Statistics Canada.

Desmond Poole, A., Sanson-Fisher, R. W., & Thompson, V. (1981). Observations on the behaviour of patients in a state mental hospital and a general hospital psychiatric unit: A comparative study. *Behaviour Research and Therapy, 19,* 125-134.

Deyo, R. (1991). The quality of life, research and care. *Annals of Internal Medicine, 114,* 695-697.

Diener, E. (1984). Subjective well-being. *Psychological Bulletin, 95,* 542-575.

Diener, E., & Emmons, R. A. (1984). The independence of positive and negative affect. *Journal of Personality and Social Psychology, 47,* 1105-1117.

DiMatteo, M. R., & Hays, R. (1981). Social support in serious illness. In B. H. Gottlieb (Ed.), *Social networks and social support* (pp. 117-148). Beverly Hills, CA: Sage.

Dixon, J. (1988). The development of an effective therapeutic recreation program. In A. H. Fine & N. M. Fine (Eds.), *Therapeutic recreation for exceptional children* (pp. 98-139). Springfield, IL: Charles C Thomas.

Dixon, J., & Welch, H. G. (1991). Priority setting: Lessons from Oregon. *Lancet, 337,* 891-894.

Dixon, R. A., & Baltes, P. (1986). Towards life-span research on the functions and pragmatics of intelligence. In R. J. Sternberg & R. K. Wagner (Eds.), *Practical intelligence: Nature and origins of competence in the everyday world* (pp. 203-235). New York: Cambridge University Press.

Dolnick, E. (1993). Deafness as culture. *The Atlantic, 272*(3), 37-53.

Donabedian, A. (1966). Evaluating the quality of medical care. *Milbank Memorial Fund Quarterly, 44,* 166-406.

Donald, C. A., & Ware, J. E. (1984). The measurement of social support. *Research in Community Mental Health, 4,* 325-370.

Dornbusch, S. M., Ritter, D. L., Leiderman, P. H., Roberts, D. F., & Fraleigh, M. J. (1987). The relation of parenting style to adolescent school performance. *Child Development, 58,* 1244-1256.

Dossa, P. A. (1989). Quality of life: Individualism or holism? A critical review of the literature. *International Journal of Rehabilitation Research, 12,* 121-136.

Dowie, J. (1991, March). *A short and slightly impolite paper about health status and health service outcome measurement.* Paper presented to Australian Institute of Health Forum, Priorities for National Health Statistics, Canberra, Australia.

Doyal, L., & Gough, I. (1991). *A theory of human need.* London: Macmillan.

Drover, G., & Kerans, P. (Eds.). (1993). *New approaches to welfare theory.* London: Edward Elgar.

Dryfoos, J. (1990). *Adolescents at risk: Prevalence and prevention.* New York: Oxford University Press.

Durkheim, E. (1951). *Suicide—A study in sociology.* New York: Macmillan.

Dworkin, R. (1977). *Taking rights seriously.* Cambridge, MA: Harvard University Press.

Dworkin, R. (1981a). What is equality: Part 1. Equality of welfare. *Philosophy and Public Affairs, 10,* 185-246.

Dworkin, R. (1981b). What is equality: Part 2. Equality of resources. *Philosophy and Public Affairs, 10,* 283-345.

Edgar, E. (1987). *Early morning thoughts on the quality of life.* Unpublished manuscript, University of Washington, Seattle.

Edgerton, R. B. (1990). Quality of life from a longitudinal research perspective. In R. L. Schalock (Ed.), *Quality of life: Perspectives and issues* (pp. 149-160). Washington, DC: American Association on Mental Retardation.

Edgerton, R. B., Bollinger, M., & Herr, B. (1984). The cloak of competence: After two decades. *American Journal of Mental Deficiency, 88,* 345-351.

Educational Testing Service. (1986). *The reading report card: Progress towards excellence in our schools.* Princeton, NJ: Educational Testing Service.

Eiseman, B. (1981). The second dimension. *Archives of Surgery, 116*(1), 11-13.

Elden, M. (1986). Socio-technical systems ideas as public policy in Norway: Empowering participation through worker-managed change. *Journal of Applied Behavioural Science, 22,* 239-255.

Elder, G. H., Jr. (1980). *Family structure and socialization.* New York: Arno.

Ellinson, J. (1979). Introduction to theme—Socio-medical health indicators. In J. Ellinson & A. E. Siegmann (Eds.), *Socio-medical health indicators* (pp. 151-175). New York: Baywood Farmingdale.

Elliot, D. (1993). Health-enhancing and health-compromising lifestyles. In S. G. Millstein, A. C. Petersen, & E. O. Nightingale (Eds.), *Promoting the health of adolescents: New directions for the twenty-first century* (pp. 119-145). New York: Oxford University Press.

Ellis, N. (1991). *Priorities in affordable public health* (A discussion paper). Sydney, Australia: New South Wales Department of Health.

Emener, W. G. (1993). Empowerment in rehabilitation: An empowerment philosophy for rehabilitation in the 20th century. In M. Nagler (Ed.), *Perspectives on disability* (2nd ed., pp. 297-305). Palo Alto, CA: Health Markets Research.

Emerson, E. B. (1985). Evaluating the impact of deinstitutionalization on the lives of mentally retarded people. *American Journal of Mental Deficiency, 90,* 277-288.

Emerson, E., & Hatton, C. (1994). *Moving out: Relocation from hospital to community.* London: Her Majesty's Stationery Office.

Emery, F. E. (1989). *Toward real democracy: Quality of working life centre.* Toronto: Ontario Ministry of Labour.

Emmons, R. A., & Diener, E. (1985). Personality correlates of subjective well-being. *Personality and Social Psychology Bulletin, 11,* 89-97.

Endicott, O. (1988). The law: Is it still a capital offence to have Down's syndrome? *Entourage, 3*(3), 17-22.

Eng, E., & Parker, E. (1994). Measuring community competence in the Mississippi Delta: The interface between program evaluation and empowerment. *Health Education Quarterly, 21,* 199-220.

Epp, J. (1986). *Achieving health for all: A framework for health promotion.* Ottawa, Ontario: Ministry of Supply and Services.

Ericsson, K. (1990). Peak performance and age: An examination of peak performance in sports. In P. Baltes & M. Baltes (Eds.), *Successful aging: Perspectives from the social sciences* (pp. 164-196). New York: Cambridge University Press.

Erikson, R. (1993). Descriptions of inequality: The Swedish approach to welfare research. In M. Nussbaum & A. Sen (Eds.), *The quality of life.* Oxford, UK: Clarendon.

Evans, D. (1994). Enhancing quality of life in the population at large. *Social Indicators Research,* *33,* 47-88.

Evans, D. R., Burns, J. E., Robinson, W. E., & Garrett, O. J. (1985). The quality of life questionnaire. *American Journal of Community Psychology, 13,* 305-322.

Evans, D. R., & Cope, W. E. (1989). *Manual for the Quality of Life Questionnaire.* Toronto: Multi-Health Systems.

Evans, D. R., Hearn, M. T., Levy, L., & Shatford, L. A. (1988, August). *Modern health technologies and quality of life: A generalizability study.* Paper presented at the meeting of the XXIV International Congress of Psychology, Sydney, Australia.

Evans, R. G., Barer, M., & Marmor, T. R. (1994). *Why are some people healthy and others not?: The determinants of health of populations.* New York: Aldine de Gruyter.

Evans, R. G., & Stoddart, G. L. (1990). Producing health, consuming health care. *Social Science and Medicine, 31,* 1347-1363.

Ewoldt, C. (1981). A psycholinguistic description of selected deaf children reading in sign language. *Reading Research Quarterly, 17,* 58-89.

Fabian, E. (1991). Using quality of life indicators in rehabilitation program evaluation. *Rehabilitation Counseling Bulletin, 34,* 344-356.

Fanning, M. F., & Emmott, S. D. (1994). *Validation of a quality of life instrument for patients with HIV Infection* (NHRDP Publication No. 6606-4334-AIDS). Ottawa, Ontario: Health & Welfare Canada.

Fanning, M. M., Emmott, S., Sherett, H., Renwick, R., Friedland, J., & Kelly, P. (1993, June). *Validation of the Fanning Quality of Life Instrument for HIV/AIDS.* Paper presented at the IX Annual International Conference on AIDS, Berlin, Germany.

Farley, J. (1979). Activities and pastimes of children and youth: Age, sex, and parental effects. *Journal of Comparative Family Studies, 10*(3), 385-410.

Felce, D. (1988). Evaluating the extent of community integration following the provision of staffed residential alternatives to institutional care. *Irish Journal of Psychology, 9,* 346-360.

Felce, D. (1989). *Staffed housing for adults with severe and profound mental handicaps: The Andover project.* Kidderminster, UK: BIMH Publications.

Felce, D., de Kock, U., & Repp, A. C. (1986). An eco-behavioural comparison of small home and institutional settings for severely and profoundly mentally handicapped adults. *Applied Research in Mental Retardation, 7,* 393-408.

Felce, D., de Kock, U., Thomas, M., & Saxby, H. (1986). Change in adaptive behaviour of severely and profoundly mentally handicapped adults in different residential settings. *British Journal of Psychology, 77,* 489-501.

Felce, D., & Perry, J. (1993). *Quality of life: A contribution to its definition and measurement.* Cardiff, Wales, UK: Mental Handicap in Wales Applied Research Unit.

Felce, D., & Perry, J. (1995). Quality of life: Its definition and measurement. *Research in Developmental Disabilities, 16,* 51-74.

Feldman, S., & Elliot, G. (Eds.). (1990). *At the threshold: The developing adolescent.* Cambridge, MA: Harvard University Press.

Ferrans, C., & Powers, M. (1992). Psychometric assessment of the quality of life index. *Research in Nursing and Health, 15*(1), 29-38.

Ferrel, M. (1989). Community recreation. *Entourage, 4*(1), 1-7.

Fine, A. H. (1987, July). *Repressing handicapism: Educating others in understanding and accepting disabled persons.* Paper presented at the International Symposium on Disability Education, Jerusalem.

Fine, A. H. (1988). *Community adjustment and the mentally retarded.* Unpublished grant proposal, California Department of Developmental Disabilities, Sacramento.

Fine, A. H. (1991, May). *Recreation: Community integration and quality of life.* Paper presented at the 114th Annual Meeting of the American Association on Mental Retardation, Atlanta, GA.

Fine, A. H. (1992, May). *Friendship and community living.* Paper presented at the 115th Annual Meeting of the American Association on Mental Retardation, Crystal City, VA.

Fine, A. H. (1994). Life, liberty and choices: A commentary of leisure's values in life. *Journal on Developmental Disabilities, 3*(2), 16-28.

Fine, A. H., & Fine, N. (1988). *Therapeutic recreation for exceptional children: Let me in, I want to play.* Springfield, IL: Charles C Thomas.

Fitzpatrick, R., & Albrecht, G. (1994). The plausibility of quality-of-life measures in different domains of health care. In L. Nordenfelt (Ed.), *Concepts and measurement of quality of life in health care* (pp. 201-227). Dordrecht, Netherlands: Kluwer.

Flanagan, J. (1978). A research approach to improving our quality of life. *American Psychologist, 33,* 138-147.

Flanagan, J. C. (1982). Measurement of quality of life: Current state of the art. *Archives of Physical Medicine and Rehabilitation, 63,* 56-59.

Flax, M. J. (1972). *A study in comparative urban indicators: Conditions in 18 large metropolitan areas.* Washington, DC: Urban Institute.

Fleishman, J., & Fogel, B. (1994). Coping and depressive symptoms among people with AIDS. *Health Psychology, 13,* 156-169.

Fletcher, S. (1986). *Cost and financing of long-term care in Canada.* Paper presented at the meeting of the American Association of Retired Persons, U.S.—Canadian Expert Group on Policies for Midlife and Older Women, Washington, DC.

Flynn, M. (1989). *Independent living for adults with a mental handicap: A place of my own.* London: Cassel.

Folkman, S., Chesney, M., & Christopher-Richards, A. (1994). Stress and coping in caregiving partners of men with AIDS. *Psychiatric Clinics of North America, 1,* 35-53.

Folkman, S., Chesney, M., Pollack, L., & Coates, T. (1993). Stress, coping, and depressive mood in human immunodeficiency virus-positive and -negative gay men in San Francisco. *Journal of Nervous and Mental Disease, 181,* 409-416.

Folkman, S., & Lazarus, R. S. (1988). *Ways of Coping Questionnaire manual.* Palo Alto, CA: Consulting Psychologists Press.

Forcese, D., & Richer, S. (1973). *Social research methods.* Englewood Cliffs, NJ: Prentice Hall.

Ford, J. (1993). *Hard of hearing people's experiences in community and culture.* Unpublished manuscript.

Fougeyrollas, P. (1992). Explanatory models of the consequences of disease and trauma: The handicaps creation process. *Proceedings of an International Symposium on Research Into Functional Limitations and Their Social Consequences (OPHQ)* (pp. 14-27). Montreal: Canadian Society for the ICIDH.

Fox, J. (1984). *Linear statistical models and related methods.* New York: John Wiley.

Franklin, J. L., Simmons, J., Solovitz, B., Clemons, J. R., & Miller, G. F. (1986). Assessing quality of life of the mentally ill: A three-dimensional model. *Evaluation and the Health Professions, 9,* 376-388.

Franklin, U. (1990). *The real world of technology.* Concord, Ontario: Anansi.

Freidson, E. (1972). *Profession of medicine.* New York: Dodd, Mead.

Freire, P. (1968). *Pedagogy of the oppressed.* New York: Seabury.

Freire, P., & Macedo, D. (1987). *Literacy: Reading the word & the world.* Boston: Bergin & Garvey.

Frey, W. D. (1984). Functional assessment in the 1980s: A conceptual enigma, a technical challenge. In A. S. Halpern & M. J. Furher (Eds.), *Functional assessment in rehabilitation* (pp. 11-43). Baltimore: Brookes.

Frick, D. (1986). *The quality of urban life.* New York: Walter de Gruyter.

Friedland, J., Renwick, R., & McColl, M. (in press). Coping and social support as determinants of quality of life in HIV/AIDS. *AIDS Care.*

Friedmann, J. (1992). *Empowerment: The politics of alternative development.* Oxford, UK: Blackwell.

Furnham, A., & Pendred, J. (1983). Attitudes toward the mentally and physically disabled. *British Journal of Medical Psychology, 56,* 170-187.

Gannon, J. (1989). *The week the world heard Gallaudet.* Washington, DC: Gallaudet University Press.

Gardell, B. (1982). Scandinavian research on stress in the workplace. *International Journal on Health Services, 12*(1), 31-41.

Gardner, J. F., & Chapman, M. S. (1993). *Developing staff competencies for supporting people with developmental disabilities: An orientation handbook* (2nd ed.). Baltimore: Brookes.

Gardner, W. H. (1966). Adjustment problems of laryngectomized women. *Archives of Otolaryngology, 83,* 31-42.

Gergen, K. J. (1986). Correspondence versus autonomy in the language of understanding human action. In D. W. Fiske & R. A. Shweder (Eds.), *Metatheory in social science: Pluralism and subjectivities* (pp. 136-162). Chicago: University of Chicago Press.

Gerson, G., Ibrahim, H., deVries, J., Eisen, G., & Lollar, S. (1991). *Understanding leisure: An interdisciplinary approach.* Dubuque, IA: Kendall Hunt.

Gibbons, J. H. (1982). *Technology and handicapped people.* Washington, DC: Office of Technology Assessment.

Glaser, B. G., & Strauss, A. L. (1967). *The discovery of grounded theory: Strategies for qualitative research.* New York: Aldine de Gruyter.

Gloerson, B., Kendall, J., Gray, P., McConnell, S., Turner, J., & Lewkowicz, J. (1993). The phenomena of doing well in people with AIDS. *Western Journal of Nursing Research, 15,* 44-58.

Goffman, E. (1963). *Stigma: Notes on the management of spoiled identity.* Englewood Cliffs, NJ: Prentice Hall.

Gold, D. (1989). Putting leisure into life. *Entourage, 4*(1), 10-11.

Goode, D. A. (1988). *Discussing quality of life: Framework and findings of the work group on quality of life.* Valhalla, NY: Mental Retardation Institute.

Goode, D. A. (1990a). Measuring the quality of life of persons with disabilities: Some issues and suggestions. *AAMR News and Notes, 3*(2), 6-7.

Goode, D. A. (1990b). Thinking about and discussing quality of life. In R. L. Schalock (Ed.), *Quality of life: Perspectives and issues* (pp. 41-57). Washington, DC: American Association on Mental Retardation.

Goode, D. A. (1991, May). *Quality of life research: A change agent for persons with disabilities.* Paper presented to the American Association on Mental Retardation National Meeting Round Table Program, Washington, DC.

Goode, D. A. (1994a). *A world without words: The social construction of children born deaf and blind.* Philadelphia: Temple University Press.

Goode, D. A. (Ed.). (1994b). *Quality of life for persons with disabilities: International perspectives and issues.* Cambridge, MA: Brookline.

Goode, D. A. (1994c). Quality of life policy: Some issues and implications of a generic social policy concept for people with developmental disabilities. *European Journal on Mental Disability, 1,* 38-45.

Goode, D. A. (1994d, December). *Quality of life (QOL) as international disability policy: Implications for European research.* Paper presented at the First European Conference on Quality of Life, European Definitions of Quality of Life: Towards a Synthesis, Copenhagen, Denmark.

Goode, D. A. (1994e). The national quality of life for persons with disabilities project: A quality of life agenda for the United States. In D. Goode (Ed.), *Quality of life for people with disabilities: International perspectives and issues* (pp. 139-161). Cambridge, MA: Brookline.

Goode, D. A., & Hogg, J. (1994). Towards an understanding of holistic quality of life in persons with profound intellectual and multiple disabilities. In D. Goode (Ed.), *Quality of life for persons with disabilities: International perspectives and issues* (pp. 197-207). Cambridge, MA: Brookline.

Goodinson, S. M., & Singeton, J. (1989). Quality of life: A critical review of current concepts, measures and their clinical implications. *International Journal of Nursing Studies, 26,* 327-341.

Goodkin, K., Blaney, N. T., Feaster, D., Fletcher, M. A., Baum, M. K., Mantero-Atienza, E., Klimas, N. G., Millon, C., Szapocznik, J., & Eisdorfer, C. (1992). Active coping style is associated with natural killer cell cytotoxicity in asymptomatic HIV-1 seropositive homosexual men. *Journal of Psychosomatic Research, 36*(7), 635-650.

Goodman, R., Steckler, A., Hoover, S., & Schwartz, R. (1993). A critique of contemporary community health promotion approaches: Based on a qualitative review of six programs in Maine. *American Journal of Health Promotion, 7,* 208-220.

Goundry, S., Peters, Y., & Currie, R. (1994). *Income security reform from a disability equality perspective: Proposals for an analytic framework.* Winnipeg, Manitoba: Canadian Disability Rights Council.

Government of Ontario. (1993). *Partnerships in long-term care: A policy framework.* Toronto: Queen's Printer for Ontario.

Graetz, B. (1993). Health consequences of employment and unemployment: Longitudinal evidence for young men and women. *Social Science and Medicine, 36,* 715-724.

Green, K. L., & Johnson, J. V. (1990). The effects of psychosocial work organization on patterns of cigarette smoking among male chemical plant employees. *American Journal of Public Health, 80,* 1368-1371.

Green, L. W., & Kreuter, M. W. (1991). *Health promotion planning: An educational and environmental approach.* Mountain View, CA: Mayfield.

Green, T. H. (1964). Liberal legislation and freedom of contract. In J. R. Rodman (Ed.), *The political theory of T. H. Green: Selected writings* (pp. 43-74). New York: Appleton-Century-Crofts.

Greenawalt, K. (1983). How empty is the idea of equality. *Columbia Law Review, 83,* 1167-1185.

Greenblatt, M., Becerra, R. M., & Serafetinides, E. A. (1982). Social networks and mental health: An overview. *American Journal of Psychiatry, 139,* 977-984.

Greenfield, S. (1989). The state of outcome research: Are we on target? *New England Journal of Medicine, 320,* 1142-1143.

Greer, S. (1984). The psychological dimension in cancer treatment. *Social Science and Medicine, 18,* 345-349.

Guba, E. (1990). The alternative paradigm dialogue. In E. Guba (Ed.), *The paradigm dialogue* (pp. 17-27). Newbury Park, CA: Sage.

Guba, E., & Lincoln, Y. (1989). *Fourth generation evaluation.* Newbury Park, CA: Sage.

Gunn, M. (1989). Sexual abuse and adults with mental handicap: Can the law help? In H. Brown & A. Craft (Eds.), *Thinking the unthinkable: Papers on sexual abuse and people with learning difficulties* (pp. 51-73). London: FPA Education Unit.

Gutek, B. A., Allen, H., Tyler, T. R., Lau, R. R., & Majchrzak, A. (1983). The importance of internal referents as determinants of satisfaction. *Journal of Community Psychology, 11,* 111-120.

Habermas, J. (1984). *The theory of communicative action* (Vol. 1). London: Heinemann.

Hadley, J. (1982). *More medical care, better health?* Washington, DC: Urban Institute.

Halpern, A. (1993). Quality of life as a conceptual framework for evaluating transition outcomes. *Exceptional Children, 59,* 486-498.

Halpern, A. (1994). Quality of life for students with disabilities in transition from school to adulthood. In D. Romney, R. Brown, & P. Fry (Eds.), *Social Indicators Research, 33,* 193-236.

Halpern, A. S., Nave, G., Close, D. W., & Wilson, D. (1986). An empirical analysis of the dimensions of community adjustment for adults with mental retardation in semi-independent living programs. *Australia and New Zealand Journal of Developmental Disabilities, 12*(3), 147-157.

Halpern, C. R. (1992). The political economy of mind-body health. *American Journal of Health Promotion, 6,* 288-291.

Hamburg, D., Elliot, G., & Parron, D. (Eds.). (1982). *Health and behaviour: Frontiers of research in the biobehavioural sciences.* Washington, DC: National Academy Press.

Hammarstrom, A. (1990). Youth unemployment and health: Results from a five year follow-up study. In K. Hurrelman & F. Losel (Eds.), *Health hazards in adolescence* (pp. 131-148). New York: Walter de Gruyter.

Hancock, T. (1994). A healthy and sustainable community: The view from 2020. In C. M. Chu & R. Simpson (Eds.), *Ecological public health: From vision to practice.* Toronto: University of Toronto Centre for Health Promotion, and ParticipACTION.

Hansell, S., & Mechanic, D. (1990). Parent and peer effects on adolescent health behavior. In K. Hurrelman & F. Losel (Eds.), *Health hazards in adolescence* (pp. 43-66). New York: Walter de Gruyter.

Harner, C. J., & Heal, L. W. (1993). The multifaceted lifestyle satisfaction scale (MLSS): Psychometric properties of an interview schedule for assessing personal satisfaction of adults with limited intelligence. *Research in Developmental Disabilities, 14,* 221-236.

Harris, M. (1990). *Unholy orders.* Toronto: Penguin.

Hartup, H. W. (1983). Peer relations. E. M. Heatherington (Ed.), *Handbook of child psychology: Vol. 4. Socialization, personality and social development* (4th ed., pp. 103-196). New York: John Wiley.

Havighurst, R. J. (1953). *Human development and education.* New York: Longmans, Green.

Havlik, R. J., Liu, B. M., & Kovar, M. G. (1987). *Health statistics on older persons, United States, 1986: Vital and health statistics, Series 3* (No. 25, DHHS Publication No. PHS 87-1409, National Center for Health Statistics, Public Health Service). Washington, DC: Government Printing Office.

Hawkridge, D., Vincent, T., & Hale, G. (1985). *New information technology in the education of disabled children and adults.* San Diego, CA: College-Hill.

Heal, L. W., & Chadsey-Rusch, J. (1985). The lifestyle satisfaction scale (LSS): Assessing individuals' satisfaction with residence, community setting and associated services. *Applied Research in Mental Retardation, 6,* 475-490.

Health and Welfare Canada. (1974). *A new perspective on the health of Canadians.* Ottawa, Ontario: Ministry of Supply and Services.

Health and Welfare Canada. (1988). *Mental health for Canadians: Striking a balance.* Ottawa, Ontario: Ministry of Supply and Services.

Health and Welfare Canada. (1994). *Children and youth with a hearing loss: Promoting mental health.* Ottawa, Ontario: Health and Welfare Canada.

Heilbroner, R. (1992). *Twenty-first century capitalism.* Concord, Ontario: Anansi.

Herbert, C., & Milsum J. (1990). *Measuring health: The documentation and evaluation of measures currently used to measure well-being.* Vancouver: University of British Columbia, Department of Health Promotion.

Hier, S. J., Korboot, P. J., & Schweitzer, R. D. (1990). Social adjustment and symptomatology in two types of homeless adolescents: Runaways and throwaways. *Adolescence, 25,* 761-771.

Hollandsworth, J. G., Jr. (1988). Evaluating the impact of medical treatment on the quality of life: A 5-year update. *Social Science Medicine, 26,* 425-434.

Hopkins, A. (Ed.). (1992). *Measures of the quality of life and uses to which such measures may be put.* London: Royal College of Physicians.

Hopkins, N., & Emler, N. (1990). Social network participation and problem behavior in adolescence. In K. Hurrelman & F. Losel (Eds.), *Health hazards in adolescence* (pp. 385-408). New York: Walter de Gruyter.

Horowitz, F. (Ed.). (1989). Children and their development: Knowledge base, research agenda, and social policy application [Special issue]. *American Psychologist 44*(2), 95-490.

House, J. S., Strecher, V., Metzner, M., & Robbins, C. (1986). Occupational stress and health among men and women in the Tecumseh community health study. *Journal of Health and Social Behavior, 27,* 62-77.

Howe-Murphy, R., & Charboneau, B. G. (1987). *Therapeutic recreation intervention: An ecological perspective.* Englewood Cliffs, NJ: Prentice Hall.

Humphries, T. (1977). *Communicating across cultures (deaf/hearing) and language learning.* Unpublished doctoral dissertation, Union Graduate School, Cincinnati, OH.

Hunt, S. M., McEwan, J., & McKenna, S. P. (1985). Social inequalities and perceived health. *Effective Health Care, 2,* 151-160.

Hunt, S. M., McKenna, S. P., McEwen, J., Williams, J., & Papp, E. (1981). The Nottingham health profile: Subjective health status and medical consultations. *Social Science and Medicine, 15A,* 221-229.

Hurrelman, K., & Losel, F. (1990). Basic issues and problems of health in adolescence. In K. Hurrelman & F. Losel (Eds.), *Health hazards in adolescence* (pp. 1-24). New York: Walter de Gruyter.

Hutchinson, P., & Lord, J. (1979). *Recreation integration: Issues and alternatives in leisure services and community involvement.* Ottawa, Ontario: Leisurability.

Ignatieff, M. (1984). *The needs of strangers.* London: Hogarth.

Institute of Medicine. (1988). *Homelessness, health, and human needs.* Washington, DC: National Academy Press.

Isaacs, B., Percival, S., Gombay, B., & Perlman, N. (1994). A social context for understanding quality of life. *Journal on Developmental Disabilities, 3*(2), 45-58.

Iso-Ahola, S. (1980). *The psychology of leisure and recreation.* Dubuque, IA: William C. Brown.

Iso-Ahola, S. (1984). Social Psychological foundations of leisure and resultant implications for leisure counseling. In E. T. Dowd (Ed.), *Leisure counseling: Concepts and applications* (pp. 97-120). Springfield, IL: Charles C Thomas.

Israel, B., Checkoway, B., Schulz, A., & Zimmerman, M. (1994). Health education and community empowerment: Conceptualizing and measuring perceptions of individual, organizational and community control. *Health Education Quarterly, 21,* 149-170.

Israel, B. A., House, J. S., Schurman, S. J., Heaney, C. A., & Mero, R. P. (1989). The relation of personal resources, participation, influence, interpersonal relationships and coping strategies to occupational stress, job strains and health: A multivariate analysis. *Work and Stress, 3*(2), 163-194.

Jackson, J. (1969). Factors of the treatment environment. *Archives of General Psychiatry, 21,* 39-45.

Jacobs, L. (1974). *A deaf adult speaks out.* Washington, DC: Gallaudet College Press.

James, T. N., & Brown, R. I. (1992). *Prader-Willi syndrome: Home, school and community.* London: Chapman & Hall.

Jankey, S. G. (1992). *Optimism, perceived control, and sense of coherence and their relationship to quality of life.* Unpublished master's thesis, York University, Toronto.

Jemmott, J. B., & Locke, S. E. (1984). Psychosocial factors, immunologic mediation and human susceptibility to infectious diseases: How much do we know? *Psychological Bulletin, 95*(1), 78-108.

Jenkins, J., Felce, D., Lunt, B., & Powell, E. (1977). Increasing engagement in activity of residents in old people's homes by providing recreational materials. *Behaviour Research and Therapy, 15,* 429-434.

Jessor, R. (1984). Adolescent development and behavioral health. In J. D. Matarazzo, S. M. Weiss, J. A. Herd, & N. E. Miller (Eds.), *Behavioral health: A handbook of health enhancement and disease prevention* (pp. 69-90). New York: John Wiley.

Jessor, R. (1993). Successful adolescent development among youth in high-risk settings. *American Psychologist, 48,* 117-126.

Jessor, R., Donovan, J. E., & Costa, F. (1990). Perceived life chances, and adolescent health behavior. In K. Hurrelman & F. Losel (Eds.), *Health hazards in adolescence* (pp. 25-42). New York: Walter de Gruyter.

Jette, A. M. (1980). Functional status index: Reliability of a chronic disease evaluation instrument. *Archives of Physical Medicine and Rehabilitation, 61,* 395-401.

Johnson, J. A., & Jaffe, E. (1989). *Health promotion and prevention programs: Models of occupational therapy practice.* New York: Haworth.

Johnson, J. V., & Johansson, G. (Eds.). (1991). *The psychosocial work environment: Work organization, democratization and health.* Amityville, NY: Baywood.

Johnson, R., Johnson, D., Wang, M., & Smiciklas-Wright, H. (1994). Characterizing nutrient intakes of adolescents by sociodemographic factors. *Journal of Adolescent Health, 15*(2), 149-154.

Jones, J. M., Levine, I. S., & Rosenberg, A. A. (1991). Homelessness research, services, and social policy. *American Psychologist, 46,* 1109-1111.

Jongbloed, L., & Crichton, A. (1990). A new definition of disability: Implications for rehabilitation practice and social policy. *Canadian Journal of Occupational Therapy, 57,* 32-38.

Jöreskog, K. G., & Sörbom, D. (1983). *LISREL V and VI: Analysis of linear structural relationships by maximum likelihood and least squares methods: User's guide* (2nd ed.). Mooresville, IN: Scientific Software.

Kabanoff, B. (1982). Occupational and sex differences in leisure needs and leisure satisfaction. *Journal of Occupational Behavior, 3,* 233-245.

Kablaoui, B., & Pautler, A. (1991). The effects of part-time work experience on high school students. *Journal of Career Development, 17,* 195-211.

Kando, T. (1980). *Leisure and popular culture in transition.* St. Louis: C. V. Mosby.

Kannapell, B. (1985). *Language choice reflects identity choice: A sociolinguistic study of deaf college students.* Unpublished doctoral dissertation, Georgetown University, Washington, DC.

Kaplan, G., & Hahn, M. P. (1989). Is there a role for prevention among the elderly? Epidemiological evidence from the Alameda County study. In M. Ory & K. Bond (Eds.), *Aging and health care: Social science and policy perspectives* (pp. 27-51). New York: Routledge.

Kaplan, R. M., Anderson, J. P., Wu, A. W., Mathews, W. C., Kozin, F., & Orenstein, D. (1989). The quality of well-being scale: Applications in AIDS, cystic fibrosis, and arthritis. *Medical Care, 27*(Suppl. 3), S27-S43.

Kaplan, R. M., & Bush, J. W. (1982). Health-related quality of life measurement for evaluation research and policy analysis. *Health Psychology, 1,* 61-80.

Karasek, R. (1989). The political implications of psychosocial work redesign: A model of the psychosocial class structure. *International Journal of Health Sciences, 13,* 481-508.

Karasek, R., & Theorell, T. (1990). *Healthy work: Stress, productivity and the reconstruction of working life.* New York: Basic Books.

Kearns, R. A., Smith, C. J., & Abbott, M. W. (1991). Another day in paradise? Life on the margins in urban New Zealand. *Social Science and Medicine, 33,* 369-379.

Keith, K., Schalock, R., & Hoffman, K. (1986). Quality of life: Measurement and programmatic implication. *Region V mental retardation series.* Nebraska City: Nebraska City.

Kelloway, E. K., & Barling, J. (1991). Job characteristics, role stress and mental health. *Journal of Occupational Psychology, 64,* 291-304.

Kerlinger, F. (1986). *Foundations of behavioral research.* New York: Holt, Rinehart & Wilson.

Kerr, N. (1977). Understanding the process of adjustment to disability. In J. Stubbins (Ed.), *Social and psychological aspects of disability: A handbook for practitioners* (pp. 305-316). Baltimore: University Park.

Kerr, N., & Meyerson, L. (1987). Independence as a goal and value of people with physical disabilities: Some caveats. *Rehabilitation Psychology, 32*(3), 173-180.

Kiecolt-Glaser, J. K., & Glaser, R. (1986). Psychological influences on immunity. *Psychosomatics, 27,* 621-624.

Kiell, N. (1964). *The universal experience of adolescence.* Boston: Beacon.

Kilian, A. (1988). Conscientisation: An empowering non-formal education approach for community health workers. *Community Development Journal, 23,* 117-123.

Kitzhaber, J. (1994). A healthier approach to health care. *Issues in Science and Technology, 7,* 59-65.

Klassen, D., Hornstra, R. K., & Anderson, P. B. (1975). Influence of social desirability on symptom and mood reporting in a community survey. *Journal of Consulting and Clinical Psychology, 45,* 448-452.

Kliegl, R., Smith, J., & Baltes, P. B. (1989). Testing the limits and the study of adult age differences in cognitive plasticity of a mnemonic skill. *Developmental Psychology, 25,* 247-256.

Klitzman, S., House, J. S., Israel, B. A., & Mero, R. P. (1990). Work, stress, nonwork stress, and health. *Journal of Behavioural Medicine, 13,* 221-243.

Knapczyk, D. R., & Yoppi, J. O. (1975). Development of cooperative and competitive play responses in developmentally disabled children. *American Journal on Mental Deficiency, 80,* 245-255.

Knapp, M., Cambridge, P., Thomason, C., Beecham, J., Allen, C., & Darton, R. (1992). *Care in the community: Challenge and demonstration.* Aldershot, UK: Ashgate.

Kobasa, S. (1979). Stressful life events, personality and health: An inquiry into hardiness. *Journal of Personality and Social Psychology, 37,* 1-11.

Koff, T. (1988). *New approaches to health care for an aging population.* San Francisco: Jossey-Bass.

Kolodny, H., & Stjernberg, T. (1986). The change process of innovative work designs: New design and redesign in Sweden, Canada and the U.S. *Journal of Applied Behavioural Science, 22,* 287-301.

Korthright, K., & Ford, J. (1993, Winter). *The hard of hearing community, its cultural aspects and its educational implications.* Symposium conducted at the Deaf Studies Class, York University, Toronto.

Kozma, A., & Stones, M. J. (1978). Some research issues in the psychological well-being of the aged. *Canadian Psychological Review, 19,* 241-249.

Kozma, A., Stones, M. J., & McNeil, J. (1991). *Psychological well-being in later life.* Toronto, Ontario: Buttersworths.

Kraft, P., & Rise, J. (1995). Prediction of attitudes towards restrictive AIDS policies: A structural equation modelling approach. *Social Science and Medicine, 40,* 711-718.

Kretschmer, R., & Kretschmer, L. W. (1990). Language. *Volta Review, 4*(6), 56-71.

Kuyek, J., & Labonté, R. (1994, November). *From power-over to power-with: Transforming professional practice.* Paper presented at the Ontario Public Health Association, Toronto.

Kymlicka, W. (1989). *Liberalism, community, and culture.* Oxford, UK: Clarendon.

Labonté, R. (1986). Social inequality and healthy public policy. *Health Promotion, 3,* 341-351.

Labonté, R. (1993). *Health promotion and empowerment: Practice frameworks* (Issues in Health Promotion Monograph Series). Toronto, Ontario: University of Toronto, Centre for Health Promotion, and ParticipACTION.

Labonté, R. (1994). Health promotion and empowerment: Reflections on professional practice. *Health Education Quarterly, 21,* 253-268.

Labonté, R., & Robertson, A. (in press). Delivering the goods, showing our stuff: The case for a constructivist paradigm for health promotion research and practice. *Health Education Quarterly.*

Lachman, M. (1986). Personal control in later life: Stability, change, and cognitive correlates. In M. Baltes & P. Baltes (Eds.), *The psychology of control and aging* (pp. 207-236). Hillsdale, NJ: Lawrence Erlbaum.

Lakin, K. C., Bruininks, R. H., & Larson, S. A. (1991). The changing face of residential services. In L. Rowitz (Ed.), *Mental retardation in the year 2000* (pp. 197-247). Berlin, Germany: Springer-Verlag.

Lalonde, M. (1974). *A new perspective on the health of Canadians.* Ottawa, Ontario: Health and Welfare Canada.

Land, K. C. (1975). Social indicator models: An overview. In K. C. Land & S. Spilerman (Eds.), *Social indicator models* (pp. 5-36). New York: Russell Sage.

Landesman, S. (1986). Quality of life and personal life satisfaction: Definition and measurement issues. *Mental Retardation, 24,* 141-143.

Landesman-Dwyer, S. (1986). Living in the community. *American Journal of Mental Deficiency, 86,* 223-234.

Landesman-Dwyer, S., Berkson, G., & Romer, D. (1979). Affiliation and friendship of mentally retarded residents in group homes. *American Journal of Mental Deficiency, 83,* 571-580.

Lane, H. (1989). *When the mind hears.* New York: Vintage.

Lane, H. (1992). *The mask of the benevolence.* New York: Knopf.

Lapoint, A., Askew, J., & Mead, N. (1992). *Learning science.* Princeton, NJ: Educational Testing Service.

Lapoint, A., Mead, J., & Askew, J. (1992). *Learning mathematics.* Princeton, NJ: Educational Testing Service.

Larson, J. S. (1991). *The measurement of health.* New York: Greenwood.

Law Reform Commission of Canada. (1979). *Sterilization: Implications for mentally retarded and mentally ill persons.* Ottawa, Ontario: Ministry of Supply and Services.

Lawton, M. P. (1991). A multidimensional view of quality of life in frail elders. In J. Birren, J. Lubben, J. Rowe, & D. Deutchman (Eds.), *The concept and measurement of quality of life in the frail elderly* (pp. 3-27). New York: Academic Press.

Lazarus, R. S., & Folkman, S. (1984). *Stress, appraisal and coping.* New York: Springer.

Leal Ocampo, R. (1995). Stronger families—Stronger societies. In Roeher Institute (Ed.), *As if children mattered: Perspectives on children, rights and disability.* North York, Ontario: Roeher Institute.

Leigh, I. W., & Stinson, M. S. (1991). Social environments, self-perceptions, and identity of hearing impaired adolescents. *Volta Review, 93*(5), 253-265.

Leiss, W. (1978). *Limits to satisfaction: Needs and commodities.* London: Boyars.

Lennerlof, L. (1988). Learned helplessness at work. *International Journal of Health Services, 18,* 207-222.

Lennon, M. C., Martin, J. L., & Dean, L. (1990). The influence of social support on AIDS-related grief reaction among gay men. *Social Science and Medicine, 31,* 477-484.

Lerner, M. (1986). *Surplus powerlessness.* Oakland, CA: Institute for Labor and Mental Health.

Lerner, M. J., & Simmons, C. H. (1966). The observer's reaction to an "innocent victim": Compassion or rejection? *Journal of Personality and Social Psychology, 4,* 203-210.

Létourneau, P. Y. (1993). The psychological effects of aphasia. In D. Lafond, Y. Joanette, J. Ponzio, R. DeGiovani, & M. T. Sarno (Eds.), *Living with aphasia* (pp. 65-85). San Diego, CA: Singular.

Lewis, S., & Lyon, L. (1986). The quality of community and the quality of life. *Sociological Spectrum, 6,* 397-410.

Liberman, R. A., de Risi, W. J., King, L. W., Eckman, T. A., & Wood, D. (1974). Behavioral measurement in a community health center. In P. O. Davidson, F. W. Clark, & L. A. Hamerlynck (Eds.), *Evaluation of behavioral programs in community, residential and school settings* (pp. 103-139). Champaign, IL: Research Press.

Lichty, J., & Johnson, P. (1992). Client intervention: Another team's experience. In R. Brown, M. Bayer, & P. Brown (Eds.), *Empowerment and developmental handicaps: Choices and quality of life* (pp. 63-74). London: Captus.

Lincoln, Y. S., & Guba, E. (1985). *Naturalistic inquiry.* Newbury Park, CA: Sage.

Lindstrom, B. (1992). Quality of life: A model for evaluating health for all. *Soz Praventivmed, 37,* 301-306.

Lindstrom, B. (1994). *The essence of existence: On the quality of life of children in the Nordic countries.* Goteborg, Sweden: Nordic School of Public Health.

Lindstrom, B., & Eriksson, B. (1993a). Quality of life among children in the Nordic countries. *Quality of Life Research, 2,* 23-32.

Lindstrom, B., & Eriksson, B. (1993b). Social paediatrics: Quality of life for children with disabilities. *Soz Praventivmed, 38,* 83-89.

Lineberry, R., Mandel, A., & Shoemaker, P. (1974). *Community indicators: Improving communities management.* Austin: University of Texas Press.

Ling, D., & Ling, A. (1978). *Aural habilitation: The foundations of verbal learning in hearing-impaired children.* Washington, DC: Alexander Graham Bell Association for the Deaf.

Linn, L. S., Gelberg, L., & Leake, B. (1990). Substance abuse and mental health status of homeless and domiciled low-income users of a medical clinic. *Hospital and Community Psychiatry, 41,* 306-310.

Liu, B. C. (1976). *Quality of life indicators in U.S. metropolitan areas: A statistical analysis.* New York: Praeger.

Livneh, H. (1988). Rehabilitation goals: Their hierarchical and multifaceted nature. *Journal of Applied Rehabilitation Counselling, 19*(3), 12-18.

Loew, F., & Rapin, C. H. (1994). The parodoxes of quality of life and its phenomenological approach. *Journal of Palliative Care, 10,* 37-41.

Loomes, G., & McKenzie, L. (1990). The scope and limitations of QALY measures. In S. Baldwin, C. Godfrey, & C. Propper (Eds.), *Quality of life: Perspectives and policies* (pp. 84-102). London: Routledge.

Lord, J. (1992, May). *Personal empowerment and active living.* Paper presented at the International Conference on Physical Activity, Fitness, and Health, Toronto, Ontario.

Lord, J., & Farlow, D. (1990). A study of personal empowerment: Implications for health promotion. *Health Promotion, 29*(2), 2-8.

Lorimer, J. (1994). Excellence & equity in education. *CAUT Bulletin, 41*(8), 24.

Loscocco, K. A., & Spitze, G. (1990). Working conditions, social support, and well-being of female and male factory workers. *Journal of Health and Social Behaviour, 31,* 313-327.

Lowe, K., & de Paiva, S. (1988). Canvassing the views of people with a mental handicap. *Irish Journal of Psychology, 9,* 220-234.

Lowe, K., & de Paiva, S. (1991). *NIMROD: An overview.* London: Her Majesty's Stationery Office.

Lubin, R. A., Schwartz, A. A., Zigman, W. B., & Janicki, M. P. (1982). Community acceptance of residential programs for developmentally disabled persons. *Applied Research in Mental Retardation, 3,* 191-200.

Lubitz, J., & Prihooda, R. (1983). *Use and costs of Medicare services in the last years of life* (DHHS Publication No. PHS 84-1232, National Centre for Health Statistics, Public Health Service). Washington, DC: Government Printing Office.

Luckasson, R., Coulter, D. L., Polloway, S., Reiss, S., Schalock, R. L., Snell, M. E., Spitalnik, D. M., & Stark, J. A. (1992). *Mental retardation: Definition, classification, and systems of supports* (9th ed.). Washington, DC: American Association on Mental Retardation.

Lukes, S. (1980). Socialism and equality. In J. Sterba (Ed.), *Justice: Alternative political perspectives* (pp. 211-230). Belmont, CA: Wadsworth.

MacFarlane, C., Brown, R. I., & Bayer, M. B. (1989). Quality of life. In R. I. Brown, M. B. Bayer, & C. MacFarlane (Eds.), *Rehabilitation programmes: Performance and quality of life of adults with developmental handicaps* (pp. 56-67). Toronto: Lugus.

Mahoney, F. I., & Barthel, D. W. (1965). Functional evaluation: The Barthel index. *Maryland State Medical Journal, 14,* 61-65.

Malbraith, L. (1982). A conceptual and research strategy for the study of ecological aspects of quality of life. *Social Indicators Research, 10,* 133-157.

Mann, J., Tarantola, D., & Netter, T. (Eds.). (1994). *AIDS in the world: A global report.* Cambridge, MA: Harvard University Press.

Marcelissen, F. H. G., Winnubst, J. A. M., Buunk, B., & de Wolff, C. J. (1988). Social support and occupational stress: A causal analysis. *Social Science and Medicine, 26,* 365-373.

Marinoble, R., & Hegenauer, J. (1988). *Quality of life for individuals with disabilities: A conceptual framework.* Sacramento: California State Department of Education.

Marlett, N. J. (1976). *Adaptive functioning index.* Calgary, Alberta: Vocational and Rehabilitation Research Institute.

Martinez, C. (1990). A dream for myself. In R. Schalock (Ed.), *Quality of life: Perspectives and issues* (pp. 3-8). Washington, DC: American Association on Mental Retardation.

Mason, D. (1990). *Visual/gestural and aural/oral bilingualism: A phenomenological study on bilingualism and deafness.* Unpublished doctoral dissertation, University of Alberta, Edmonton.

Mason, D. (1994a). Bilingual/bicultural education for the deaf is appropriate. In G. Bunch & M. Bibby (Eds.), *ACEHI monograph series* (No. 2, pp. 1-33). Toronto: York University Press.

Mason, D. (1994b). *What do teacher preparation programmes offer North America?* Unpublished manuscript, York University, Toronto.

Mathison, S. (1991). What do we know about internal evaluation? *Evaluation and Program Planning, 14,* 159-165.

McCarthy, B., & Hagan, J. (1991). Homelessness: A criminogenic situation? *British Journal of Criminology, 31,* 393-410.

McColl, M., & Rosenthal, C. (1994). A model of resource needs of aging spinal cord injured men. *International Medical Society of Paraplegia, 32,* 261-270.

McComas, J., & Carswell, A. (1994). A model for action in health promotion: A community experience. *Canadian Journal of Rehabilitation, 7,* 257-265.

McConkey, R., Naughton, M., & Nugent, U. (1983). Community contacts of adults who are mentally handicapped. *Mental Handicap, 11,* 57-59.

McConkey, R., Walsh, P. N., & Conneally, S. (1993). Neighbours' reactions to community services: Contrasts before and after services open in their locality. *Mental Handicap Research, 6,* 131-141.

McDowell, I., & Newell, C. (1987). *Measuring health: A guide to rating scales and questionnaires.* New York: Oxford University Press.

McFadden, D. L., & Burke, E. P. (1991). Developmental disabilities and the new paradigm: Direction for the 1990s. *Mental Retardation, 29,* iii-vi.

McGrew, K. S., & Bruininks, R. H. (1992). A multidimensional approach to the measurement of community adjustment. In M. Hayden & B. Avery (Eds.), *Community living for persons with mental retardation and related conditions* (pp. 124-141). Baltimore: Brookes.

McKnight, J. (1987, Winter). Regenerating community. *Social Policy,* pp. 54-58.

McNeil, B. J., Weichselbaum, R., & Parker, S. G. (1982). On the elicitation of preference for alternative therapies. *New England Journal of Medicine, 306,* 1259-1262.

McPherson, G. (1990). Are you ready for the revolution? *Canadian Journal of Rehabilitation, 3,* 1-5.

McQueen, D. (1994). Health promotion research in Canada: A European/British perspective. In A. Pederson, M. O'Neill, & I. Rootman (Eds.), *Health promotion in Canada: Provincial, national, and international perspectives.* Toronto: W. B. Saunders.

Mechanic, D. (1986). Role of social factors in health and well-being: Biopsychosocial model from a social perspective. *Integrative Psychiatry, 4,* 2-11.

Meenan, R. F., German, P. M., Mason, J. H., & Dunaif, R. (1982). The arthritis impact measurement scale: Further investigations of a health status measure. *Arthritis and Rheumatology, 25,* 1048-1053.

Meredith, C. N., & Dwyer, J. T. (1991). Nutrition and exercise: Effects on adolescent health. *Annual Review of Public Health, 12,* 309-333.

Merleau-Ponty, J. (1968). *The visible and invisible.* Evanston, IL: Northwestern University Press.

Merton, R. K. (1967). *On theoretical sociology.* New York: Free Press.

Metellus, J., Lefebvre-des-Noettes-Gisquet, V., & Vendeuvre, I. (1993). The physical experience. In D. Lafond, Y. Joanette, J. Ponzio, R. DeGiovani, & M. T. Sarno (Eds.), *Living with aphasia* (pp. 53-63). San Diego, CA: Singular.

Meyer, L. H., Peck, C. A., & Brown, L. (Eds.). (1990). *Critical issues in the lives of people with severe disabilities.* Baltimore: Brookes.

Michalos, A. C. (1986). Job satisfaction, marital satisfaction, and the quality of life: A review and a preview. In F. M. Andrews (Ed.), *Research on the quality of life* (pp. 57-82). Ann Arbor, MI: Institute for Social Research.

Milbrath, L. W. (1979). Policy relevant quality of life research. *Annals of the American Academy of Political and Social Science, 444,* 33-45.

Milburn, N., & D'Ercole, A. (1991). Homeless women: Moving toward a comprehensive model. *American Psychologist, 46,* 1161-1169.

Miles, I. (1985). *Social indicators for human development.* London: Frances Pinter.

Miller, L., & Davey, R. (1994, November). *A description and evaluation of Barkuma's linkworker service.* Paper presented to the Australian Society for the Study of Intellectual Disability, Newcastle, New South Wales, Australia.

Millstein, S. G., & Litt, I. F. (1990). Adolescent health. In S. Feldman & G. Elliot (Eds.), *At the threshold: The developing adolescent* (pp. 431-456). Cambridge, MA: Harvard University Press.

Millstein, S. G., Petersen, A. C., & Nightingale, E. O. (Eds.). (1993). *Promoting the health of adolescents: New directions for the twenty-first century.* New York: Oxford University Press.

Minister of Health and Welfare on Child Sexual Abuse in Canada. (1990). *Reaching for solutions* (Cat. No. H74-28/1990E). Ottawa, Ontario: Ministry of Supply and Services.

Ministry of Health. (1991). *Healthy elderly: Principles and program strategies.* Toronto: Ministry of Health, Public Health Branch.

Minkler, M. (1990). Improving health through community organization. In K. Glanz, F. Lewis, & B. Rimer (Eds.), *Health behavior and health education: Theory, research and practice* (pp. 47-62). San Francisco: Jossey-Bass.

Mishra, R. (1990). *The welfare state in capitalist society: Policies of retrenchment and maintenance in Europe, North America and Australia.* Toronto: University of Toronto Press.

Momeni, J. (Ed.). (1990). *Homelessness in the United States.* New York: Praeger.

Mondros, J., & Wilson, S. (1994). *Organizing for power and empowerment.* New York: Columbia University Press.

Moore, D. (1992, October). *The remarkable phenomenon of deaf bilingualism and biculturalism and its incorporation in deaf education.* A symposium conducted at the meeting of the WHIN Conference, Madison, WI.

Moos, R. (1974). *The social climate scales: An overview.* Palo Alto, CA: Consulting Psychologists Press.

Morgan, G. (1991). Advocacy as a form of social science. In P. Harries-Jones (Ed.), *Making knowledge count: Advocacy and social science* (pp. 223-231). Montreal: McGill-Queen's University Press.

Morris, D. (1967). *The naked ape: A zoologist's study of the human animal.* London: Cape.

Morris, D. (1971). *The human zoo.* New York: Bantam.

Morriss, P. (1987). *Power: A philosophical analysis.* Manchester, UK: Manchester University Press.

Murrell, S. A., & Norris, F. H. (1983). Quality of life as the criterion for need assessment and community psychology. *Journal of Community Psychology, 11,* 88-97.

Muthen, B. O. (1987). *LISCOMP: Analysis of linear structural equations with a comprehensive measurement model: A program for advanced research.* Mooresville, IN: Scientific Software.

Muthny, F. A., Koch, U., & Stump, S. (1990). Quality of life in oncology patients. *Psychotherapy and Psychosomatics, 54,* 145-160.

Naess, S. (1987). *Quality of life research: Concepts, methods, and applications.* Oslo, Norway: Institute of Applied Social Research.

Namir, S., Wolcott, D., Fawzy, F., & Alumbaugh, M. (1990). Implications of different strategies for coping with AIDS. In L. Temoshack & A. Baum (Eds.), *Psychological perspectives on AIDS* (pp. 173-190). Hillsdale, NJ: Lawrence Erlbaum.

National Council of Welfare. (1994). *Poverty profile update for 1991.* Ottawa, Ontario: National Council of Welfare.

National Council on the Aging. (1975). *Codebook for the "myth and reality of aging."* Durham, NC: Duke University, Center for the Study of Aging.

Navarro, V. (1977). *Health and medical care in the U.S.: A critical analysis.* Farmingdale, NY: Baywood.

Nelson, E. C., & Berwick, D. M. (1989). The measurement of health status in clinical practice. *Medical Care, 27,* 577-590.

Neugarten, B., Havighurst, R., & Tobin, S. (1961). The measurement of life satisfaction. *Journal of Gerontology, 16,* 134-143.

New South Wales Office on Social Policy. (1994). *Quality of life: A social policy approach.* Sydney, Australia: NSW Government Social Policy Directorate.

Nordenfelt, L. (1994). Quality of life as a new goal for medicare and health care. In L. Norderfelt (Ed.), *Concepts and measurement of quality of life in health care* (pp. 1-15). Dordrecht, Netherlands: Kluwer.

Nordlohne, E., & Hurrelman, K. (1990). Health impairment, failure in school, and the use and abuse of drugs. In K. Hurrelman & F. Losel (Eds.), *Health hazards in adolescence* (pp. 149-166). New York: Walter de Gruyter.

Novak-Amado, A. (1993). Steps for supporting community connections. In A. Novak-Amado (Ed.), *Friendships and community connections between people with and without developmental disabilities* (pp. 299-326). Baltimore: Brookes.

Nozick, R. (1974). *Anarchy, state and utopia.* New York: Basic Books.

O'Brien, S. J., & Vertinsky, P. A. (1991). Unfit survivors: Exercise as a resource for aging women. *The Gerontologist, 31,* 347-357.

O'Connor, L. (1994). *Characteristics of sociodramatic play of hard-of-hearing children and its relationship to language development.* Unpublished master's thesis, York University, Toronto.

O'Donnell, M. (1986, Summer). Definition of health promotion. *American Journal of Health Promotion,* pp. 4-5.

Office of Technology Assessment. (1991). *Adolescent health* (3 volumes). Washington, DC: Office of Technology Assessment.

O'Leary, A. (1985). Self-efficacy and health. *Behaviour Research and Therapy, 23,* 437-451.

Oliver, C. (1986). Self-concept assessment. *Mental Handicap, 14,* 24-25.

Oliver, M. (1989). The sound and political context of educational policy: The case of special needs. In L. Barton (Ed.), *The politics of special education needs* (pp. 13-31). London: Falmer.

Oliver, M. (1990). *The politics of disablement.* London: Macmillan.

Olsen, M., & Marger, M. (Eds.). (1993). *Power in modern societies.* San Francisco: Westview.

Ontario Children's Health Study. (1989). *Summary of findings.* Toronto: Government of Ontario.

O'Reilly-Fleming, T. (1993). *Down and out in Canada: Homeless Canadians.* Toronto: Canadian Scholar's Press.

Ostrow, D., Monjan, A., Joseph, J., VanRaden, M., Fox, R., Kingsley, L., Dudley, J., & Phair, J. (1989). HIV-related symptoms and psychological functioning in a cohort of homosexual men. *American Journal of Psychiatry, 146,* 737-742.

Ouellette-Kuntz, H. (1989). *A pilot study in the use of the quality of life interview schedule with emphasis on intra- and inter-rater agreement.* Master's thesis, Queen's University, Kingston, Ontario.

Ouellette-Kuntz, H. (1990). A pilot study in the use of the quality of life interview schedule. *Social Indicators Research, 23,* 283-298.

Padden, C., & Humphries, T. (1988). *Deaf in America: Voices from a culture.* Cambridge, MA: Harvard University Press.

Painter, B., & Smith, T. J. (1986). Benefits of a participatory safety and hazard management program in a British Columbia forestry and logging organization. In O. Brown, Jr., & H. W. Hendrick (Eds.), *Human factors in organizational design and management* (Vol. 2, pp. 279-290). Amsterdam: Elsevier.

Paproski, M. (1988). Quality of life: A parent's perspective. *Proceedings of the 2nd Annual 1988 Refresher Course in the Developmental Disability Field.* Kingston, Ontario: Developmental Consulting Program.

Parmenter, T. (1988). An analysis of the dimensions of quality of life for people with physical disabilities. In R. Brown (Ed.), *Quality of life for handicapped people* (pp. 7-36). London: Croom Helm.

Parmenter, T. R. (1992). Quality of life of people with developmental disabilities. In N. W. Bray (Ed.), *International review of research in mental retardation* (Vol. 18, pp. 160-172). New York: Academic Press.

Parmenter, T. R. (1994). Quality of life as a construct and measurable entity. *Social Indicators Research, 33,* 9-46.

Pateman, C. (1970). *Participation and democratic theory.* Cambridge, UK: Cambridge University Press.

Pathway to integration, final report, mainstream 1992 (Report to Ministers of Social Services on the Federal/Provincial/Territorial Review of Services Affecting Canadians With Disabilities, Canadian Government Publication No. H74-53/1993E). (1993). Ottawa, Ontario: Government Printing Office.

Patrick, D. L., & Erickson, P. (1993). Assessing health-related quality of life for clinical decision-making. In S. R. Walker & R. M. Rosser (Eds.), *Quality of life assessment: Key issues in the 1990's* (pp. 11-63). London: Kluwer.

Pederson, A., O'Neill, M., & Rootman, I. (Eds.). (1994). *Health promotion in Canada: Provincial, national, and international perspectives.* Toronto: W. B. Saunders.

Pelletier, K. R. (1992). Mind-body health: Research, clinical, and policy applications. *American Journal of Health Promotion, 6,* 345-358.

Penning, M., & Chappell, N. (1993). Age-related differences. In T. Stephens & D. Graham (Eds.), *Canada's health promotion survey 1990: Technical report* (pp. 247-262). Ottawa, Ontario: Ministry of Supply and Services.

Perry, J., & Felce, D. (1995). Objective assessments of quality of life: How much do they agree with each other? *Journal of Community and Applied Social Psychology, 5,* 1-19.

Perry-Hunnicut, C., & Newman, C. (1993). Adolescent dieting practices and nutrition knowledge. *Health Values: The Journal of Health Behavior, Education, and Promotion, 17,* 35-40.

Petersen, A. C. (1988). Adolescent development. In M. R. Rosenzweig (Ed.), *Annual review of psychology* (pp. 583-607). Palo Alto, CA: Annual Reviews.

Pettis, K. W., & Hughes, R. D. (1985). Sexual victimization of children: Implications for educators. *Behavioral Disorders, 10*(3), 175-182.

Pfeffer, R. I., Kurosaki, T. T., Chance, J. M., Filos, S., & Bates, D. (1984). Use of the mental function index in older adults: Reliability, validity, and measurement of change over time. *American Journal of Epidemiology, 120,* 922-935.

Picherack, F. G. (1988). Health promotion and AIDS: Challenge to primary care. *Hygiene, 7*(2), 23-27.

Pittock, F., & Potts, M. (1988). Neighbourhood attitudes to people with a mental handicap: A comparative study. *British Journal of Mental Subnormality, 34,* 35-46.

Pliskin, J. S., Shepard, D. S., & Weinstein, M. C. (1980). Utility functions for life years and health status. *Operations Research, 28,* 206-224.

Prizant, B. M., Audet, L., Burke, G., Hummel, L., Maher, S., & Theodore, G. (1990). Communication disorders and emotional/behavioral disorders in children. *Journal of Speech and Hearing Disorders, 55,* 179-192.

Prizant, B. M., & Meyer, E. C. (1993). Socioemotional aspects of language and social-communication disorders in young children and their families. *American Journal of Speech-Language Pathology, 2*(3), 56-71.

Qualter, T. (1986). *Conflicting political ideas in liberal democracies.* Agincourt, Ontario: Methuen.

Rabinow, P. (Ed.). (1984). *The Foucault reader.* New York: Pantheon.

Rabkin, J., Remien, R., Katoff, L., & Williams, J. (1993). Resilience in adversity among long-term survivors of AIDS. *Hospital and Community Psychiatry, 44*(2), 162-167.

Raeburn, J., & Rootman, I. (1995). *People-centred health promotion: Theory and practice for students, professionals, and community workers.* Manuscript submitted for publication.

Rahe, R. H. (1975). Epidemiological studies of life change and illness. *International Journal of Psychiatry in Medicine, 6*(1/2), 133-146.

Ramund, B., & Stensman, R. (1988). Quality of life and evaluation of functions among severely impaired mobility and non-disabled controls. *Scandinavian Journal of Psychology, 29*(3/4), 137-144.

Raphael, D., Brown, I., & Renwick, R. (1993). *The quality of life profile: Seniors' version.* Toronto: University of Toronto, Centre for Health Promotion.

Raphael, D., Brown, I., Renwick, R., & Rootman, I. (1994a). *Quality of life and health promotion: Implications of a new model of quality of life.* Toronto: University of Toronto, Centre for Health Promotion.

Raphael, D., Brown, I., Renwick, R., & Rootman, I. (1994b). *Quality of life theory and assessment: What are the implications for health promotion?* Toronto: University of Toronto, Centre for Health Promotion, and ParticipACTION.

Raphael, D., Brown, I., Renwick, R., & Rootman, I. (in press). Assessing the quality of life of persons with disabilities: Description of a new model, measuring instruments, and initial findings. *International Journal of Disability, Development, and Education.*

Raphael, D., & McClelland, B. (1994). *Prospectus: Using the quality of life profile: Seniors version in public health activities.* North York, Ontario: North York Community Health Promotion Research Unit.

Raphael, D., Renwick, R., & Brown, I. (1993). Studying the lives of persons with developmental disabilities: Methodological lessons from the quality of life project. *Journal on Developmental Disabilities, 2*(2), 30-49.

Raphael, D., Robinson, G., Renwick, R., & Cho, S. (1994). *The development and application of community-level quality of life indicators.* Unpublished manuscript, University of Toronto, Centre for Health Promotion.

Raphael, D., Rukholm, E., Brown, I., & Bailey, N. (1995). *The quality of life profile: Adolescent version.* Toronto: University of Toronto, Centre for Health Promotion.

Rappaport, J. (1987). Terms of empowerment/examplars of prevention: Towards a theory for community psychology. *American Journal of Community Psychology, 15,* 121-148.

Rawls, J. A. (1971). *A theory of justice.* Cambridge, MA: Harvard University Press.

Raynes N. V., Pratt, M. W., & Roses, S. (1979). *Organisational structure and the care of the mentally retarded.* London: Croom Helm.

Reiss, S. (1988). *Test manual for the Reiss screen for maladaptive behavior.* Orland Park, IL: International Diagnostic Systems.

Rennie, D. L., Phillips, J. R., & Quartaro, G. K. (1988). Grounded theory: A promising approach to conceptualization in psychology? *Canadian Psychologist, 29*(2), 21-30.

Renwick, R. (1993). An holistic conceptual approach to quality of life [Abstract]. *Canadian Journal of Occupational Therapy, 60,* 14.

Renwick, R., Brown, I., & Raphael, D. (1994). Quality of life: Linking a conceptual approach to service provision. *Journal on Developmental Disabilities, 3,* 32-44.

Renwick, R., Rudman, D., Brown, I., & Raphael, D. (1994). *The quality of life profile: Version for persons with physical disabilities.* Toronto: University of Toronto, Centre for Health Promotion.

Renzulli, J. S., & McGreevy, A. (1986). Twins included and not included in special programs for the gifted. *Roeper Review, 9,* 120-127.

Richardson, J. (1992). Cost-utility analysis in health care: Present status and future issues. In J. Daly, I. McDonald, & E. Willis (Eds.), *Researching health care: Designs, dilemmas, disciplines* (pp. 21-44). London: Tavistock/Routledge.

Riddington, J. (1989). *Different therefore unequal: Employment and women with disabilities* (Position paper). Vancouver, BC: DAWN Canada.

Rife, J. C., First, R. J., Greenlee, R. W., Miller, L. D., & Feichter, M. A. (1991). Case management with homeless mentally ill people. *Health & Social Work, 16,* 58-67.

Rinear, E. E. (1985). Sexual assault and the handicapped victim. In A. W. Burgess (Ed.), *Rape and sexual assault* (pp. 139-145). New York: Garland.

Rioux, M. H. (1991). Exchanging charity for rights: A challenge for the 1990's. *Entourage, 6*(2), 3.

Rioux, M. H. (1994). Towards a concept of equality of well-being: Overcoming the social and legal construction of inequality. *Canadian Journal of Law and Jurisprudence, 7,* 127-147.

Rioux, M. H., & Bach, M. (Eds.). (1994). *Disability is not measles: New research paradigms in disability.* North York, Ontario: Roeher Institute.

Rioux, M. H., & Crawford, C. (1994). *Canadian disability resource program: Offsetting costs of disability and assuring access to disability-related supports.* North York, Ontario: Roeher Institute.

Risley, T. R., & Cataldo, M. F. (1973). *Planned activity check: Materials for training observers.* Lawrence, KS: Center for Applied Behavior Analysis.

Ritter-Brinton, K., & Stewart, D. (1992). Hearing parents and deaf children: Some perspectives on sign communication and service delivery. *American Annals of the Deaf, 137*(2), 85-91.

Robertson, A. (1990). The politics of Alzheimer's disease: A case study in apocalyptic demography. *International Journal of Health Services, 20,* 429-442.

Robinson, J. P. (1977). *How Americans use their time: A social psychological analysis of everyday behavior.* New York: Praeger.

Rodin, J. (1986a). Aging and health: Effects of the sense of control. *Science, 233,* 1271-1276.

Rodin, J. (1986b). Health, control, and aging. In M. Baltes & P. Baltes (Eds.), *The psychology of control and aging* (pp. 139-166). Hillsdale, NJ: Lawrence Erlbaum.

Roeher Institute. (1988). *Income insecurity: The disability income system in Canada.* North York, Ontario: Roeher Institute.

Roeher Institute. (1992). *On target: Canada's employment-related programs for persons with disabilities.* North York, Ontario: Roeher Institute.

Roeher Institute. (1993). *Social well-being: A paradigm for reform.* North York, Ontario: Roeher Institute.

Roessler, R. T. (1990). A quality of life perspective on rehabilitation counseling. *Rehabilitation Counseling Bulletin, 34,* 82-90.

Romney, D. M., Brown, R. I., & Fry, P. S. (Eds.). (1994). *Improving the quality of life: Recommendations for people with and without disabilities.* Dordrecht, Netherlands: Kluwer.

Rootman, I., & Raeburn, J. (1994). The concept of health. In A. Pederson, M. O'Neill, & I. Rootman (Eds.), *Health promotion in Canada: Provincial, national and international perspectives* (pp. 56-71). Toronto: W. B. Saunders.

Rootman, I., Raphael, D., Renwick, R., Brown, I., Friefeld, S., Garber, M., & Talbot, Y. (1995). *Quality of life project reliability/validity and pilot study: Manual for administering the quality of life instrument package.* Toronto: University of Toronto, Centre for Health Promotion, and Ministry of Community and Social Services, Government of Ontario.

Rootman, I., Raphael, D., Shewchuk, D., Renwick, R., Friefeld, S., Garber, M., Talbot, Y., & Woodill, D. (1992a). *Development of an approach and instrument package to measure quality of life of persons with developmental disabilities.* Toronto: University of Toronto, Centre for Health Promotion.

Rootman, I., Raphael, D., Shewchuk, D., Renwick, R., Friefeld, S., Garber, M., Talbot, Y., & Woodill, G. (1992b). *Highlights from the development of an approach and instrument package to measure quality of life of persons with developmental disabilities.* Toronto: University of Toronto, Centre for Health Promotion.

Rosander, A. C. (1991). *Deming's 14 points applied to services.* Milwaukee, WI: ASQC Quality Press.

Rosenberg, R. D., & Rosenstein, E. (1980). Participation and productivity: An empirical study. *Industrial and Labor Relations Review, 33,* 355-367.

Roth, W. (1983). Handicap as a social construct. *Society, 20*(3), 56-61.

Rowe, J. W., & Kahn, R. L. (1987). Human aging: Usual and successful. *Science, 237,* 143-149.

Rudman, D., Renwick, R., Raphael, D., & Brown, I. (1995). The quality of life profile for adults with physical disabilities [Abstract]. *Canadian Journal of Occupational Therapy, 62,* 25.

Ruedrich, S. (1994, September/October). Psychopathology and DSM-IV. *Habilitative Health Care Newsletter,* pp. 84-86.

Rustin, L., & Kuhr, A. (1989). *Social skills and the speech impaired.* Philadelphia: Taylor & Francis.

Rutter, M., Maughan, B., Mortimore, P., & Ouston, J. (1979). *Fifteen thousand hours: Secondary schools and their effects upon children.* Cambridge, MA: Harvard University Press.

Rybash, J. M., Hoyer, W. J., & Rodin, P. A. (1986). *Adult cognition and aging: Developmental changes in processing, knowing, and thinking.* Elmsford, NY: Pergamon.

Rybczynski, W. (1991). *Waiting for the weekend.* New York: Penguin.

Sackett, D. L., & Torrance, G. W. (1978). The utility of different health states as perceived by the general public. *Journals of Chronic Diseases, 31,* 697-704.

Safire, W., & Safire, L. (1989). *Words of wisdom.* New York: Simon & Schuster.

Sahlin, I. G. (1992). Defining homelessness. *Sociologisk-Forskning, 29*(2), 51-71.

Sartorius, N. (1992). Rehabilitation and quality of life. *Hospital and Community Psychiatry, 43,* 1180-1181.

Sass, R. (1989). The implications of work organizations for occupational health policy: The case of Canada. *International Journal of Health Services, 19,* 157-173.

Saxby, H., Thomas, M., Felce, D., & de Kock, U. (1986). The use of shops, cafes and public houses by severely and profoundly mentally handicapped adults. *British Journal of Mental Subnormality, 32,* 69-81.

Sayer, A. (1984). *Method in social science: A realist approach.* London: Hutchinson.

Scambler, G. (1987). Habermas and the power of medical expertise. In G. Scambler (Ed.), *Sociological theory and medical sociology* (pp. 165-193). New York: Methuen.

Schabas, R. (1992). *Opportunities for health.* Toronto, Ontario, Canada: Ministry of Health.

Schaie, K. W. (1990). The optimization of cognitive functioning in old age: Predications based on cohort-sequential and longitudinal data. In P. Baltes & M. Baltes (Eds.), *Successful* aging: Perspectives from the social sciences (pp. 94-117). New York: Cambridge University Press.

Schalock, R. L. (1990a). Attempts to conceptualize and measure quality of life. In R. L. Schalock (Ed.), Quality of life: Perspectives and issues (pp. 141-148). Washington, DC: American Association on Mental Retardation.

Schalock, R. L. (Ed.). (1990b). Quality of life: Perspectives and issues. Washington, DC: American Association on Mental Retardation.

Schalock, R. L. (1990c). Where do we go from here? In R. Schalock (Ed.), Quality of life: Perspectives and issues. Washington, DC: American Association on Mental Retardation.

Schalock, R. L. (1991, May). The concept of quality of life in the lives of persons with mental retardation. Paper presented at the 15th Annual Meeting of the American Association on Mental Retardation, Washington, DC.

Schalock, R. L. (1994a). The concept of quality of life and its current applications in the field of mental retardation/developmental disabilities. In D. Goode (Ed.), Quality of life for persons with disabilities: International perspectives and issues (pp. 266-284). Cambridge, MA: Brookline.

Schalock, R. L. (1994b). Promoting quality through quality enhancement techniques and outcome base evaluation. Journal on Developmental Disabilities, 3(2), 1-16.

Schalock, R. L. (1994c). Quality of life, quality enhancement and quality assurance: Implications for program planning and evaluation in the field of mental retardation and developmental disabilities. Evaluation and Program Planning, 17, 121-131.

Schalock, R. L. (in press). Outcome based evaluation: Application to special education, mental health and disability programs. New York: Plenum.

Schalock, R. L., & Genung, L. T. (1993). Placement from a community-based mental retardation program: A 15-year follow-up. American Journal of Mental Retardation, 98, 400-407.

Schalock, R. L., & Harper, R. S. (1978). Placement from community-based mental retardation programs: How well do clients do? American Journal of Mental Deficiency, 83, 240-247.

Schalock, R. L., Harper, R. S., & Carver, S. (1981). Independent living placement: Five years later. American Journal of Mental Deficiency, 86, 170-177.

Schalock, R. L., & Keith, K. D. (1993). Quality of life questionnaire. Worthington, OH: IDS.

Schalock, R. L., Keith, K. D., & Hoffman, K. (1990). Quality of life questionnaire: Standardization manual. Hastings: Mid-Nebraska Mental Retardation Services.

Schalock, R. L., Keith, K. D., Hoffman, K., & Karan, O. C. (1989). Quality of life: Its measurement and use. Mental Retardation, 27, 25-31.

Schalock, R. L., & Kiernan, W. E. (1990). Habilitation planning for adults with disabilities. New York: Springer-Verlag.

Schalock, R. L., Lemanowicz, J. A., Conroy, J. W., & Feinstein, C. S. (1994). A multivariate investigative study of the correlates of quality of life. Journal of Developmental Disabilities, 3(2), 59-73.

Schalock, R. L., & Lilley, M. A. (1986). Placement from community-based mental retardation programs: How well do clients do after 8 to 10 years? American Journal of Mental Deficiency, 90, 669-676.

Scheier, M. F., & Carver, C. S. (1985). Optimism, coping, and health: Assessment and implications of generalized outcome expectancies. Health Psychology, 4, 219-247.

Scherer, M. J. (1988). Assistive device utilization and quality-of-life in adults with spinal cord injuries or cerebral palsy. Journal of Applied Rehabilitation Counselling, 19(2), 21-30.

Schipper, H. (1983). Why we measure quality of life? Canadian Medical Association, 128, 1367-1370.

Schipper, H., Clinch, J., & Powell, V. (1990). Definitions and conceptual issues. In B. Spilker (Ed.), *Quality of life assessments in clinical trials* (pp. 11-24). New York: Raven.

Schipper, H., & Levitt, M. (1985). Measuring quality of life: Risks and benefits. *Cancer Treatment Reports, 69,* 1115-1123.

Schmitz, K. (1993, Fall). Between two worlds: Postlingually deaf people search for a cultural identity. *NTID Focus,* pp. 14-17.

Schneller, R. (1988). Video watching and its societal functions for small town adolescents in Israel. *Youth and Society, 19,* 441-459.

Schuessler, K. F., & Fisher, G. A. (1985). Quality of life research and sociology. *Annual Review of Sociology, 11,* 129-149.

Schumacher, M., Olschewski, M., & Schulgen, G. (1991). Assessment of quality of life in clinical trials. *Statistics in Medicine, 10,* 1915-1930.

Schwarzer, R., & Leppin, A. (1990). Social support, health, and health behavior. In K. Hurrelman & F. Losel (Eds.), *Health hazards in adolescence* (pp. 363-384). New York: Walter de Gruyter.

Selai, C., & Rosser, R. (1993). The role of quality of life measurement in psychiatry. *Current Medical Literature: Psychiatry, 4*(3), 67-71.

Seligman, M. (1975). *Helplessness: On depression, development and death.* San Francisco: Freeman.

Selnow, G. W., & Reynolds, H. (1984). Some opportunity costs of television watching. *Journal of Broadcasting, 28,* 315-322.

Sen, A. (1980). Plural utility. *Proceedings of the Aristotelian Society, 81,* 193-218.

Senior Citizen's Consumers' Alliance on Long-Term Care. (1992). *Consumer report on long-term care.* Toronto: Author.

Senn, C. Y. (1988). Vulnerable: Sexual abuse and people with an intellectual handicap. *Monographs of the Family Violence Prevention Division of Health and Welfare Canada* (No. ED 302 975). Downsview, Ontario: G. Allan, Roeher Institute.

Seton, F. R. (1993). Statement of Rehabilitation International. *International Rehabilitation, 43,* 10.

Shadish, W. R., & Bootzin, R. R. (1984). The social integration of psychiatric patients in nursing homes. *American Journal of Psychiatry, 141,* 1203-1207.

Shain, M. (1990). *The right of employees to participate in the organization and design of work.* Unpublished doctoral dissertation, University of Toronto.

Shain, M. (1990/91). My work makes me sick: Evidence and health promotion implications. *Health Promotion, 29*(3), 11-12.

Shain, M. (1992). *Labour law is a hazard to your health: Implications for reform* (Issues in Health Promotion Series, #1). Toronto: University of Toronto, Centre for Health Promotion.

Shain, M. (1993). The wellness audit: Key concepts and tools for occupational health and safety professionals. In F. Makdessian (Ed.), *Workplace audit series: How to conduct audits in hygiene safety environments and wellness* (pp. 32-41). Don Mills, Ontario: Occupational Health & Safety Canada, Southam Information and Technology Group.

Shanks, J. (1979). Development of the feminine voice and refinement of the esophageal voice. In R. Keith & F. Darley (Eds.), *Laryngectomy rehabilitation* (pp. 367-378). Houston, TX: College-Hill.

Shea, S., Basch, C., Lantigua, R., & Wechsler, H. (1992). The Washington Heights-Inwood healthy heart program: A third generation community-based cardiovascular disease prevention program in a disadvantaged urban setting. *Preventive Medicine, 21,* 203-217.

Shea, W. R. (1976). The quest for a high quality of life. In J. Farlow & W. R. Shea (Eds.), *Values and quality of life* (pp. 1-5). New York: Service History Publications.

Shehadeh, V., & Shain, M. (1990). *Influences on wellness in the workplace: A multivariate approach* (Health and Welfare Canada Technical Report). Ottawa, Ontario: Supply and Services Canada.

Sherbourne, C. D., Meredith, L. S., Rogers, W., & Ware, J. E., Jr. (1992). Social support and stressful life events: Age differences in their effects on health-related quality of life among the chronically ill. *Quality of Life Research, 1,* 235-246.

Sigelman, C., Schoenrock, C., Winer, J., Spanhel, C., Hromas, S., Martin, P., Budd, E., & Bensberg, G. (1981). Issues in interviewing mentally retarded persons: An empirical study. In R. Bruininks, C. Meyers, B. Sigford, & K. Lakin (Eds.), *Deinstitutionalization and community adjustment of mentally retarded people* (pp. 114-129). Washington, DC: American Association on Mental Deficiency.

Silbereisen, R., Schonpflug, U., & Albrecht, H. T. (1990). Smoking and drinking: Prospective analyses in German and Polish adolescents. In K. Hurrelman & F. Losel (Eds.), *Health hazards in adolescence* (pp. 167-192). New York: Walter de Gruyter.

Simmons, H. (1982). *From asylum to welfare.* Toronto: Roeher Institute.

Slevin, M. L., Plant, H., Lynch, D., Drinkwater, J., & Gregory, W. M. (1988). Who should measure quality of life, the doctor or the patient? *British Journal of Cancer, 57,* 109-112.

Smith, D., & Theberge, N. (1987). *Why people recreate.* Champaign, IL: Life Enhancement Publications.

Smith, L. (1986). A new paradigm for equality rights. In L. Smith, G. Côté-Harper, R. Elliot, & M. Seydegart (Eds.), *Righting the balance: Canada's new equality rights* (pp. 351-407). Saskatoon, Saskatchewan: Canadian Human Rights Reporter.

Smull, M. W., & Danehey, A. J. (1993). The challenges of the 90's: Increasing quality while reducing costs. In V. J. Bradley, J. W. Ashbaugh, & B. Blaney (Eds.), *Creating individual supports for people with developmental disabilities: A mandate for change at many levels* (pp. 140-154). Baltimore: Brookes.

Sobsey, D. (1988). Sexual offenses and disabled victims: Research and implications. *Vis-à-Vis: A National Newsletter on Family Violence, 6*(4), 2-3.

Sobsey, D. (1994). *Violence and abuse in the lives of people with disabilities: The end of silent acceptance?* Baltimore: Brookes.

Soderfeldt, B. (1991). Cochlear implants and the deaf community. *A Deaf American Monograph, 41*(1-2), 141-143.

Soldo, B. J., & Manton, K. G. (1985). Changes in the health status and service needs of the oldest old: Current patterns and future trends. *Milbank Memorial Fund Quarterly, 63,* 286-323.

Spector, P. E. (1986). Perceived control by employees: A meta-analysis of studies concerning autonomy and participation at work. *Human Relations, 39,* 1005-1016.

Spilker, B. (1990). *Quality of life in clinical trials.* New York: Raven.

Spitzer, W. O., Dobson, A. J., Hall, J., Chesterman, E., Levi, J., Shepherd, R., Battista, R. N., & Catchlove, B. R. (1981). Measuring the quality of life of cancer patients. *Journal of Chronic Diseases, 34,* 585-597.

Staley, J. (1994). Cochlear implants: Are they magic? *Communication Exchange: An Information Resource for Speech-Language and Hearing Professionals in Schools, 5*(1), 2-3.

Stam, H., Koopmans, J. P., & Mathieson, C. M. (1991). The psychosocial impact of a laryngectomy: A comprehensive assessment. *Journal of Psychosocial Oncology, 9*(3), 37-58.

Starhawk. (1987). *Truth or dare.* New York: Harper & Row.

Statistics Canada. (1992). *The labour force* (Catalogue #71-001). Ottawa, Ontario: Statistics Canada (Household Surveys Division).

Steinberg, L., Fegley, S., & Dornbusch, S. (1993). Negative impact of part time work on adolescent adjustment: Evidence from a longitudinal study. *Developmental Psychology, 29,* 171-180.

Stensman, R. (1985). Severely mobility-disabled people assess the quality of their lives. *Scandinavian Journal of Rehabilitation Medicine, 17*(2), 87-99.

Steptoe, A., & Appels, A. (1989). *Stress, personal control and health.* Chichester, UK: Wiley.

Stewart-Muirhead, E. (1994). "Fixing" deafness: Ethical issues in cochlear implantation. *Bioethics Bulletin, 6*(4), 1-4.

Stokols, D. (1992). Establishing and maintaining healthy environments: Toward a social ecology of health promotion. *American Psychologist, 47,* 6-22.

Stones, M. L., & Kozma, A. (1980). Issues relating to the usage of conceptualizations of mental constructs employed by gerontologists. *International Journal of Ageing and Human Development, 11,* 269-281.

Stuifbergen, A. K., & Becker, H. A. (1994). Predictors of health-promoting lifestyles in persons with disabilities. *Research in Nursing and Health, 17,* 3-13.

Stull, D. E. (1987). Conceptualizations and measurement of well-being: Implications for policy evaluation. In E. F. Borgatta & R. J. V. Montgomery (Eds.), *Critical issues in ageing policy* (pp. 53-90). Newbury Park, CA: Sage.

Sullivan, E. (1984). *A critical psychology: Interpretation of the personal world.* New York: Plenum.

Sundram, C. J. (1984). Obstacles to reducing patient abuse in public institutions. *Hospital and Community Psychiatry, 35*(3), 238-243.

Superintendent of Family & Child Service v. R. D. & S. D. et al. [1983] 3 W.W.R. 597 (B.C. Provincial Court, 1983); 3 W.W.R. 618 (B.C. Supreme Court, 1983).

Sutherland, N. (1976). *Children in English-Canadian society.* Toronto: University of Toronto Press.

Sutter, P., & Meyeda, T. (1979). *Characteristics of the treatment environment: MR/DD community home manual.* Pomona, CA: Lantermann Developmental Center.

Takanishi, R. (Ed.). (1993a). Adolescence [Special issue]. *American Psychologist, 48*(2).

Takanishi, R. (1993b). The opportunities of adolescence—Research, interventions, and policy: Introduction to the special issue. *American Psychologist, 48,* 85-87.

Tarnopolsky, W. S. (1982). The equality rights. In W. S. Tarnopolsky & G. Beaudoin (Eds.), *The Canadian charter of rights and freedoms: Commentary* (pp. 395-441). Toronto: Carswell.

Tarnopolsky, W. S., & Pentney, W. F. (Eds.). (1985). *Discrimination and the law in Canada: Including equality rights under the charter* (Fifth cumulative supplement). Don Mills, Ontario: Richard De Boo.

Taylor, C. (1992). *Multiculturalism and "the politics of recognition": An essay.* Princeton, NJ: Princeton University Press.

Taylor, S. J. (1994). In support of research on quality of life, but against QOL. In D. Goode (Ed.), *Quality of life for persons with disabilities: International perspectives and issues* (pp. 260-265). Cambridge, MA: Brookline.

Taylor, S., & Bogdan, R. (1981). A qualitative approach to the study of community adjustment. In R. Bruininks, C. Meyers, B. Sigford, & K. Lakin (Eds.), *Deinstitutionalization and community adjustment of mentally retarded people* (pp. 71-81). Washington, DC: American Association on Mental Deficiency.

Taylor, S., & Bogdan, R. (1990). Quality of life and the individual's perspective. In R. Schalock & M. Begab (Eds.), *Quality of life: Perspectives and issues* (pp. 27-40). Washington, DC: American Association on Mental Retardation.

Teague, M. L., Cipriano, R. E., & McGhee, V. L. (1990). Health promotion as a rehabilitation service for people with disabilities. *Journal of Rehabilitation, 56,* 52-56.

Tesh, S. (1988). *Hidden arguments: Political arguments and disease prevention policy.* New Brunswick, NJ: Rutgers University Press.

QUALITY OF LIFE, HEALTH, REHABILITATION

Tiggeman, M., & Winefield, A. H. (1984). The effects of unemployment on the mood, self-esteem, locus of control and expressive affect of school-leavers. *Journal of Occupational Psychology, 57,* 33-42.

Tilson, H., & Spilker, B. (1990). Quality of life bibliography and indexes. *Medical Care, 28* (Suppl. 12).

Timmer, D. A. (1988). Homelessness as deviance: The ideology of the shelter. *Free Inquiry in Creative Sociology, 16*(1), 163-170.

Timmons, V. (in press). Quality of life and teenagers with special needs. In R. I. Brown (Ed.), *Issues in quality of life.* Toronto: Captus.

Tinsley, H., & Johnson, T. (1984). A preliminary taxonomy of leisure activities. *Journal of Leisure Research, 16,* 234-244.

Torrance, G. W. (1976). Social preferences for health states: An empirical evaluation of three measurement techniques. *Socio-Economic Planning Sciences, 3,* 129-136.

Torrance, G. W. (1982). Multiattribute utility theory as a method of measuring social preferences for health states in long-term care. In R. L. Kane & R. A. Kane (Eds.), *Values and long-term care* (pp. 127-156). Lexington, MA: Lexington Books.

Torres, R. T. (1992). Improving the quality of internal evaluation: The evaluator as consultant-mediator. *Evaluation and Program Planning, 14,* 189-198.

Townsend, E. (1993). Occupational therapy's social vision. *Canadian Journal of Occupational Therapy, 60,* 174-184.

Turner, J., Frankel, B., & Levin, D. (1983). Social support: Conceptualization, measurement and implications for mental health. *Research in Community and Mental Health, 3,* 67-111.

Turner, J., & Noh, S. (1988). Physical disability and depression: A longitudinal analysis. *Journal of Health and Social Behaviour, 29,* 23-37.

Turner, R. R. (1990). Rehabilitation. In B. Spilker (Ed.), *Quality of life assessments in clinical trials* (pp. 247-267). New York: Raven.

United Nations. (1983). *World programme of action concerning disabled persons.* New York: Author.

U.S. Department of Health and Human Services. (1991). *Healthy people 2000.* Washington, DC: Author.

U.S. Department of Health, Education, and Welfare. (1969). *Toward a social report.* Washington, DC: Government Printing Office.

Van Riper, C., & Emerick, L. (1984). *Speech correction* (7th ed.). Englewood Cliffs, NJ: Prentice Hall.

van Vliet, W. (1989). The limits of social research. *Society, 26*(3), 16-20.

Vash, C. L. (1981). *The psychology of disability.* New York: Springer.

Veatch, R. (1986). *The foundations of justice: Why the retarded and the rest of us have claims to equality.* New York: Oxford University Press.

Veenhoven, R. (1984). *Conditions of happiness.* Hingham, MA: Kluwer.

Velde, B. (in press). Relationships of leisure and quality of life. In R. I. Brown (Ed.), *Issues in quality of life.* Toronto: Captus.

Vogt, J. F., & Hunt, B. D. (1988, May). What really goes wrong with participative work groups? *Training and Development Journal,* pp. 96-100.

Von Neumann, J., & Morgenstern, O. (1944). *Theory of games and economic behavior.* Princeton, NJ: Princeton University Press.

Wade, C., & Travis, C. (1990). *Psychology* (2nd ed.). New York: Harper & Row.

Wadsworth, Y. (1991). *Everyday evaluation on the run.* Melbourne, Australia: Action Research Issues Association.

Waldo, D., & Lazenby, H. (1984, Fall). Demographic characteristics and health care use and expenditures by the aged in the United States. *Health Care Financing Review, 6,* 1-49.

Wallerstein, N. (1992). Powerlessness, empowerment and health: Implications for health promotion programs. *American Journal of Health Promotion, 6,* 197-205.

Wallerstein, N., & Bernstein, E. (1988). Empowerment education: Freire's ideas adapted to health education. *Health Education Quarterly, 15,* 379-394.

Ward, N. (1990). Reflections on my quality of life: Then and now. In R. Schalock (Ed.), *Quality of life: Perspectives and issues* (pp. 9-16). Washington, DC: American Association on Mental Retardation.

Ware, J. E. (1991). Measuring functioning, well-being, and other generic health concepts. In D. Osoba (Ed.), *Effects of cancer on quality of life* (pp. 8-23). Boca Raton, FL: CRS.

Ware, J. E. (1993). Measuring patients' views: The optimum outcome measure. *British Medical Journal, 306,* 1429-1430.

Wartenberg, T. (1990). *The forms of power: From domination to transformation.* Philadelphia: Temple University Press.

Warwick, R. (1994). *Jones memorial lecture in deafness: Between two worlds: A hard of hearing perspective.* Edmonton, Alberta: Western Canadian Centre of Specialization in Deafness.

Weber, K. (1994, May). Is the integration movement destroying itself? *Journal: A Newsletter for Teachers, 5*(2), 1-4.

Weiler, R., Sliepcevich, E. M., & Sarvela, P. D. (1993). Development of the adolescent health concerns inventory. *Health Education Quarterly, 20,* 569-583.

Weiler, R., Sliepcevich, E. M., & Sarvela, P. D. (1994). Adolescents' concerns as reported by adolescents, teachers, and parents. *Health Values: The Journal of Health Behavior, Education, and Promotion, 18,* 50-62.

Weinberg, N. (1984). Physically disabled people assess the quality of their lives. *Rehabilitation Literature, 45,* 12-15.

Weinberg, N., & Williams, J. (1978). How the physically disabled perceive their disabilities. *Journal of Rehabilitation, 44*(3), 31-33.

Weiss, C. H., & Bucuvalis, M. J. (1977). The challenge of social research to decision making. In C. H. Weiss (Ed.), *Using social research in public policy making* (pp. 213-233). Lexington, MA: Lexington Books.

Weitz, R. (1989). Uncertainty and the lives of persons with AIDS. *Journal of Health and Social Behavior, 30,* 270-281.

Whitbourne, S. K. (1985). *The aging body.* New York: Springer.

White, C., & Janson, P. (1986). Helplessness in institutional settings: Adaptation or iatrogenic disease? In M. Baltes & P. Baltes (Eds.), *The psychology of control and aging* (pp. 297-314). Hillsdale, NJ: Lawrence Erlbaum.

White, S. (1988). *The recent work of Jürgen Habermas: Reason, justice, and modernity.* New York: Cambridge University Press.

Wiedenfeld, S. A., O'Leary, A., Bandura, A., Brown, S., Levine, S., & Raska, K. (1990). Impact of perceived self-efficacy in coping with stressors on components of the immune system. *Journal of Personality and Social Psychology, 59,* 1082-1094.

Wilbur, R. (1987). *American Sign Language: Linguistic and applied dimensions.* Toronto: College-Hill.

Wilkin, D., Hallam, L., & Dogett, M. (1992). *Measuring need and outcome for primary health care.* Oxford, UK: Oxford University Press.

Williams, A. (1988). Economics and the rational use of medical technology. In F. F. H. Rutter & S. J. Reiser (Eds.), *The economics of medical technology* (pp. 75-95). Berlin: Springer.

Williams, B. (1962). The idea of equality. In P. Laslett & W. G. Runciman (Eds.), *Philosophy, politics and society* (2nd ed., pp. 110-131). Oxford, UK: Basil Blackwell.

Wilson, D., & Hare, A. (1990). Health care screening for people with mental handicap living in the community. *British Medical Journal, 301,* 1379-1380.

Wilson, J. (1983). *Social theory.* Englewood Cliffs, NJ: Prentice Hall.

Wolcott, D. (1986, August). Psychosocial aspects of acquired immune deficiency syndrome and the primary care physician. *Annals of Allergy, 57,* 95-102.

Wolfensberger, W. (1972). *Normalization: The principle of normalization in human services.* Toronto: National Institute of Mental Retardation.

Wolfensberger, W. (1983). Social role valorization: A proposed new term for the principle of normalization, *Mental Retardation, 21,* 234-239.

Wolfensberger, W. (1994). Let's hang up "quality of life" as a hopeless term. In D. Goode (Ed.), *Quality of life for persons with disabilities: International perspectives and issues* (pp. 285-321). Cambridge, MA: Brookline.

Wood, R., & Steere, D. (1992). Evaluating quality in supported employment: The standards of excellence for employment support services. *Journal of Vocational Rehabilitation 2*(2), 35-45.

Wood-Dauphinée, S., & Kuchler, T. (1992). Quality of life as a rehabilitation outcome: Are we missing the boat? *Canadian Journal of Rehabilitation, 6,* 3-12.

Wood-Dauphinée, S., & Williams, J. I. (1987). Reintegration to normal living as a proxy to quality of life. *Journal of Chronic Disease, 40,* 491-499.

Woodill, G. (1992). *Independent living and participation in research: A critical analysis.* Toronto: Centre for Independent Living in Toronto.

Woodill, G. (1994). The social semiotics of disability. In M. Rioux & M. Bach (Eds.), *Disability is not measles: New research paradigms in disability* (pp. 201-226). North York, Ontario: Roeher Institute.

Woodill, G., Renwick, R., Brown, I., & Raphael, D. (1994). Being, belonging, becoming: An approach to the quality of life of persons with developmental disabilities. In D. Goode (Ed.), *Quality of life for persons with disabilities: International perspectives and issues* (pp. 57-74). Cambridge, MA: Brookline.

World Health Organization. (1948). *Charter.* Geneva: Author.

World Health Organization. (1980a). *International classification of diseases (9th review).* Geneva: Author.

World Health Organization. (1980b). *International classification of impairments, disabilities, and handicaps.* Geneva: Author.

World Health Organization. (1984). *Health promotion: A discussion document on the concepts and principles.* Copenhagen: Author, Regional Office for Europe.

World Health Organization. (1986). *Ottawa charter for health promotion.* Ottawa, Ontario: Canadian Public Health Association.

Wright, B. A. (1983). *Physical disability: A psychosocial approach* (2nd ed.). New York: Harper & Row.

Wyngaarden, M. (1981). Interviewing mentally retarded persons: Issues and strategies. In R. Bruininks, C. Meyers, B. Sigford, & K. Lakin (Eds.), *Deinstitutionalization and community adjustment of mentally retarded people* (pp. 107-113). Washington, DC: American Association on Mental Deficiency.

Yalnizian, A. (1993). *Defining social security, defining ourselves: Why we need to change our thinking before it's too late.* Ottawa, Ontario: Canadian Centre for Policy Alternatives.

Young, I. M. (1990). *Justice and the politics of difference.* Princeton, NJ: Princeton University Press.

Zaner, R. (1981). *The context of self: A phenomenological inquiry using medicine as a clue.* Athens: Ohio University Press.

Zaslow, M. J., & Takanishi, R. (1993). Priorities for research on adolescent development. *American Psychologist, 48,* 185-192.

Zautra, A., Beier, E., & Cappel, L. (1977). The dimensions of life quality in a community. *American Journal of Community Psychology, 5,* 85-97.

Zautra, A., & Goodhart, D. (1979). Quality of life indicators: A review of the literature. *Community Mental Health Review, 4*(1), 1-10.

Zautra, A., & Hempel, A. (1984). Subjective well-being and physical health: A narrative literature review with suggestions for future research. *International Journal of Aging and Human Development, 19*(2), 95-110.

Zeithaml, V. A., Parasuraman, A., & Berry, L. C. (1990). *Delivering quality service: Balancing customer perceptions and expectations.* New York: Free Press.

Zigler, E., & Balla, D. (1977). Impact of institutional experience on the behaviour and development of retarded persons. *American Journal of Mental Deficiency, 82,* 1-11.

Zola, I. (1981). Communication barriers between the able-bodied and the handicapped. *Archives of Physical Medicine and Rehabilitation, 62,* 355-359.

Zola, I. K. (1994). Towards inclusion: The role of people with disabilities in policy and research issues in the United States: A historical and political analysis. In M. H. Rioux & M. Bach (Eds.), *Disability is not measles: New research paradigms in disability* (pp. 49-66). North York, Ontario: Roeher Institute.

Index

About the Editors

Rebecca Renwick, Ph.D., is Associate Professor in the Department of Occupational Therapy and the Graduate Department of Rehabilitation Science at the University of Toronto. She is also Codirector of the Quality of Life Research Unit at the Centre for Health Promotion, University of Toronto. She has a Ph.D. in psychology from the University of Lancaster, UK, and is a graduate of the program in occupational therapy and physiotherapy at the University of Toronto.

Her research and publications focus on quality of life for persons with and without disabilities as well as related issues, such as coping, social support, and inclusion in community life. Part of the research program she has carried out, in collaboration with a multidisciplinary group of investigators from the Quality of Life Research Unit, has concentrated on the development of a conceptual model of quality of life and instrumentation based on this model. Her research on quality of life for persons with disabilities has included several populations—namely, individuals with physical and sensory disabilities, persons who are HIV-positive, and adults with developmental disabilities.

Ivan Brown, Ph.D. (special education), is Senior Researcher at the University of Toronto's Centre for Health Promotion. He has worked in the fields of education and developmental disabilities. His recent research interests include quality of life for people with developmental disabilities, quality of family life, and barriers to education for people with physical disabilities.

Mark Nagler, Ph.D. (sociology), is Associate Professor in the Department of Sociology at the University of Waterloo. His research focuses on disability-related issues, medical sociology, and race and ethnic relations. He works with parents and various groups on contemporary concerns in his disability-related research.

About the Contributors

Michael Bach, M.E.S. (environmental studies), is currently Senior Researcher with the Roeher Institute and Assistant Professor Faculty of Environmental Studies at York University. He conducts research on public policy as it affects persons with disabilities and in the area of human rights and disability.

J. David Baker, LL.M. (law), is a founder and the current Executive Director of the Advocacy Resource Centre for the Handicapped (ARCH) in Toronto, Ontario, Canada. He is an internationally recognized lawyer and advocate for the rights of persons with disabilities.

Roy I. Brown, Ph.D. (psychology), is Foundation Professor and Dean of the School of Special Education and Disability Studies at Flinders University of South Australia. His research focuses on longitudinal studies of persons with intellectual disabilities.

Hy Day, Ph.D. (psychology), is Professor Emeritus with the Department of Psychology, York University, and a rehabilitation psychologist in private practice. His current research is on quality of life for people with disabilities and methods of assessing the impact of assistive devices.

Ron Draper, B.A., is an Associate of the Centre for Health Promotion at the University of Toronto. He was the primary organizer of the First (1986) and Second (1988) International Conferences on Health Promotion as well as the recipient of the Defries Award, the Canadian Public Health Association's highest honor for outstanding contributions to the field of public health.

David Felce, Ph.D. (community medicine), is Professor of Research in Learning Disabilities, Department of Psychological Medicine, at the University of Wales College of Medicine. He is also Director of the Welsh Centre for Learning Disabilities, Applied Research Unit, and he conducts evaluation research on services for persons with developmental disabilities.

Aubrey H. Fine, Ed.D. (school psychology), is currently Professor in the School of Education and Integrative Studies at California State Polytechnic University and Director for the Center for Special Populations. His research is on friendship skills development and community adjustment of persons with developmental disabilities.

Judith Friedland, Ph.D. (special education), is Associate Professor and Chair of the Department of Occupational Therapy at the University of Toronto as well as Associate Professor in the Department of Psychiatry. Her clinical work and research focuses on psychosocial adjustment to disability and the effectiveness of social support.

Sharon Friefeld, M.A. (special education), is a doctoral candidate in applied psychology and Assistant Professor in the Department of Occupational Therapy at the University of Toronto. She is a researcher in child development, especially the functional implications of disability on day-to-day performance.

Sharon G. Jankey, M.A. (psychology), is a doctoral candidate in clinical psychology at York University. She is conducting research on quality of life and rehabilitation as well as coping with chronic illness.

Ronald Labonté, M.A. (communications), is a doctoral candidate in sociology at York University in addition to being a community health consultant. He currently teaches in the graduate Health Promotion Program at the University of Toronto and consults health authorities in Canada, the United States,

Australia, New Zealand, and Latin America, and consults with the World Health Organization and UNICEF.

David G. Mason, Ph.D. (educational psychology), is Assistant Professor and Director of the Teacher Preparation Program in the Education of Deaf and Hard-of-Hearing Students at York University. His research is in the area of sociocultural aspects of deafness, particularly deaf bilingualism (American Sign Language and English) and deaf biculturalism (deaf and hearing cultures).

Bruce McCreary, M.D. (psychiatry), is Associate Professor and Chairman of the Division of Developmental Disabilities, Department of Psychiatry, Queen's University. He specializes in professional training and manpower in the field of developmental disabilities, neuropsychiatric genetics, and quality of life.

Eva R. McPhail, M.Ed. (early childhood education), is a doctoral candidate in applied psychology at the University of Toronto. She is researching the development, care, and education of young infants and children, including those deemed exceptional. She has a son with significant disabilities.

Bernard M. O'Keefe, Ph.D. (communication disorders), is Associate Professor in the Department of Speech Pathology at the University of Toronto. His research is on psychosocial effects of communication aids on users and their speaking partners, essential features of voice output in the mainstream classroom, and integration of individuals who use communication aids into the mainstream classroom.

Hélène Ouellette-Kuntz, M.Sc. (community health and epidemiology), is Assistant Professor in the Department of Community Health and Epidemiology, Queen's University, and Epidemiologist with Ongwanada Resource Centre. She specializes in research on quality of life, health promotion, and permanency planning.

Trevor R. Parmenter, Ph.D. (education), is Professor in the School of Education and Director of the Unit for Community Integration Studies at Macquarie University, Sydney, Australia. His research is on inclusion of persons with disabilities in community life.

Jonathan Perry, M.Sc. (psychology), is currently with the Department of Psychological Medicine, University of Wales College of Medicine, Welsh

Centre for Learning Disabilities, Applied Research Unit. He conducts evaluation research on services for persons with developmental disabilities.

John M. Raeburn, Ph.D. (psychology), is Associate Professor and Head of Behavioural Science for the Department of Psychiatry and Behavioural Science, School of Medicine, University of Auckland. He is also Chairman of the Mental Health Foundation in New Zealand. His research is on community-based health promotion and mental health promotion.

Dennis Raphael, Ph.D. (educational psychology), is Associate Professor in the Department of Behavioural Science and an Associate Director of the Masters of Health Science Program in Health Promotion at the University of Toronto. He is also Codirector of the Quality of Life Research Unit, Centre for Health Promotion, University of Toronto. His research is on quality of life and health promotion—specifically, quality of life of persons with disabilities, older adults, and adolescents.

Marcia H. Rioux, Ph.D. (jurisprudence and social policy), is Executive Director of the Roeher Institute and Assistant Professor in Environmental Studies at York University. She conducts research on social policy and disability.

Irving Rootman, Ph.D. (sociology), is Director of the Centre for Health Promotion and Professor in the Department of Preventative Medicine and Biostatistics at the University of Toronto. His research is on community health promotion, quality of life, evaluation methods in health promotion, and smoking policy research.

Robert L. Schalock, Ph.D. (psychology), is Professor and Chairman of the Department of Psychology at Hastings College. He specializes in program development and evaluation and quality of life for persons with disabilities.

Martin Shain, S.J.D. (jurisprudence), is Senior Scientist and Head of the Workplace Program for the Addiction Research Foundation and Centre for Health Promotion at the University of Toronto. He is also Assistant Professor in the Department of Behavioural Science at the University of Toronto. His research is focused on health promotion and protection in the workplace.